NEUROFIBROMATOSIS

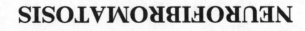

ANNALS OF THE NEW YORK ACADEMY OF SCIENCES
Volume 486

NEUROFIBROMATOSIS

Edited by Allan E. Rubenstein, Richard P. Bunge,
and David E. Housman

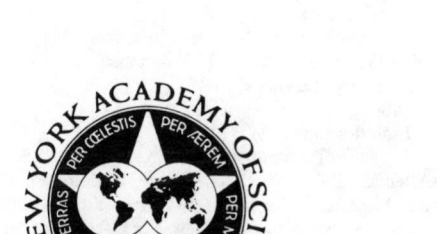

The New York Academy of Sciences
New York, New York
1986

Library of Congress Cataloging in Publication Data

Neurofibromatosis.

(Annals of the New York Academy of Sciences, ISSN 0077-8923 ; vol. 486)
The results of a conference held from May 22 to May 24, 1985, in New York, N.Y., sponsored by the New York Academy of Sciences.
Bibliography: p.
Includes index.
1. Neurofibromatosis—Congresses. I. Rubenstein, Allen E., 1944-   II. Bunge, Richard P., 1933-
III. Housman, David E.   IV. New York Academy of Sciences.
V. Series: Annals of the New York Academy of Sciences; v. 486.
Q11.N5 vol. 486   500s   86-33322
[RC280.N4]   [616.99′28]
ISBN 0-89766-367-5
ISBN 0-89766-368-3 (pbk.)

PCP
Printed in the United States of America
ISBN 0-89766-367-5 (Cloth)
ISBN 0-89766-368-3 (Paper)
ISSN 0077-8923

ANNALS OF THE NEW YORK ACADEMY OF SCIENCES

Volume 486
December 31, 1986

NEUROFIBROMATOSIS[a]

Editors and Conference Organizers
ALLAN E. RUBENSTEIN, RICHARD P. BUNGE, and DAVID E. HOUSMAN

CONTENTS

[a]This volume is the result of a conference entitled Neurofibromatosis held from May 22 to May 24, 1985 in New York, N.Y., sponsored by The New York Academy of Sciences and through a special grant from the National Neurofibromatosis Foundation.

Funding for this conference was provided through a special grant from:

- THE NATIONAL NEUROFIBROMATOSIS FOUNDATION

Neurofibromatosis

A Review of the Clinical Problem

ALLAN E. RUBENSTEIN

Department of Neurology
Mount Sinai School of Medicine
One Gustave Levy Place
New York, New York 10029

Neurofibromatosis (NF) is one of the most common single-gene disorders to affect the nervous system, with an estimated incidence of 1 in 3000 live births.[1] There is no known racial, ethnic, or geographic predilection for the disorder, though few epidemiologic data, are available from other than the United States and western Europe.[2] Frederick von Recklinghausen, a German pathologist, first correctly identified the neural origin of the most common lesion in NF, the neurofibroma, in 1882[3] (FIGURE 1). Though several other scientists previously described what we now know to be NF prior to von Recklinghausen's contribution, his correct identification of the pathologic nature of the neurofibroma has led to the disorder also being known as von Recklinghausen's disease (FIGURE 2).

CLASSIFICATION AND DIAGNOSIS OF NF

The major manifestations of NF involve the skin and the nervous and skeletal systems. The gene for NF appears to be inherited as an autosomal dominant. Previous kindred studies have demonstrated almost 100% penetrance of the gene with a great degree of variability of expression.[4] Most large series of NF, including ours, have a spontaneous mutation rate of approximately 50%, a rate high enough to seriously question the single-gene etiology of the typical form of the disorder. At the present time there is no biomarker for the gene for NF; the diagnosis is made purely on clinical grounds.[5] A recent working group established by the National Institutes of Health to establish diagnostic criteria for all forms of NF led to a classification of NF into two forms: (1) *von Recklinghausen NF* refers to the typical form of the disorder as described by von Recklinghausen, with multiple café-au-lait spots and multiple dermal neurofibromas (FIGURE 3). (2) *Bilateral acoustic NF* refers to a less common form of the disorder in which the predominant manifestations are bilateral acoustic neuromas and occasionally other brain and spinal cord tumors. Multiple dermal neurofibromas and multiple café-au-lait spots are uncommonly present.[6,7] Not all patients with signs of the disorder will fulfill these criteria. Segmental NF refers to individuals in whom signs of the disorder are confined to a specific body segment.

1

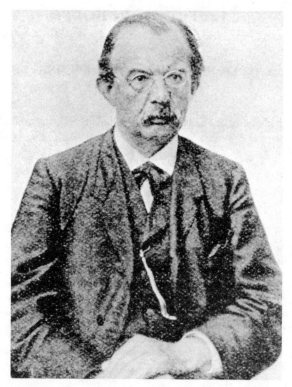

FIGURE 1. Friedrich Daniel von Recklinghausen (1833-1910). (Courtesy of the National Library of Medicine.)

It has been suggested that this may represent a somatic mutation and may therefore not be heritable.[8] However, we have evaluated two kindreds in which segmental signs of the disorder were transmitted in an autosomal dominant manner.[9]

Von Recklinghausen's NF is considered to be present in an individual with two of the following criteria, provided no other disease accounts for the findings:

1. On examination in room light, at least five café-au-lait macules over 5 mm in greatest diameter, if prepubertal; six café-au-lait macules over 15 mm in greatest diameter.
2. Based on clinical or histological grounds, two or more neurofibromas of any type, or one plexiform neurofibroma.
3. Multiple freckles in the axillary or inguinal regions (FIGURE 4).
4. Sphenoid wing dysplasia or congenital bowing or thinning of long bone cortex, with or without pseudoarthrosis.
5. Bilateral optic nerve gliomas.

6. Two or more iris Lisch nodules on slit lamp examination (FIGURE 5).
7. A first-degree relative (parent, sibling, or offspring) with von Recklinghausen neurofibromatosis, by the above criteria.

Bilateral acoustic NF is considered to be present in an individual with either of the following:

1. Computer tomography (CT) or magnetic resonance imaging evidence of bilateral internal auditory canal masses, consistent with acoustic neuromas; or,
2. A first-degree relative with bilateral acoustic neurofibromatosis and one of the following:
   a. CT or magnetic resonance imaging evidence of unilateral internal auditory canal mass, consistent with acoustic neuroma.

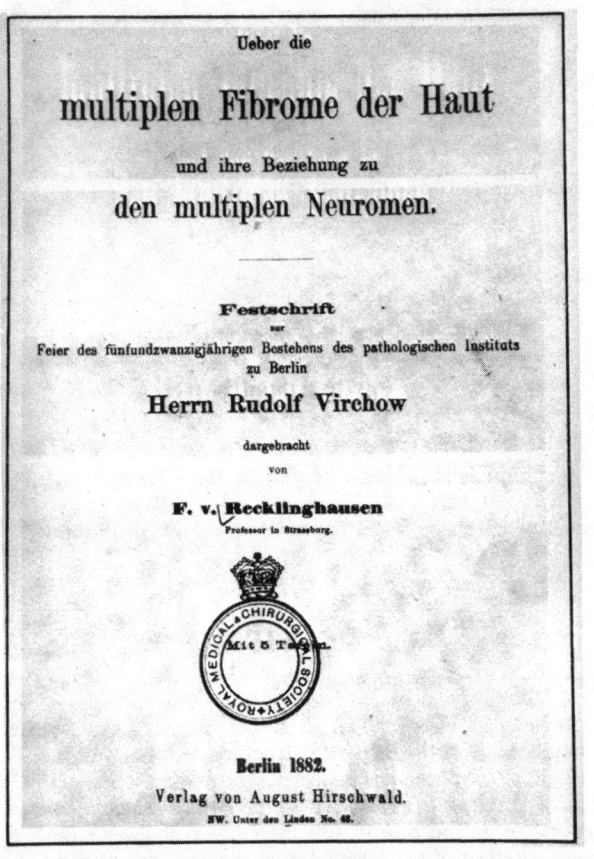

FIGURE 2. The title page of von Recklinghausen's treatise on neurofibromatosis. (Courtesy of The Royal Society of Medicine, London, England.)

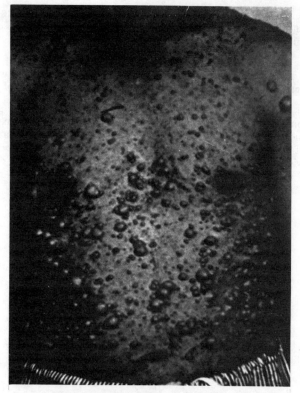

FIGURE 3. Multiple dermal neurofibromas.

b. A plexiform neurofibroma or two of the following: meningioma, glioma, neurofibroma at any site.
c. Imaging evidence of an intracranial or spinal cord tumor.

COMPLICATIONS OF NF

The earliest sign of NF is usually multiple café-au-lait spots, which may be present at birth or may become noticeable within the first five years of life. Dermal neurofibromas are usually first noticeable at puberty. The association of dermal neurofibromas with puberty, their frequent presence in the periareolar area in women, and frequent anecdotal reports of an increase in size or number of lesions during pregnancy all suggest a potential effect of sex hormones on the growth potential of these lesions.[10] Plexiform neurofibromas typically grow along major nerves, nerve roots, and in the retroperitoneal and mediastinal regions (FIGURE 6). The differences in biological behavior between dermal and plexiform tumors are summarized in TABLE 1.

TABLE 2 summarizes the types of complications we saw in the first 250 patients with NF evaluated in the Mount Sinai Neurofibromatosis Clinic. Previously published series of NF patients have frequently been biased toward those more severely affected, as in inpatient-based series, or toward patients with orthopedic problems or cancer, as in series from specialty-oriented institutions. We believe our series of outpatients, approximately evenly distributed between adults and children with NF, more accurately reflects the spectrum of the disorder.[11] Forty-one percent of our patients had no significant medical problem as a result of having the gene and came for a general evaluation and/or counseling. Thirty-five percent of patients had neurologic complications of some type, 13.2% had disfigurement requiring cosmetic surgery, 6.8% had orthopedic problems other than minimal scoliosis, and 3.6% had a neurofibrosarcoma.

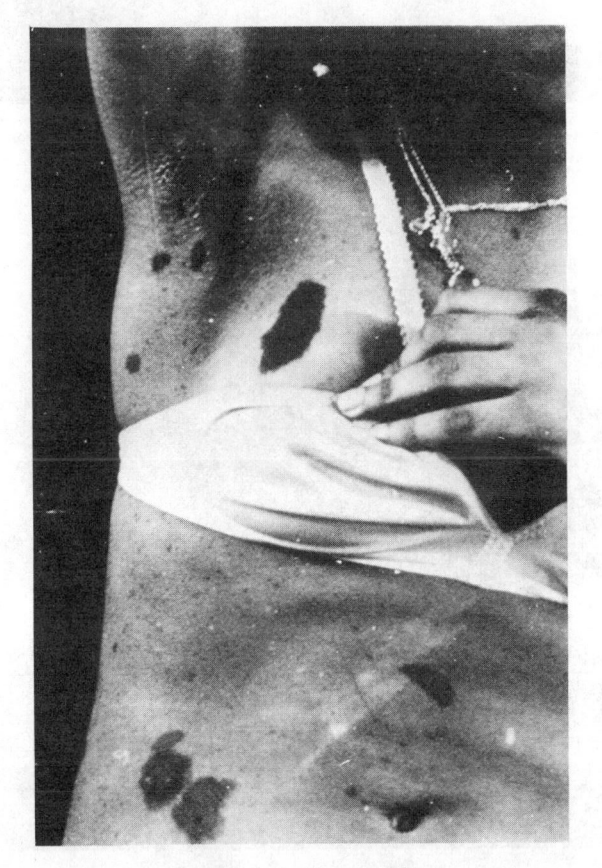

FIGURE 4. Axillary freckling.

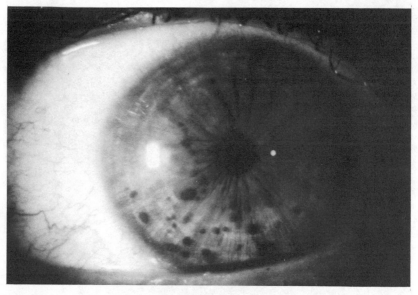

FIGURE 5. Multiple iris nodules (Lisch spots). Slit lamp examination is required to distinguish iris nodules from normal iris freckling.

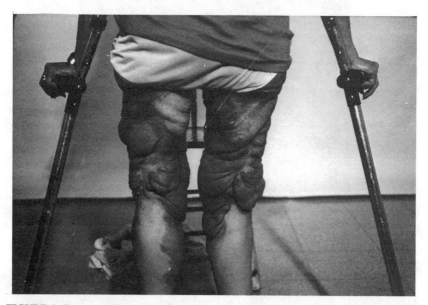

FIGURE 6. Extensive bilateral plexiform neurofibromas with associated soft tissue hypertrophy and overlying pigmentation.

TABLE 1. Differences between Neurofibroma Types

	Dermal	Plexiform
Location	Superficial, unrelated to major nerves	Subcutaneous or deep, often along major nerves
Number	Usually multiple	Usually single
Age of onset	Usually puberty	Pre- or postpubertal
Malignant degeneration	0	5%
Regional hypertrophy	Absent	Frequent
Overlying pigmentation	Absent	Common

NEUROLOGIC COMPLICATIONS

TABLE 3 lists the neurologic complications in our series. The most common neurologic problem was learning disability; almost as common was idiopathic megalencephaly in the absence of hydrocephalus. There was no relation between the presence of learning disability and megalencephaly.[12] Acoustic neuromas invariably presented in the second decade of life or later, while optic gliomas frequently presented in the first decade of life. There have been suggestions that optic gliomas in NF may be relatively benign, similar to hamartomas in their growth potential.[13] We have seen patients with relatively static optic gliomas over decades and patients with extremely aggressive lesions. A recent study has suggested that cerebellar astrocytomas may be unusually aggressive in NF.[14] Our experience with astrocytomas of this area in NF tends to confirm this impression. We have seen two patients with lifelong constipation due to megacolon secondary to neurofibromatous changes in the autonomic innervation of the colon, a phenomenon observed by several others.[15,16] Contrary to previous claims made that constipation is common in patients with NF, a symptomatic survey of our clinic population found no increase in this problem compared to patients' closest unaffected relatives.[17] We additionally saw two patients who presented as adults with anterior sacral and lateral thoracic meningocoeles (FIGURE 7).[18] We consider meningocoeles unlikely to be coincidental to the problem of NF. A separate study found 78% of patients with lateral thoracic meningocoeles to have NF.[19] Meningocoeles in NF may be due to progressive dural ectasia of the spinal cord, a phenomenon we have frequently noted in NF.

TABLE 2. Types of Complications in 250 Patients with von Recklinghausen's Neurofibromatosis

	Number	Percent
Asymptomatic	102	41
Neurologic	88	35.2
Disfigurement	33	13.2
Orthopedic	17	6.8
Sarcoma	9	3.6

TABLE 3. Neurologic Complications in 250 Patients with von Recklinghausen's Neurofibromatosis

	Number
Learning disability	29
Megalencephaly	20
Brain tumors	18
Acoustic Neuroma	5
Optic gioma	5
Meningioma	3
Astrocytoma	2
Other glial tumors	3
Primary seizure disorder	11
Spinal cord/root neurofibroma	14
Mental retardation	9
Aqueductal stenosis	2
Agenesis sphenoid wing	3
Megacolon	2
Meningocoele	2
Hyptertrophic neuropathy	1

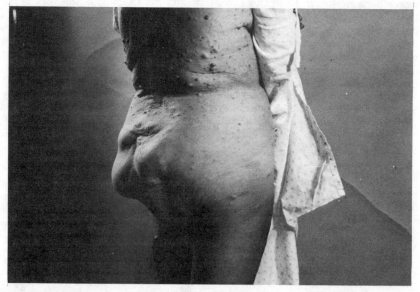

FIGURE 7. Sixty-eight-year-old woman with von Recklinghausen's neurofibromatosis and fluctuant sacral mass with adult onset presentation. Myelography demonstrated large anterior sacral meningocoele.

ORTHOPEDIC COMPLICATIONS

Skeletal problems in NF have been reviewed extensively by Holt,[20] Crawford,[21] and others. Scoliosis is by far the most common skeletal problem. The scoliosis in NF typically involves five vertebrae or less and causes a sharp, angular curve which is frequently associated with a cervical kyphosis (FIGURE 8).

Anterolateral bowing of the tibia and ulna is a congenital deformity which can lead to a fracture that frequently fails to heal, causing pseudoarthrosis (FIGURE 9). Localized hypertrophy of bone often occurs in an area associated with a plexiform neurofibroma. An uncommon accompaniment to hypertrophy of long bones is subperiosteal hemorrhage, which may be recurrent (FIGURE 10). Congenital agenesis of

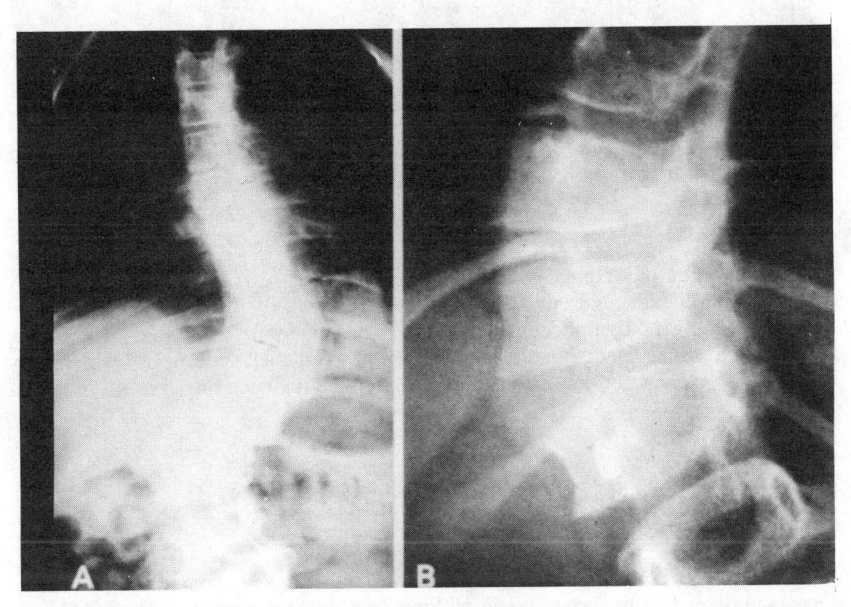

FIGURE 8. Short, angular scoliotic curve.

the lateral portion of the sphenoid wing may lead to a pulsating exophthalmos which can gradually produce optic atrophy (FIGURE 11).

CANCER IN NF

The most common malignancy in NF is neurofibrosarcoma. Malignant schwannomas are less common. Malignant degeneration occurred in 3.6% of our patients. The use of radiotherapy in treating such tumors has caused some controversy, due

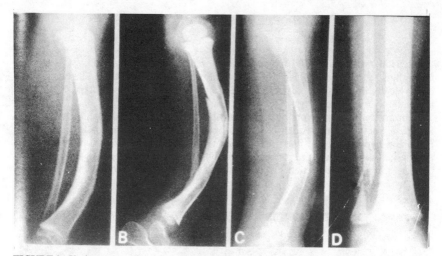

FIGURE 9. Various types of congenital bowing and pseudoarthroses of tibia and fibula in infants and young children with neurofibromatosis. Pseudoarthrosis of fibula is usually present at birth but frequently occurs later in tibia due to minor trauma. (Courtesy of Dr. John Holt.)

to the observation of secondary malignancies developing in the field of radiation.[22] A small but well-documented increase in the frequency of other cancers has been noted in NF, including nonlymphocytic leukemia[23] and rhabdomyosarcoma.[24] Cutaneous and gastrointestinal leiomyomas[25] and congenital giant melocytic nevi,[26] which may predispose to melanoma, have been observed by us in association with NF.

OTHER COMPLICATIONS OF NF

Vasculopathy is a phenomenon in NF that may be underestimated.[27] Renal artery stenosis may lead to hypertension in children; pheochromocytoma is more likely to cause hypertension in adults with NF. Cerebral vasculopathy has been reported to cause stroke syndromes in children with NF and also may be clinically inapparent.

Short stature is a phenomenon that has been increasingly recognized in children with NF in the absence of severe skeletal deformity or hypothalmic mass lesion, though both of these can also be associated with short stature in NF. Pruritus is also a problem recently recognized to be part of the spectrum of NF. Its etiology is unclear.

SUMMARY

NF is a relatively common genetic disorder which predisposes to a variety of clinical manifestations involving multiple body systems. NF poses important questions

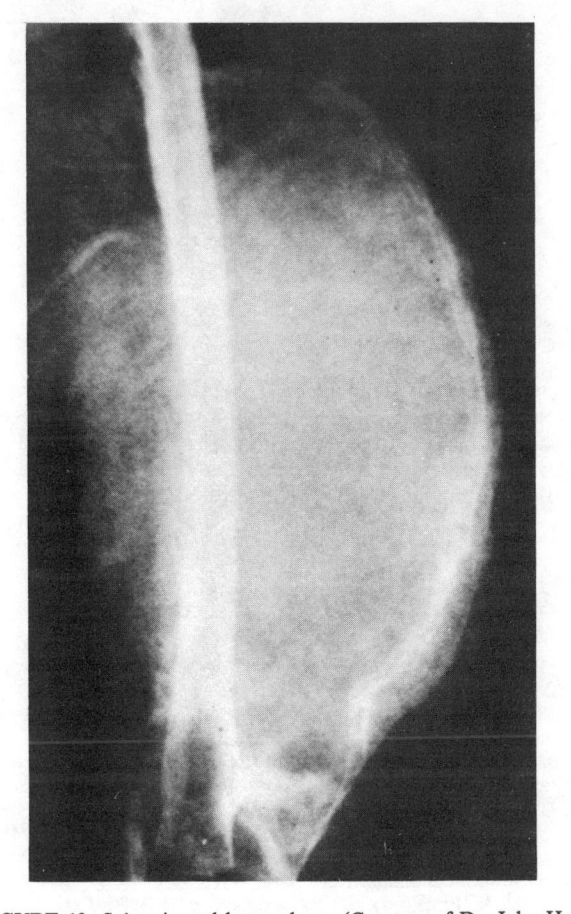

FIGURE 10. Subperiosteal hemorrhage. (Courtesy of Dr. John Holt.)

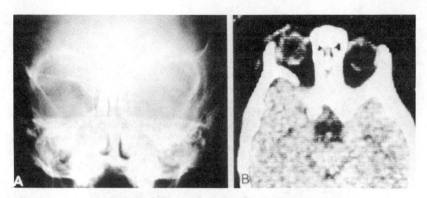

FIGURE 11. One-year-old girl with typical sphenoid dysplasia on left. (A) Enlargement of left orbit, elevation of sphenoid ridge and distortion of superior orbital fissure. (B) Computer tomography scan showing obvious exophthalmos. (Courtesy of Dr. John Holt.)

to researchers involved with developmental neurobiology, nerve regeneration and growth, the mechanism of malignant degeneration, and the use of molecular techniques to identify genetic disorders. It is hoped that this conference will bring together researchers who have developed new techniques in these areas and will encourage them to apply these techniques to the problem of NF.

REFERENCES

1. CROWE, F. W., W. J. SCHULL & J. V. NEEL. 1956. A Clinical, Pathological and Genetic Study of Multiple Neurofibromatosis. C. Thomas. Springfield, Ill.
2. SORENSEN, S. A., J. J. MULVIHILL & A. NIELSEN. 1986. Long term follow-up of von Recklinghausen's neurofibromatosis. N. Engl. J. Med. **314**(16): 1010-1015.
3. RECKLINGHAUSEN, F. 1882. Uber die multiplen Fibrome der Haut und ihre Beziehung zu d'en multiplen Neuromen. Virchow Festschrift. A. Hirschwald. Berlin, Germany.
4. CAREY, J. C., J. M. LAUB & B. D. HALL. 1978. Penetrance and variability in Neurofibromatosis: a genetic study of 60 families. Annu. Rev. Birth Defects **15**(5B): 271-282.
5. MULVIHILL, J., Ed. 1986. Neurofibromatosis Research Newsletter **2**(2): 1. The National Neurofibromatosis Foundation. New York, N.Y.
6. KANTER, W. R., R. ELDRIDGE, R. FABRICANT, et al. 1980. Central neurofibromatosis with bilateral acoustic neuroma: genetic, clinical and biochemical distinctions from peripheral neurofibromatosis. Neurology **30**: 851-859.
7. MARTUZA, R. L. & R. G. OJEMANN. 1982. Bilateral acoustic neuromas: clinical aspects, pathogenesis and treatment. Neurosurgery **10**: 1-12.
8. MILLER, N. R. & R. S. SPARKES. 1977. Segmental neurofibromatosis. Arch. Dermatol. **113**: 837-838.
9. RUBENSTEIN, A. E., J. L. BADER, A. ARON & S. WALLACE. 1983. Familial transmission of segmental neurofibromatosis. Neurology **33**(Suppl. 2): 76.
10. MARTUZA, R. L., D. T. MACLAUGHLIN & R. G. OJEMANN. 1981. Specific estradiol binding in schwannomas, meningiomas and neurofibromas. Neurosurgery **9**: 665-667.
11. RUBENSTEIN, A. E., S. WALLACE, A. ARON, et al. 1984. Neurological complications in 250 cases of neurofibromatosis. Ann. Neurol. **16**(1): 133.

12. RUBENSTEIN, A. E., R. WALLERSTEIN, A. ARON, et al. 1985. Lack of correlation of megalencephaly with learning disability in disseminated neurofibromatosis. Am. J. Hum. Genet. 37(Suppl.): 214.
13. BORIT, A. & E. P. RICHARDSON. 1982. The biology and clinical behavior of pilocytic astrocytomas of the optic pathways. Brain 105: 161-187.
14. ILGREN, E. B., L. M. KINNIER-WILSON & C. A. STILLER. Gliomas in neurofibromatosis: a series of 89 cases with evidence for enhanced malignancy in associated cerebellar astrocytomas.
15. RUBENSTEIN, A. E., L. B. COHEN, A. ARON, et al. 1984. Primary mesenteric plexus alteration as a cause of megacolon in neurofibromatosis. Neurology 34(Suppl. 1): 211.
16. FEINKAT, T., et al. 1984. Megacolon and neurofibromatosis: a neuronal intestinal dysplasia. A case report and review of the literature. Gastroenterology 86(6): 1573-1579.
17. RICCARDI, V. 1981. Von Recklinghausen neurofibromatosis. N. Engl. J. Med. 305: 1617-1627.
18. RUBENSTEIN, A. E., A. ARON & S. WALLACE. 1984. Adult presentation of meningocoeles in neurofibromatosis. Neurology 34(Suppl. 1): 168.
19. ERKULVRAWATR, S., T. E. GAMMAL, J. HAWKINS, et al. 1979. Intrathoracic meningoceles and neurofibromatosis. Arch. Neurol. 36: 557-559.
20. HOLT, J. F. 1978. Neurofibromatosis in children. Am. J. Roentgenol. 130: 615-639.
21. CRAWFORD, A. H. 1986. Neurofibromatosis in children. Acta Orthoped. Scand. 57(Suppl. 218).
22. FOLEY, F. M., J. M. WOODRUFF, F. T. ELLIS, et al. 1980. Radiation-induced malignant and atypical nerve sheath tumors. Ann. Neurol. 7: 311-318.
23. BADER, J. L. & R. W. MILLER. 1978. Neurofibromatosis and childhood leukemia. J. Pediatr. 92: 925-929.
24. MCKEEN, E. A., J. BODURTHA, A. T. MEADOWS, et al. 1978. Rhabdomyosarcoma complicating multiple neurofibromatosis. J. Pediatr. 93: 992-993.
25. RUBENSTEIN, A. E., J. L. BADER, J. PEARSON, et al. 1983. The association of smooth muscle tumors with neural crest tumors: implications for the pathogenesis of neurofibromatosis. Proc. Am. Soc. Clin. Oncol. 24: 123.
26. RUBENSTEIN, A. E., S. C. SETTZ, S. WALLACE, et al. 1985. Increased risk of congenital premalignant melanocytic nevi in neurofibromatosis. Neurology 35(Suppl. 1): 194.
27. WERTELECKI, W., D. W. SUPERNEAU, W. R. BLACKBURN, et al. 1982. Neurofibromatosis: skin hemangiomas and arterial disease. Birth Defects 18: 29-41.

The Malformative Central Nervous System Lesions in the Central and Peripheral Forms of Neurofibromatosis

A Neuropathological Study of 22 Cases

L. J. RUBINSTEIN

Division of Neuropathology
University of Virginia School of Medicine
Charlottesville, Virginia 22908

In 1822, Wishart, a Scottish surgeon, published in the *Edinburgh Medical and Surgical Journal* the first detailed description of a deaf and blind boy with multiple tumors arising in the dura and from the cranial nerve roots.[1] Similar anatomical findings have since been recorded at infrequent intervals and over the past five decades have been detailed, and the observations extended, in various reviews of the subject.[2-6] This combination of multiple central nervous system (CNS) neoplasms has therefore long been recognized as the central form of von Recklinghausen's neurofibromatosis (NF). Generally speaking, the tumors in this condition are characterized by their diversity and their multiplicity, involve predominantly the sheath cells of the cranial nerves and intrathecal spinal nerve roots, but implicate with almost equal frequency the meningeal and glial elements of the brain and spinal cord. The neoplastic profile of the disease typically consists then of multiple intracranial and intraspinal schwannomas, neurofibromas, and meningiomas, often in association with multiple spinal intramedullary ependymomas. In some cases of NF, however, the glial neoplastic process is expressed by an astrocytic glioma, either midline or hemispheric, with a predilection for the cerebellum, but most often by the development of unilateral or bilateral optic nerve gliomas. Tumors of ganglionic cells may also be found, but these are almost always of neural crest derivation and only exceptionally of central origin. These neuronal neoplasms include pheochromocytomas and, less often, peripheral ganglioneuromas and neuroblastomas.

The relationship of the central to the peripheral form of NF has always presented a challenge, and a revival of interest in the definition of the central form and in its genetic, clinical, and biochemical characteristics is evident from recent contributions to the problem.[7,8] While both forms show a Mendelian autosomal dominant pattern of inheritance, their relative incidence differs widely: the number of individuals afflicted with peripheral NF has been estimated to be over 100,000 in the United States, with a prevalence of 60 per 100,000, whereas the number of cases with the central form has been estimated to be less than 1000, with a prevalence of 0.1 per 100,000. Both forms have been linked with an increase of serum nerve growth factor (NGF) activity, but this increase may be expressed differently in each form: the antigenic activity (as measured by radioimmunoassay) has been stated to be normal in peripheral NF but increased in the central form, whereas its functional activity (as measured by radio-receptor assay) is either normal or decreased in the central form but increased in peripheral NF.[9,10] These differences have, however, not always been confirmed in other studies.[8,11]

There may be disagreement on the definition of central NF. The development of bilateral acoustic schwannomas associated with only minimal lesions elsewhere has been suggested as constituting a distinct subentity that defines the central form of NF:[7,8] in our view, such a concept is too restrictive. It is true that bilateral acoustic tumors transmitted as a Mendelian autosomal dominant trait with high penetrance and remarkably constant expressivity have been recorded in several kindreds,[7,8,12-14] but the association of VIIIth nerve tumor bilaterality with other multiple cranial nerve tumors, with multiple meningiomas, and with multiple intraaxial gliomas (especially spinal intramedullary ependymomas) evidently extends the spectrum of the disease, as shown in the reviews cited above and in the case material to be presented. Moreover, bilateral acoustic schwannomas, while an extremely frequent integral part of the picture of central NF, are not invariably present in the disease. Additional support for this view is to be found in occasional reports of kindreds in whom the development of multiple familial meningiomas has been an expression of NF inheritance.[15]

Less familiar than the strictly neoplastic manifestations of central NF are the discrete and often microscopic malformative lesions implicating the intracranial and intraspinal neural structures, to which this review will draw attention. These lesions may be grouped under the general term of hamartomas. Their interest lies in the frequency with which they are found on systematic microscopic examination and, by reason of their topographical association with other lesions that are already clearly neoplastic, in their potential significance as a source of tumor formation. They also emphasize the malformative, or dysplastic, element that seems to be at the basis of many of the tumors involving the glial, meningeal, and Schwann cell elements in NF.

In addition to the central form of NF as defined above, a variety of gliomas have been reported in patients with peripheral NF. While they do not come within the scope of this review, they are of importance in providing transitional links between the central and the peripheral form of the disease. The most frequently encountered CNS tumors in that setting are optic nerve gliomas, either unilateral or bilateral,[16-19] but the occurrence of other glioma types, in particular cerebellar astrocytomas of various degrees of malignancy[19] and cerebral glioblastomas,[20] is well documented.

The following survey reviews the chief neuropathological features of 22 autopsied cases of NF examined by us over a period of 25 years in five different institutions. Eleven of the cases represented the central form of the disease as we have defined it, and 11 examples of the peripheral form. In all cases, multiple areas from the brain and its gross lesions were available for histological study. The spinal cord was available in 19 of the 22 cases. Individual details and illustrations on 19 of these cases have previously been published in five studies.[5,21-24] Additional gross and microscopic features have also been illustrated in two comprehensive texts.[25,26]

ANALYSIS OF CASE MATERIAL AND COMMENTS

General Features

FIGURE 1 shows the ages at death of the patients in our material with each form of the disease. Most of the patients with central NF died in the second or third decade, largely by reason of the involvement of the intracranial cavity and/or spinal canal by multiple space-occupying lesions. The ages of the patients with peripheral NF are more evenly distributed.

The major causes of death of patients with peripheral NF are shown in TABLE 1. Eight of the 11 patients died as a direct or indirect result of the disease, the most frequent being a sarcomatous change in a neurofibroma.

It has long been well known that the peripheral, in particular the cutaneous, manifestations of the disease are either scanty or absent in the central form. However, small numbers of cutaneous neurofibromas or café-au-lait spots, or both, have been stated to be present in 60% of the cases with central NF.[8] More specifically, it has been estimated that six or more café-au-lait spots are found in 75% of the patients with peripheral NF and in none of those with central NF, whereas one or more café-au-lait spots are found in 94% of patients with peripheral NF and in 42% of those with central NF.[7] TABLE 2 confirms this general concept.

Many of the examples of central NF in our material had no record of any familial incidence, but investigation into the family history may not have been thorough or complete. Two of our cases, however, are of interest in illustrating the variation in the phenotypic picture that may be expressed by the NF trait. In case 12,[5] in a 14-year-old boy with a large third-ventricle astrocytoma that invaded the chiasm and both optic nerves (Reference 26, Figure 119), a few café-au-lait spots but no neurofibromas were present, but the mother harbored the classical peripheral form of NF,

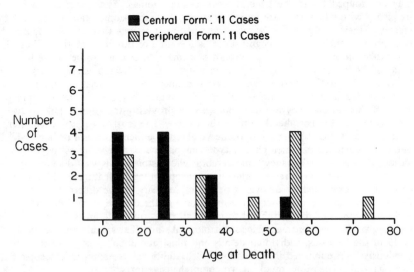

FIGURE 1. Neurofibromatosis (22 autopsied cases).

TABLE 1. Major Causes of Death in 11 Cases of Peripheral Neurofibromatosis

Neurofibrosarcoma	6
Cardiorenal complications secondary to functional pheochromocytoma	1
Hydrocephalus due to dysplastic ependymal granulations	1
Unrelated causes	3

one brother had died at the age of 14 of a cystic tumor of the posterior fossa, and another brother had been operated because of a proptosis. In case 11,[5] in a 38-year-old man with multiple cranial nerve and spinal nerve root schwannomas, multiple cranial and spinal meningiomas, and two intraspinal ependymomas, acoustic tumors had been documented in three generations of the patient's family, and his nephew had an astrocytoma of the optic nerve head.[27]

Cranial Nerve and Spinal Nerve Root Tumors

Not every case of bilateral acoustic schwannomas is necessarily an example of NF, but of the eight autopsied cases of bilateral acoustic schwannomas we have studied, seven had also other evidence of NF, predominantly of the central form. In six of these seven cases, other cranial nerve tumors were also present (TABLE 3), and multiple meningiomas were associated with six cases also (TABLE 4). In all our autopsied cases of NF in which acoustic tumors were found, these were bilateral.

Although they cannot be differentiated histologically from the peripheral schwannomas and neurofibromas that constitute the hallmark of peripheral NF, cranial and intrathecal spinal nerve root tumors, almost always multiple, are therefore characteristic of central NF (TABLE 3). When encountered in peripheral NF, they usually present as small, single, incidental lesions. However, the neoplastic manifestations of NF are so protean that every statement about this disease will carry exceptions.

Meningiomas

As shown in TABLE 4, when meningiomas are present in central NF they are almost always multiple. They involve both the cranial and the spinal compartments. Notable is the frequency of meningiomas originating from the stroma of the choroid plexuses: these tumors, which were bilateral in two of our three cases, are usually relatively small and, as reported in one of them, may show extensive calcifications (Reference 23, case 1).

Gliomas

The gliomas found in central NF are characteristic: the most frequent have been ependymomas, usually spinal and multiple, in which an association with bilateral

TABLE 2. Cutaneous Manifestations Noted in 11 Cases of Central Neurofibromatosis

Skin Lesions	Few	None
Neurofibromas	6	5
Pigmented areas	5	6
Congenital ichthyosis		1

acoustic schwannomas, with other multiple cranial and spinal nerve root schwannomas, and with multiple meningiomas constitutes the most typical picture (TABLE 4). In our material, ependymomas accounted for five of the seven cases of central neuraxial glioma associated with central NF: in four of these five cases, the ependymomas were multiple, a feature shared by most of the spinal intramedullary examples reported by others.[6] An exceptional example of bilateral retinal astrocytomas originating in the optic discs was studied by us in a 17-year-old girl with the classical multiple lesions of central NF.[22,23]

Malformative CNS Lesions in Central NF

Central NF is characterized by the very frequent presence (in 9 of our 11 cases) of malformative CNS lesions which are often distinctive. TABLE 5 presents their incidence in our material. It emphasizes the variety of the cells involved (Schwann cells, meningeal cells, endothelial cells, glial cells, and ependymocytes) and the frequent association of these usually microscopic lesions with florid neoplastic proliferations of the same or different cell elements. A close topographical relationship is often found between these microscopic dysplastic lesions and the more developed tumors involving the CNS.

These presumably hamartomatous lesions have been described, illustrated, and discussed in previous publications[5,25,26] and will therefore not be detailed here. Their significance as potential sources of neoplastic transformation in the CNS and the question of their specificity in central NF, however, merit a few comments.

The term intramedullary schwannosis has been applied to foci in the spinal cord, virtually always beneath the incoming dorsal nerve root and situated in the dorsal

TABLE 3. Cranial and Intrathecal Spinal Nerve Tumors in 22 Cases of Neurofibromatosis

	Central Form— 11 Cases (Number of Cases)	Peripheral Form— 11 Cases (Number of Cases)
Cranial nerve Tumors	8	2
Multiple	7	0
Bilateral acoustic	7	0
With other cranial nerve tumors	6	
Spinal nerve root tumors (19 cords)	9	5
Multiple	9	0

TABLE 4. Meningeal and Glial Tumors in 11 Cases of Central Neurofibromatosis

1. **Meningiomas** (cranial and spinal)	8	multiple	7	
Multiple meningiomas and bilaterial VIII nerve tumors				6
Associated with gliomas				5
Involving choroid plexuses				3
2. **Astrocytomas** of third ventricle, juvenile type			2	
3. **Ependymomas**	5	multiple	4	
Associated with bilateral VIII nerve tumors				5
Associated with multiple meningiomas				4
4. **Retinal astrocytomas** (bilateral)			1	

gray horn and its vicinity (zona terminalis of Lissauer), in which Schwann cells and reticulin fibers occupy the substance of the neural parenchyma, separating the intramedullary nerve fibers. In all our cases, this picture—when present—has been found adjacent to a schwannoma of the dorsal nerve root (Reference 26, Figure 19). It is generally assumed that in this lesion the ectopic Schwann cells have been centrally displaced in ontogenesis. In support of this hypothesis is their frequent association with other cellular ectopias, especially of ependymal cells. An alternative interpretation is that they represent attempts, within the spinal cord parenchyma, at regeneration by peripheral nervous system elements:[28] such a regenerative reaction might be related to the fact that intramedullary schwannosis is almost invariably associated with a local neoplastic lesion, such as an ependymoma, that results in focal spinal cord destruction or compression. The evidence in favor of a reactive as opposed to a dysplastic etiology has been further discussed elsewhere.[26] While we are not aware of these foci having been documented to undergo neoplastic change, they theoretically could be the source of origin of the rare intramedullary schwannomas.

Another form of schwannosis involves the perivascular sheaths of the spinal blood vessels and results in the development of microscopic neuromatous nodules which expand the perivascular spaces, especially in the ventral fissure and the gray commissure (Reference 26, Figure 24). These lesions have often been observed in various chronic (traumatic, neoplastic, degenerative, or compression-producing) lesions of the spinal cord, as well as in unselected autopsy material, and have generally been regarded as evidence of collateral regeneration from intra- or extramedullary neurites.[26] Aberrant axons may be found in these formations. While they are, therefore, not specific for NF, they often are unusually exuberant in this disease, and they originally were described in cases of central NF. They may, as seen in one of our cases and as reported by others,[29] develop into small schwannomas, and it is therefore possible that some

TABLE 5. Malformative CNS Lesions in 9/11 Cases of Central Neurofibromatosis

1. Intramedullary schwannosis	5	associated with ependymomas	5
2. Schwannosis of spinal blood vessels ("angioneuromatosis")			3
3. Meningioangiomatosis of brain or brain stem			4
4. Atypical glial cell nests	5	with meningioangiomatosis	4
5. Ependymal ectopias	5	associated with ependymomas	5
6. Hypertrophic gliosis of optic nerve			1
7. Marginal astrocytosis of spinal cord			1
8. Syringomyelia			2
9. Hydromyelia			1
10. Chiari malformation of medulla and sacral spina bifida			1

of the rare examples of so-called true central schwannomas originated from these formations.

In meningioangiomatosis, there is a proliferation of ectopic meningeal cells along the parenchymatous blood vessel walls that extends diffusely in the substance of the cerebral cortex (Reference 26, Figure 23), and occasionally in the thalamus or the cerebral peduncle. Concentric perivascular formations are found that are identical with those of a meningioma; they may include large numbers of psammoma bodies (Reference 26, Figure 22). These lesions may be multiple, as in one of our cases. In three examples they were associated with multiple meningiomas. In addition, the lesion may accompany a diffuse angiomatosis of the adjacent cortical and subcortical parenchyma, with thickening and hyalinization of the redundant blood vessel walls (Reference 26, Figure 22).

Occasionally, as in one of our cases, meningioangiomatosis of the cerebral cortex may be closely associated with an arteriovenous malformation in the overlying leptomeninges. All our four cases with this lesion also exhibited atypical glial cell nests in the cerebral cortex and basal ganglia, and occasionally in the gray matter of the spinal cord as well. The nests of atypical glia were often closely related topographically to the foci of intracortical meningioangiomatosis, therefore suggesting a dysplastic mechanism common to both, but in some examples the two types of lesion were quite independent. Although meningioangiomatosis is highly characteristic of central NF, it has, exceptionally, been found in the absence of other manifestations of the disease.[30,31]

In our material, foci of ectopic ependymal cells were most frequently found in the spinal cord, and in all these cases the patient harbored one or more spinal ependymomas. The ependymal ectopias were often situated in close proximity to the ependymomas, indicating a narrow relationship between ependymal dysplasia and tumor formation.

An association with syringomyelia, a well-documented component of NF,[32] was found in two of our cases, both of which had multiple intramedullary ependymomas.

This series does not comprise any examples of optic nerve glioma, but it includes an instance of diffuse hyperplastic gliosis of the optic nerve. The case was that of a 24-year-old woman with no cutaneous manifestations and a negative family history, and who harbored multiple neurofibromas of the cervical nerve roots and right vagus nerve: the left optic nerve and adjacent chiasm were thickened by a dense cellular pilocytic fibrillary gliosis that widely separated the nerve fibers (Reference 5, case 13). A few similar examples have been reported by others.[33] These cases are clinically asymptomatic; their distinction from an early stage of neoplasia is difficult. The question arises whether some of the optic nerve lesions demonstrated by computed tomography in approximately 10% of patients with NF who have no clinical symptoms or signs pointing to optic nerve involvement[18] could have a similar pathology. The significance and subsequent evolution of such a lesion are uncertain.

TABLE 6. Malformative (?) CNS Lesions in 5/11 Cases of Peripheral Neurofibromatosis

1. Subependymal gliofibrillary nodules	3
(causing aqueduct stenosis)	2
2. Hyperplastic (?neoplastic) proliferative gliosis	1
3. Meningoencephalic cerebellar gliosis	1
4. Micronodular vascular proliferations	1
5. Hydromyelia	1

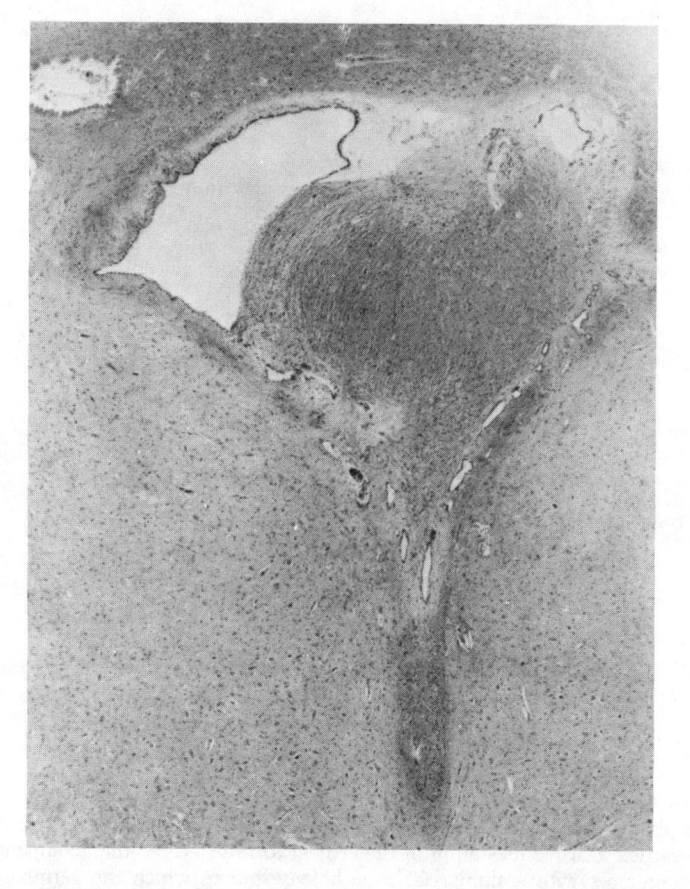

FIGURE 2. Aqueduct stenosis in a 59-year-old woman with classical peripheral NF. The lesion, which is indistinguishable from a small fibrillary pilocytic astrocytoma, did not cause internal hydrocephalus. The original contour of the partly occluded aqueduct is represented by the small slitlike cavities lined by ependymal cells. H&E × 25.

Malformative and Proliferative CNS Lesions in Peripheral NF

The presence of malformative and proliferative lesions involving the CNS was documented in 5 of our 11 patients with peripheral NF (TABLE 6). They have been the object of relatively little attention up till now.

The most frequent of these changes (found in three cases) consisted in focal cellular proliferations of fibrillated subependymal glial cells, with the development of well-defined nodules or fingerlike projections at various levels of the ventricular cavities (FIGURES 2, 3, and 4).

In two patients, these nodules produced aqueduct stenosis. One of these patients was described by Dorothy Russell in 1949 in her monograph on the pathology of

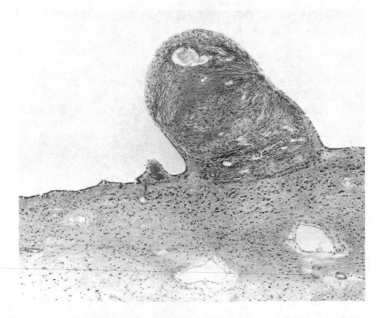

FIGURE 3. Fingerlike nodule of fibrillated glia projecting in the left lateral ventricle of a 50-year-old woman with peripheral NF. The nodule is adjacent to an old infarct showing rarefaction of the neural tissue and gliosis (lower edge of the figure). Note small ependymal granulation to the left of the larger nodule. H&E × 50.

hydrocephalus (Reference 21, case 28, Figures 28-30). Although this condition has been regarded as a manifestation of the central form of NF,[5,21] the documentation of subsequent cases with a similar CNS pathology, but in which the peripheral manifestations of NF have been conspicuous, indicates that these patients have in fact the peripheral form of the disease. Sixteen examples in which aqueductal stenosis, presumed to be due to similar polypoid ependymal granulations, resulted in hydrocephalus have recently been reviewed:[34] the ages of the patients when hydrocephalus was first detected ranged from 5 to 28 years.

The possibility, however, that an identical form of cellular proliferation resulting in aqueduct stenosis will not necessarily cause obstructive hydrocephalus is suggested by our second case, illustrated in FIGURE 2: a 59-year-old woman with the typical manifestations of peripheral NF and who died from a sarcomatous transformation of a mediastinal neurofibroma presumed to have originated from the left vagus nerve. Examination of the CNS revealed as sole lesions a small neurofibroma on a lumbar nerve root and a 2-mm-wide subependymal nodule of fibrillary glia, causing partial occlusion of the aqueduct, but no internal hydrocephalus. As shown in FIGURE 2, the original contour of the aqueduct is partly represented by small slitlike cavities lined by ependymal cells. The histological features of this glial nodule are indistinguishable from those of a subependymal pilocytic astrocytoma, but there was no clinical evidence that it was progressive. Presumably the cellular glial proliferation was self-limited in this case; whether it should be regarded as neoplastic or dysplastic is open to debate.

The third case in this series which exhibited similar multiple subependymal glio-fibrillary nodules is of interest because of their association with other glial proliferative changes within the neural parenchyma. The patient was a 50-year-old woman with multiple café-au-lait spots and movable subcutaneous nodules scattered over the face and trunk and with a strong family history of peripheral NF (her father, uncle, paternal grandfather, and daughter had multiple café-au-lait spots and subcutaneous nodules). She had been suffering for 25 years from paroxysmal hypertension, which resulted in the surgical removal of a left-sided pheochromocytoma at the age of 42. However, severe persistent hypertension of renal origin developed due to a right-sided nephro-sclerosis resulting from chronic ureteric obstruction by a small polypoid neurofibroma. Multiple episodes of cerebrovascular accidents punctuated the last three years of her life. These accidents were documented at autopsy by the presence of several small old hemorrhages and infarcts in the basal ganglia, pons, and cerebellum. Multiple polypoid projections of subependymal fibrillated glia (FIGURES 3 and 4) were found over the lateral ventricles and the walls of the aqueduct and fourth ventricle; their distribution was notable in that the segments of the ventricular ependyma that were mostly involved

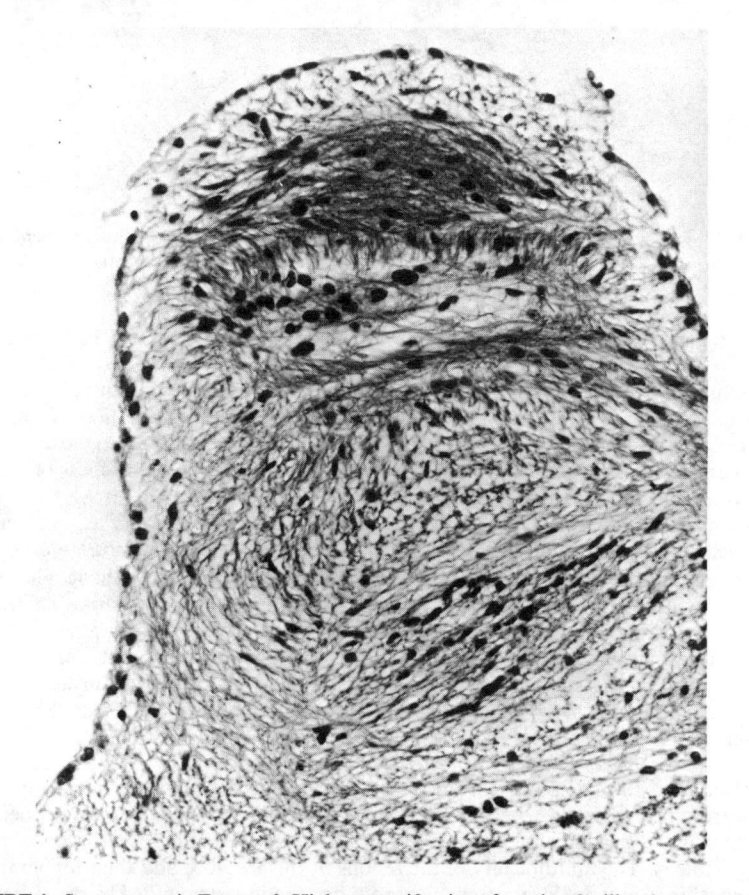

FIGURE 4. Same case as in FIGURE 3. Higher magnification of another fibrillated subependymal nodule projecting from the lateral wall of the fourth ventricle. H&E × 250.

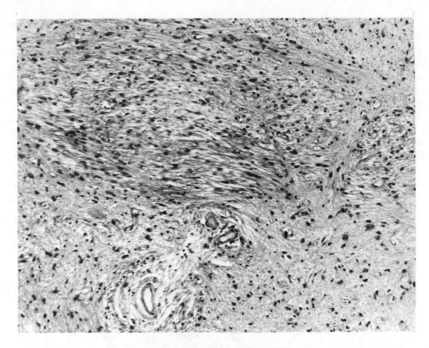

FIGURE 5. Same case as in FIGURES 3 and 4. Hyperplastic fibrillary gliosis in pontine tegmentum. Note invasion of perivascular spaces by neuroglial tissue (lower left). × 100.

were adjacent to areas of CNS gliosis in the neighborhood of old cerebrovascular infarcts.

Other hyperplastic proliferative lesions involving the glia were found in the same patient. Notable was an irregular, rather densely cellular proliferation of fibrillated pilocytic cells in the pontine tegmentum, with focal invasion of the perivascular spaces by neuroglial tissue (FIGURE 5): the cellular features, the increase in mass of the area involved, and the presence of local invasion were indistinguishable from a neoplastic process, i.e., a diffuse fibrillary astrocytoma. In the cerebellum, a marked proliferation of fibrillary glia was found to extend from the cerebellar cortex into the leptomeninges (FIGURES 6 and 7): this picture of a proliferative meningoencephalic gliosis was identical with a form of cerebellar dysplasia[35] and with some of the histological features of the cerebellar astrocytomas that are typically associated with NF,[36] as confirmed in a recent review:[19] characteristics of these cerebellar lesions are the preponderant involvement of the subpial marginal layer and their propensity to invade the subarachnoid spaces by way of multiple glial bridges. The intriguing feature about the lesion illustrated in FIGURES 6 and 7 is that it was found in the vicinity of a small old cystic cerebellar infarct.

This case then demonstrated at various levels of the CNS an unusually active proliferation of the glia which, by reason of its cellular density and the evidence of local invasion, was indistinguishable from the picture seen in diffuse or focal fibrillary astrocytomas. The multifocality of the lesions in this instance and their topographical relationship to areas of local parenchymatous destruction surrounded by reactive gliosis suggest that we might be dealing, in the setting of NF, with an abnormal proliferative response to an otherwise banal pathological condition: the unusual morphologic features, which clearly exceeded the limits of an ordinary reactive gliosis, raise the speculation of increased activity by cell growth factors in this disease, to which not only the nerve sheath elements but also the neuroglia might be responsive.

Two other findings involving the CNS in peripheral NF merit brief mention. In one of our cases, in a 15-year-old male who succumbed to a sarcomatous transformation in a cervical neurofibroma, the right occipital cortex demonstrated discrete micronodular hyperplastic foci involving the parenchymatous arterioles and capillary blood vessels, corresponding to the lesions of vascular NF, as described in the European literature.[37-39] This seldom-discussed entity has up till now been reported only in the viscera, and not in the brain. Several forms of vascular hyperplastic lesions in NF have been described. FIGURE 8 illustrates the adventitial nodular form, in which a proliferation of endothelial cells within the vasa vasorum of small-caliber arteries results in the development of glomeruli-like foci in the perivascular space. Another form, shown in FIGURE 9, consists largely in cellular hyperplasia involving the intimal and muscular medial elements of an arteriole. There is some dispute as to the histogenesis of these vascular alterations, some of which have been attributed to endothelial cells, others to smooth muscle cells, and others to perineurial cells in the vascular walls. The similarity of some of these lesions to the glomeruloid foci of

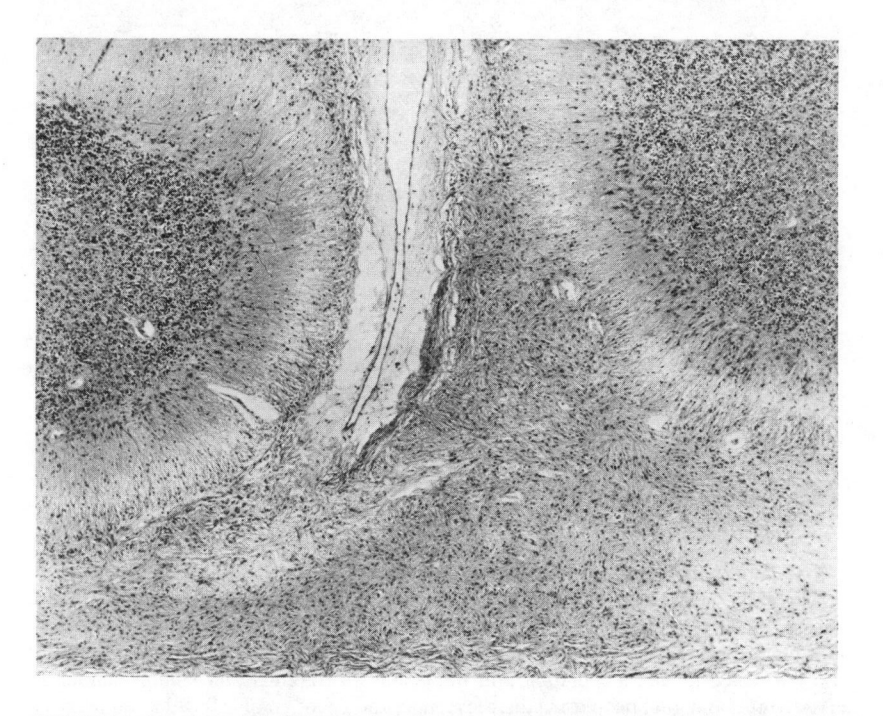

FIGURE 6. Same case as in FIGURES 3-5. Conspicuous invasion of leptomeninges by fibrillated glia originating from the superficial cerebellar cortex. The appearances are indistinguishable from those of an infiltrating cerebellar astrocytoma. PTAH × 50.

vascular endothelial proliferation found in malignant gliomas suggests to us an endothelial origin (FIGURE 8).

Hydromyelia, identified in our series in one example of central NF and one with peripheral NF, constitutes one more malformative CNS lesion that can occasionally be associated with von Recklinghausen's disease.[40]

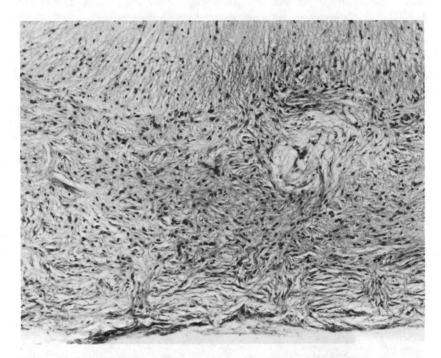

FIGURE 7. Higher magnification of FIGURE 6. The cerebellar subarachnoid space is occupied by fibrillated glial cells which have transgressed the cerebellar pia by way of glial bridges (upper right). PTAH × 150.

SUMMARY

The neuropathological features of 22 autopsied cases of NF have been reviewed, with special reference to the malformative and proliferative lesions implicating the intracranial and intraspinal neural structures. Eleven cases represented examples of the central form of the disease, and 11 examples of the peripheral form. The central form is defined by the association and multiplicity of cranial and spinal meningeal, nerve-sheath, and glial neoplasms (astrocytomas and ependymomas). Bilateral acoustic schwannomas are a frequent, but not invariable, component of the disease. Central NF is also characterized by the very frequent incidence (9 out of 11 cases) of distinctive malformative CNS lesions, which included intramedullary and perivascular schwannosis, meningioangiomatosis, discrete ependymal ectopias, atypical glial cell nests in

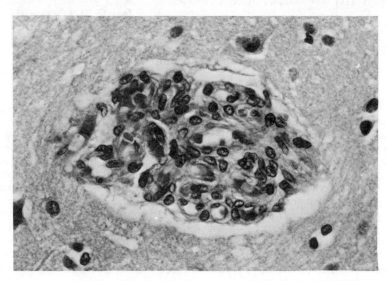

FIGURE 8. Lesion of vascular NF (adventitial nodular type) in the occipital cortex of a 15-year-old patient with peripheral NF. H&E × 500.

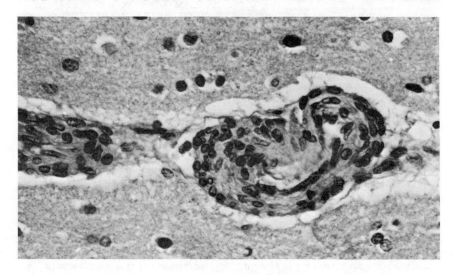

FIGURE 9. Same case as in FIGURE 8. Vascular lesion of NF (intimal and medial cellular hyperplasia) in the occipital cortex. H&E × 500.

the grey matter, and, less frequently, syringomyelia. Many of these hamartomatous changes were closely associated topographically with florid neoplastic lesions.

Five of the 11 cases of peripheral NF showed involvement of the CNS by cellular proliferative changes that included subependymal gliofibrillary nodules in 3 cases (causing aqueduct stenosis in 2, with resulting hydrocephalus in 1); hyperplastic meningoencephalic gliosis involving the pons and the cerebellum in 1 case; and micronodular capillary and arteriolar proliferations typical of the vascular form of NF in 1 case. Whereas some of the glial proliferations are probably hamartomatous in nature, others may represent an abnormal productive neuroglial response to adjacent pathological conditions, such as antecedent cerebral hemorrhage or infarct, known to stimulate a proliferative gliosis. Such a response may exhibit morphological features that are indistinguishable from those of an astrocytoma, including leptomeningeal and perivascular invasion. The incidence of proliferative CNS lesions in both the central and the peripheral form of NF indicates that the spectrum of tissues implicated extends beyond those derived solely from the neural crest.

REFERENCES

1. WISHART, J. H. 1822. Case of tumours in the skull, dura mater and brain. Edinburgh Med. Surg. J. **18:** 393-397.
2. WORSTER-DROUGHT, C., W. E. C. DICKSON & W. H. MCMENEMEY. 1937. Multiple meningeal and perineural tumors with analogous changes in the glia and ependyma (neurofibroblastomatosis). Brain **60:** 85-117.
3. LICHTENSTEIN, B. W. 1949. Neurofibromatosis (von Recklinghausen's disease of the nervous system). Arch. Neurol. Psychiatry **62:** 822-839.
4. RUSSELL, D. S. & L. J. RUBINSTEIN. 1959. Pathology of Tumours of the Nervous System. 1st edit.: 31-37. Edward Arnold. London, England.
5. RUBINSTEIN, L. J. 1963. Tumeurs et hamartomes dans la neurofibromatose centrale. *In* Les Phakomatoses Cérébrales. L. Michaux & M. Feld, Eds.: 427-451. SPEI Editeurs. Paris, France.
6. RODRIGUEZ, H. A. & M. BERTHRONG. 1966. Multiple primary intracranial tumors in von Recklinghausen's neurofibromatosis. Arch. Neurol. **14:** 467-475.
7. KANTER, W. R., R. ELDRIDGE, R. FABRICANT, J. C. ALLEN & T. KOERBER. 1980. Central neurofibromatosis with bilateral acoustic neuroma: genetic, clinical and biochemical distinctions from peripheral neurofibromatosis. Neurology **30:** 851-859.
8. ELDRIDGE, R. 1981. Central neurofibromatosis with bilateral acoustic neuroma. Adv. Neurol. **29:** 57-65.
9. FABRICANT, R. N., G. J. TODARO & R. ELDRIDGE. 1979. Increased levels of a nerve-growth-factor cross-reacting protein in "central" neurofibromatosis. Lancet **1:** 4-7.
10. FABRICANT, R. N. & G. J. TODARO. 1981. Increased serum levels of nerve growth factor in von Recklinghausen's disease. Arch. Neurol. **38:** 401-405.
11. RIOPELLE, R. J., V. M. RICCARDI, S. FAULKNER & M. C. MARTIN. 1984. Serum neuronal growth factor levels in von Recklinghausen's neurofibromatosis. Ann. Neurol. **16:** 54-59.
12. GARDNER, W. J. & O. TURNER. 1940. Bilateral acoustic neurofibromas. Further clinical and pathologic data on hereditary deafness and Recklinghausen's disease. Arch. Neurol. Psychiatry **44:** 76-99.
13. MOYES, P. D. 1968. Familial bilateral acoustic neuroma affecting 14 members from four generations. J. Neurosurg. **29:** 78-82.
14. ALLIEZ, J., J.-L. MASSE & B. ALLIEZ. 1975. Tumeurs bilatérales de l'acoustique et maladie de Recklinghausen observées daus plusieurs générations. Rev. Neurol. **131:** 545-558.
15. DELLEMAN, J. W., J. G. Y. DEJONG & G. M. BLEEKER. 1978. Meningiomas in five members of a family over two generations, in one member simultaneously with acoustic neurinomas. Neurology **28:** 567-570.

16. DAVIS, F. A. 1940. Primary tumors of the optic nerve (a phenomenon of Recklinghausen's disease). A clinical and pathologic study with a report of four cases and a review of the literature. Arch. Ophthalmol. New Ser. **23**: 735-821, 957-1018.
17. BORIT, A. & E. P. RICHARDSON, JR. 1982. The biological and clinical behaviour of pilocytic astrocytomas of the optic pathways. Brain **105**: 161-187.
18. LEWIS, R. A., L. P. GERSON, K. A. AXELSON, V. M. RICCARDI & R. P. WHITFORD. 1984. von Recklinghausen neurofibromatosis. II. Incidence of optic gliomata. Ophthalmologica **91**: 929-935.
19. ILGREN, E. B., L. M. KINNIER-WILSON & C. A. STILLER. 1985. Gliomas in neurofibromatosis: a series of 89 cases with evidence of enhanced malignancy in associated cerebellar astrocytomas. In Pathology Annual, Part 1. S. C. Sommers, P. P. Rosen & R. E. Fechner, Eds. **20**: 331-358. Appleton-Century-Crofts. Norwalk, Conn.
20. MANUELIDIS, E. E. & G. B. SOLITARE. 1971. Glioblastoma multiforme. In Pathology of the Nervous System. J. Minckler, Ed. **2**: 2026-2071. McGraw-Hill. New York, N.Y.
21. RUSSELL, D. S. 1949. Observations on the Pathology of Hydrocephalus. Special Report Series No. 265: 48-50. Medical Research Council. H. M. Stationery Office. London, England.
22. SARAN, N. & F. C. WINTER. 1967. Bilateral gliomas of the optic discs associated with neurofibromatosis. Am. J. Ophthalmol. **64**: 607-612.
23. ZATZ, L. M. 1968. Atypical choroid plexus calcification associated with neurofibromatosis. Radiology **91**: 1135-1139.
24. MACAULAY, R. A. A. 1978. Neurofibrosarcoma of the radial nerve in von Recklinghausen's disease with metastatic angiosarcoma. J. Neurol. Neurosurg. Psychiatry **41**: 474-478.
25. RUBINSTEIN, L. J. 1972. Tumors of the central nervous system. In Atlas of Tumor Pathology. 2nd series, fascicle 6. Armed Forces Institute of Pathology. Washington, D.C.
26. RUSSELL, D. S. & L. J. RUBINSTEIN. 1977. Pathology of Tumours of the Nervous System. 4th edit.: 48-55. Edward Arnold. London, England.
27. STALLARD, H. B. 1938. A case of intraocular neuroma (von Recklinghausen's disease) of the left optic nerve head. Br. J. Ophthalmol. **22**: 11-18.
28. HORI, A. 1973. Über intraspinale Schwannosen der Zona terminalis (Lissauer). (Formes frustes der Neurofibromatose Recklinghausen oder 'reaktiv'?). Acta Neuropathol. **25**: 89-94.
29. LAMBERS, K. & J. C. ORTIZ DE ZARATE. 1952. Zentral und periphere Neurofibromatose unter besonderer Berücksichtung ihrer Beziehungen zur hypertrophischen Neuritis. Dtsch. Z. Nervenheilkd. **169**: 284-307.
30. KASANTIKUL, V. & W. J. BROWN. 1981. Meningioangiomatosis in the absence of von Recklinghausen's disease. Surg. Neurol. **15**: 71-75.
31. HALPER, J., B. W. SCHEITHAUER & H. OKAZAKI. 1985. Meningioangiomatosis: report of three cases with associated Alzheimer's neurofibrillary change. Lab. Invest. **52**: 27A.
32. POSER, C. M. 1956. The Relationship between Syringomyelia and Neoplasm. Charles C. Thomas. Springfield, Ill.
33. SPENCER, W. H. & A. BORIT. 1967. Diffuse hyperplasia of the optic nerve in von Recklinghausen's disease. Am. J. Ophthalmol. **64**: 638-642.
34. HORWICH, A., V. M. RICCARDI & U. FRANCKE. 1983. Aqueductal stenosis leading to hydrocephalus—an unusual manifestation of neurofibromatosis. Am. J. Med. Genet. **14**: 577-581.
35. WALKER, A. E. 1941. Astrocytosis arachnoideae cerebelli. A rare manifestation of von Recklinghausen's neurofibromatosis. Arch. Neurol. Psychiatry **45**: 520-532.
36. DE AJURIAGUERRA, J., M. DAVID & F. HAGUENAU. 1955. Gliose méningo-cérébelleuse et maladie de Recklinghausen. Rev. Neurol. **93**: 645-655.
37. REUBI, F. 1944. Les vaisseaux et les glandes endocrines dans la neurofibromatose. Schweiz. Z. Pathol. Bakteriol. **7**: 168-236.
38. FEYRTER, F. 1949. Über die vasculäre Neurofibromatose, nach Untersuchungen am menschlichen Magen-Darmschlauch. Virchows Arch. **317**: 221-265.
39. MIKUZ, G., G. WEISER & A. PROPST. 1975. Vascular neurofibromatosis. Pathol. Microbiol. **43**: 195-198.
40. HEFFNER, R. R., JR. 1969. Hydromyelia in von Recklinghausen's disease with neurofibrosarcoma. Conn. Med. **33**: 311-313.

On the Natural History of von Recklinghausen Neurofibromatosis

SVEN ASGER SØRENSEN,[a] JOHN J. MULVIHILL,[b]
AND ARNE NIELSEN[a]

[a]Institute of Medical Genetics
The Panum Institute
Blegdamsvej 3
DK-2200 Copenhagen N, Denmark
[b]Clinical Genetics Section
Clinical Epidemiology Branch
National Cancer Institute
Landow Building, Room 8C41
Bethesda, Maryland 20892

INTRODUCTION

With an occurrence of about 1 in 3000 live births,[1] neurofibromatosis is one of the most frequent monogenic inherited disorders. Since von Recklinghausen made the disease a nosologic entity 100 years ago,[2] it has been established that it is inherited as an autosomal dominant trait, that it affects various organs and tissues, and that manifestations vary greatly, even within families.[3] There is also evidence that cancer is associated with neurofibromatosis.[1,4-9] But little is known about the natural history of von Recklinghausen disease.

A nationwide cohort of patients with neurofibromatosis was investigated by Borberg in Denmark about 40 years ago.[10] In order to study the natural history of the disease, we followed up this cohort. The purpose of this paper is to report on the survival and causes of death in the cohort as well as on the incidence and types of neoplasms.

METHODS

The cohort followed up comprises 212 cases of neurofibromatosis. Among these, 84 were probands who consisted of nearly all the patients with the disorder hospitalized in Denmark during the 20-year period from January 1, 1924 to January 1, 1944. The remaining 128 patients were relatives to 35 of the probands. The other 49 probands probably represent new mutations, as there were no proved cases of neurofibromatosis among their relatives.

Borberg's original material was lost but fortunately, in his thesis, Borberg gave the hospital and patient number for each proband so it was possible to identify them at each hospital and then to reconstruct each family through the different national vital records. Except for two relatives who emigrated to the United States, we succeeded in identifying each patient and obtaining vital data for each of these. Thus, the follow-up rate was 99%.

Death certificates were obtained for all dead patients. For those patients we had information about hospitalization, we reviewed hospital records and, when available, also records on postmortem examinations including microscopical descriptions of tumors. To obtain data on the occurrence and types of tumors in the cohort, all 212 patients were searched for at the Danish Cancer Registry. As tumors we considered all malignant neoplasms, as well as benign neoplasms of the central nervous system, but not neurofibromas.

Survival was estimated by standard life-table methods.[11] The numbers of expected neoplasms were determined by applying the age-, year-, and sex-specific incidence rates of the Danish Cancer Registry[12-15] to the corresponding numbers of years at risk, beginning at January 1, 1944. The analysis included 1694 person-years of follow-up for probands and 2145 person-years for the relatives. The strength of association was measured by the ratio of observed cases to expected cases and is referred to as the relative risk.

RESULTS

The distribution of ages at death (FIGURE 1) covers a wide range. Compared to the general population, there is a marked shift in mortality from old age to childhood and middle age. Female neurofibromatosis patients seemed to have a higher mortality in childhood and the reproductive years than males had.

When our follow-up closed on June 1, 1983, 26 of the 36 male probands and 34 of the 40 female probands alive at January 1, 1944 had died. The mean age ± standard deviation (SD) at death for male probands was 57.4 ± 12.7 and for female probands 56.5 ± 20.0. Among the relatives known to have neurofibromatosis and alive at January 1, 1944, 24 of 31 males and 29 of 48 females were dead. The mean age at death for male and female relatives was 67.2 ± 18.9 and 69.7 ± 15.9, respectively.

The survival rates of patients with neurofibromatosis who were alive on January 1, 1944 were compared with the survival rates that would have been expected if their year-, age-, and sex-specific death rates had been those of the general population. Lowered survival rates were encountered for probands as well as for relatives. Survival was significantly worse than that of the general population, and was worse among probands than among relatives. The lowest survival rate was observed in female probands, whereas female relatives with neurofibromatosis had a survival rate just slightly lower than that of the general population.

The causes of death among the 113 patients who died after January 1, 1944 are shown in TABLE 1 from which it appears that the causes of death were as those of the general population. Thus, 77% of the deaths were due to cancer, myocardial infarction, cerebrovascular accidents, and pneumonia. The three cases of death in status epilepticus and the one case of hemorrhage of a pheochromocytoma are probably associated with the patients' neurofibromatosis.

Among those patients who had been hospitalized after January 1, 1944, only four had been hospitalized because of neurofibromatosis. Two had undergone neurosurgery because of neurofibromas in the spinal cord, one was described as having a monstrous plexiform neurofibroma of the face, and the fourth patient had been hospitalized several times for removal of neurofibromas. The remaining causes of hospitalization were very heterogenous, representing most of the common diseases in the general population. Besides tumors, no particular disease appeared with an increased frequency in comparison to the general population. Lung diseases, comprising chronic bronchitis,

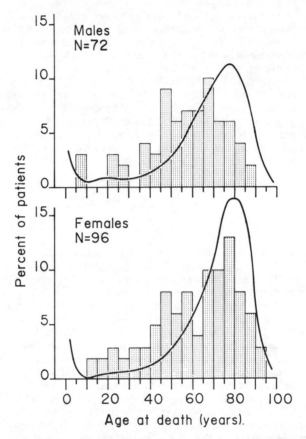

FIGURE 1. Distributions of ages at death of neurofibromatosis patients. Single line represents relative proportions of ages at death in the general Danish population in 1973-1977.

emphysema, and bronchiectasis, were encountered in 10% of the hospitalized patients. Examination of hospital records revealed that 11 patients suffered from epilepsy. Five of these cases were not reported by Borberg,[10] which indicates that epilepsy in these patients developed in middle age or later.

TABLE 2 shows the number of patients with neurofibromatosis who developed a tumor after January 1, 1944. Comparison with the expected numbers calculated from national incidence rates reveals that tumors were more frequent in probands than in

TABLE 1. Causes of Death in 113 Patients with Neurofibromatosis

	Females		Males		Total		
	Probands	Relatives	Probands	Relatives	Females	Males	Male & Female
Malignancy	12	7	9	3	19	12	31
Heart attack	7	7	6	6	14	12	26
Cerebrovascular attack	6	6	1	3	12	4	16
Pneumonia	1	4	6	3	5	9	14
Embolus of pulmonary artery	1	2	1		3	1	4
Epileptic state	2			1	2	1	3
Suicide	1			2	1	2	3
Accident	1		1	1	1	2	3
Pulmonary tuberculosis		1		1	1	1	2
Uremia				2		2	2
Hemorrhage of pheochromocytoma			1			1	1
Hemothorax			1			1	1
Respiratory insufficiency				1		1	1
Hepatic coma		1			1		1
Ileus	1				1		1
Hyperpyrexia	1				1		1
Thyrotoxic crisis		1			1		1
Extrauterin pregnancy	1				1		1
Uncertain (found dead)				1		1	1
	$\overline{34}$	$\overline{29}$	$\overline{26}$	$\overline{24}$	$\overline{63}$	$\overline{50}$	$\overline{113}$

TABLE 2. Neurofibromatosis Patients with Tumors, by Sex and Proband Status

	Males			Females			Total		
	Number	(%)	Relative Risk (CI)[a]	Number	(%)	Relative Risk (CI)[a]	Number	(%)	Relative Risk (CI)[a]
Probands alive January 1, 1944									
observed	14	(39)	3.5 (1.9; 5.9)	20	(50)	4.4 (2.7; 6.8)	34	(45)	4.0 (2.8; 5.6)
expected	4.0			4.5			8.5		
Relatives alive January 1, 1944									
observed	4	(13)	0.9 (0.3; 2.3)	15	(31)	1.9 (1.1; 3.1)	19	(24)	1.5 (0.9; 2.4)
expected	4.4			7.9			12.3		
Total cohort									
observed	18	(27)	2.1 (1.3; 3.4)	35	(40)	2.8 (2.0; 3.9)	53	(34)	2.5 (1.9; 3.3)
expected	8.4			12.4			20.8		

[a] 95% confidence interval for relative risk.

relatives with neurofibromatosis. Tumors arose in 45% of probands but only 24% of relatives, similar to the national lifetime rates in Denmark. The relative risk for probands was significantly high at 4.0 (confidence interval: 2.8; 5.6) while it was insignificantly increased at 1.5 (confidence interval: 0.9; 2.4) for relatives. Among the two sexes, females had relatively more tumors than did males and only females had a statistically increased excess of tumors among the relatives.

The median age at diagnosis of tumor in the total neurofibromatosis cohort was 55 years compared with 68 years (1973-1977) in the general population (FIGURE 2). The shift was even greater for central nervous system (CNS) tumors with a median of 23 years, and for the few peripheral nervous system tumors, 44 years. In the general Danish population, 24% of all CNS tumors occurred under age 40 years. In the cohort, 76% were diagnosed by that age.

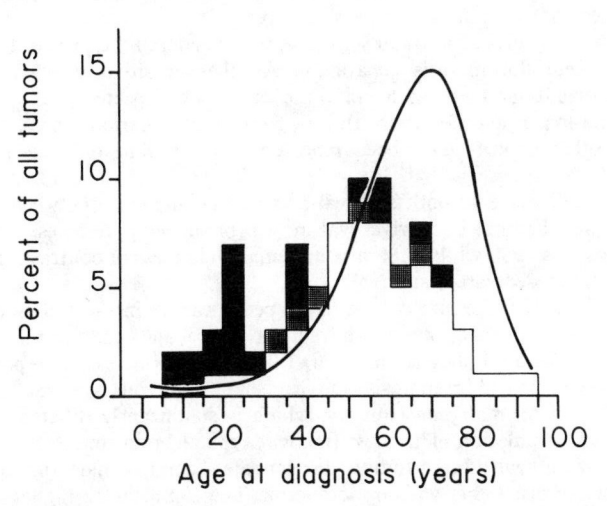

FIGURE 2. Distribution of ages at diagnosis of tumors in neurofibromatosis. Tumor type: black areas, central nervous system; cross-hatched areas, peripheral nervous system; white area; other. Single line represents relative proportions of ages at diagnosis of tumors in the general Danish population in 1973-1977.

The number of tumors in the total cohort was 84: 21 were localized in the central nervous system, 6 in the peripheral nervous system, and the remaining 57 occurred outside the nervous system. Among the tumors of the central nervous system, 19 were histologically documented; 16 of these (84%) were gliomas, two were meningiomas, and 1 a malignant neurolemmoma. The neoplasms of the peripheral nervous system were 4 neurosarcomas, 1 neuromyxoma, and 1 neurinoma of the acoustic nerve.

The tumors outside the nervous system were of different types, some of which occurred with unusual frequency: 12 stomach cancers, 3 pheochromocytomas, 2 osteosarcomas of the maxillary bone, 4 ovarian cancers, and only 2 cases of lung cancer.

Sixteen second primary tumors were encountered. As a second cancer develops in 4% of patients with one cancer in the general population,[16] only two to three cases of secondary primaries were expected among the 70 patients who developed a cancer in the neurofibromatosis cohort. The second tumors occurred all but one in probands and were diagnosed from 0 to 22 years after the first tumor. All but one patient with optic glioma had a second nervous system tumor, including one pheochromocytoma.

DISCUSSION

Because of the great variation of manifestation in neurofibromatosis, ascertainment bias is a serious problem in studies of the disease and may distort the true picture of for instance the natural history of the disorder. The almost complete cohort we have followed up has, like other series, the bias of hospital selection. When Borberg selected his material,[10] he identified the patients by searching hospital records for admission. The probands in his—and our—material are therefore expected to have been so seriously affected that hospitalization was required.

To circumvent the bias of hospital selection, we considered the probands' relatives suffering from neurofibromatosis separately. As these relatives were ascertained through the probands and not as hospitalized cases, we expected that they would express the variation in manifestation, that is, from mild to serious cases.

Studies of other cohorts have been reported,[1,17,18] but none of these have been followed up.

We found a difference in both survival and cancer incidence between probands and relatives. The difference in survival was most pronounced in females: the survival among probands was 15% while 41% among female relatives. In contrast, males had almost identical, but decreased, survival.

About one-third of the entire cohort developed a cancer in the follow-up period of four decades. Again, cancer was more frequent in probands than in relatives. The total relative risk of 2.5 (confidence interval: 1.9; 3.3) confirms earlier reports on an association between neurofibromatosis and cancer.[1,4-9] Nervous system tumors accounted for 47% of all malignant tumors, which is significantly different from the 2% in the general population. The most frequent type of brain tumor was glioma.

Nine of 21 patients with brain tumors developed a second primary tumor. Among these were 5 of the 6 patients with optic glioma. The significantly higher incidence of second primaries in neurofibromatosis in comparison with the general population is a further support to an association between neurofibromatosis and cancer. Second tumors were also more frequent in probands (18%) than in relatives (1%).

The common types of tumors in the general population were also seen in the neurofibromatosis cohort, but with unusual frequency. For instance, there were only two cases of lung cancer in men and seven cases of ovarian cancer in five women.

Two main conclusions can be drawn from our study: a reduction in survival and an increase in the risk of cancer in females. These conclusions are based on the findings among relatives with neurofibromatosis since these, as mentioned before, are expected to reflect more accurately the natural history of neurofibromatosis.

REFERENCES

1. CROWE, F. W., W. J. SCHULL & J. V. NEEL. 1956. A Clinical, Pathological and Genetic Study of Multiple Neurofibromatosis. Charles C. Thomas. Springfield, Ill.
2. VON RECKLINGHAUSEN, F. 1882. Ueber die multiplen Fibrome der Haut und Ihre Beziehung zu den multiplen Neuromen. August Hirschwald. Berlin, Germany.

3. RICCARDI, V. M. 1981. von Recklinghausen neurofibromatosis. N. Engl. J. Med. **305:** 1617-1627.

4. HOSOI, K. 1931. Multiple neurofibromatosis (von Recklinghausen's disease) with special reference to malignant transmission. Arch. Surg. **22:** 258-281.

5. SANDS, M. J., M. T. MCDONOUGH, A. M. COHEN, H. L. RUTENBERG & J. W. EISNER. 1975. Fatal malignant degeneration in multiple neurofibromatosis. J. Am. Med. Assoc. **233:** 1381-1382.

6. KNIGHT, W. A., W. K. MURPHY & J. A. GOTTLIEB. 1973. Neurofibromatosis associated with malignant neurofibromas. Arch. Dermatol. **107:** 747-750.

7. D'AGOSTINO, A. N., E. H. SOULE & R. H. MILLER. 1963. Sarcomas of the peripheral nerves and somatic soft tissues associated with multiple neurofibromatosis (von Recklinghausen's disease). Cancer **16:** 1015-1017.

8. BRASFIELD, R. D. & T. K. DAS GUPTA. 1972. von Recklinghausen's disease: a clinico-pathological study. Ann. Surg. **175:** 86-104.

9. HOPE, D. G. & J. J. MULVIHILL. 1981. Malignancy in neurofibromatosis. Adv. Neurol. **29:** 33-56.

10. BORBERG, A. 1951. Clinical and genetic investigations into tuberous sclerosis and Recklinghausen's neurofibromatosis: contribution to elucidation of interrelationship and eugenics of the syndromes. Acta Psychiatr. Neurol. **71**(Suppl.): 1-239.

11. ARMITAGE, P. 1971. Statistical Methods in Medical Research. Blackwell. Oxford, England.

12. CLEMMESEN, J. 1964. Statistical Studies in Malignant Neoplasms. II. 1943-1957. Munksgaard. Copenhagen, Denmark.

13. CLEMMESEN, J. 1969. Statistical Studies in Malignant Neoplasms. III. 1958-1962. Munksgaard. Copenhagen, Denmark.

14. CLEMMESEN, J. 1974. Statistical Studies in Malignant Neoplasms. IV. Lung-Bladder Ratio: Denmark 1943-67. Munksgaard. Copenhagen, Denmark.

15. CLEMMESEN, J. 1977. Statistical Studies in Malignant Neoplasms. V. Trends and Risks: Denmark 1943-77. Munksgaard. Copenhagen, Denmark.

16. STORM, H. H., O. M. JENSEN, M. EWERTZ, E. LYNGE, J. H. OLSEN, G. SCHOU & A. ØSTERLIND. 1985. Summary: multiple primary cancers in Denmark, 1943-80. Nat. Cancer Inst. Monogr. **68:** 411-430.

17. SAVICKY, V. A. & A. N. TJEREPOU. 1972. Recklinghausen's Neurofibromatosis. Medicina. Moscow, USSR.

18. SAMUELSSON, B. 1981. Neurofibromatosis (v. Recklinghausen's disease): a clinical-psychiatric and genetic study. Dr. Med. Thesis. University of Gothenburg. Gothenburg, Sweden.

Neurofibromatosis

A Genetic Epidemiologist's Point of View

JOHN J. MULVIHILL

Clinical Genetics Section
Clinical Epidemiology Branch
National Cancer Institute
Landow Building, Room 8C41
Bethesda, Maryland 20892

Human genetics is defined as the study of variation and heredity in man; epidemiology is the study of the distribution and determinants of human disease.[1] Therefore, genetic epidemiology is the study of variation and heredity in the distribution and determinants of human disease. An alternate definition of genetic epidemiology is the study of the etiology, distribution, and control of disease in relatives and inherited causes of disease in populations.[2]

As research on neurofibromatosis enters its second century, interdisciplinary studies are finally under way, supplementing and, one may hope, surpassing the endless reports on clinical manifestations. Besides cellular and molecular biology, one research approach that should expedite insight into neurofibromatosis involves the tool called genetic epidemiology. Contrasting the goals and methods of epidemiology and human genetics might clarify these definitions and identify what one discipline might teach the other.

SIMILARITIES

Both disciplines address variation within human populations; the fields would not exist if human beings were not different from one another in stature, intelligence, disease, etc. Each science relies extensively on statistics and has, in turn, stimulated developments in biostatistics to attack problems such as multiple determinants and confounding factors in the same population and clustering in time and space or within families. For both disciplines, the natural phenomenon of twinning and multiple births provides a special tool for distinguishing intrinsic and extrinsic determinants. Other areas of joint interest include variation by ethnicity, sex, and family occurrence. In practice, differences in these features are often cited as evidence for environmental causes by epidemiologists and for inherited factors by geneticists, especially if cultural inheritance is included. At times, both interpretations may be correct.

DISSIMILARITIES

As a science, genetics represents a body of knowledge about genes. In contrast, the core of epidemiology is methodologic; its body of knowledge comprises ways of understanding disease. The concern of epidemiology is human disease, that is, differences in health. Epidemiologists tend to dichotomize traits, especially disease versus nondisease. Population geneticists often study continuous variation in traits that need not be matters of health; in fact, they typically examine quantitative variations within the normal population (e.g., finger dermal ridge counts). Unlike the fairly monolithic discipline of epidemiology, medical genetics has fragmented in recent years to encompass areas that sometimes communicate poorly: cytogenetics, metabolic genetics, behavioral genetics, population genetics, and statistical genetics.

LESSONS FROM GENETICS FOR EPIDEMIOLOGISTS

The first message is that there are genes. Geneticists quickly turn to laboratory methodologies to clarify clinical observations, whereas epidemiologists in general are slow to do so; they must count and analyze, things they do very well.

Present-day epidemiologists have focused on the environmental antecedents of disease and have neglected single-gene traits like neurofibromatosis. Clearly, there are time-dependent manifestations of the neurofibromatosis gene. In other words, because the clinical picture changes with age, environmental factors must interact with the mutant gene. Epidemiologists might help search for such factors. Four obvious issues that would benefit from epidemiologic expertise are the age of onset of various features, the age of progression of features, inter- and intrafamilial variations, and possible hormonal influences. The latter includes the "maternal effect," namely, whether or not offspring are more severely affected when they inherit the gene from their mothers than when they represent new mutations or inheritance from affected fathers. J. C. Carey explains these and other genetic questions in detail (this volume).

LESSONS FROM EPIDEMIOLOGY FOR GENETICISTS

Origin of the Danish Follow-up

To my thinking, the follow-up study by the Danish cohort of neurofibromatosis is an example of effective genetic epidemiology. The collaboration began at a coffee break in 1979 at Chateaux Ripaille, on the French coast of Lake Geneva, where one of a series of three-day meetings was being held by the Committee of Epidemiology of the International Commission for Protection Against Environmental Mutagens and Carcinogens. The committee's task was to write working papers on how epidemiologists might document germ cell mutations in human beings.[3] One of the seven men on the committee was Johannes Clemmeson (FIGURE 1), an engaging Danish pathologist, who, in 1943, founded what became the world's most famous cancer registry. Since I was in the midst of preparing a monograph on neurofibromatosis,[4] I asked Dr. Clemmeson if he knew Dr. Alan Borberg (FIGURE 2) and his monograph on neurofibromatosis and tuberous sclerosis.[5] Dr. Clemmeson said he thought Borberg was a psychiatrist; he said the name rang a bell and that he would follow up.

As it turned out, Dr. Borberg had died that very month at age 66 years. He had done his M.D. thesis in Kemp's Institute of Medical Genetics, University of Copenhagen. It happened that the first statistician in Clemmeson's Danish Cancer Registry, Mr. Arne Nielson, was currently in the Institute for Medical Genetics. Dr. Clemmeson called Mr. Nielson, who approached Dr. S. Asger Sørensen, who called Dr. Borberg's widow. She said she had just discarded her husband's papers! Fortunately, the original monograph gave, for each proband, the initials, hospital of ascertainment, and hospital chart number.[5] So it was possible for Dr. Sørensen to track down all 212 patients in the series, except the two who moved to the United States, where I subsequently failed to find them.

The points in this story are these: design, data, denominator.

Design of Clinical Studies

In epidemiological terms, the Danish study has the many advantages of a retrospective cohort study (or a longitudinal study). The statistical methods for handling such data were well in hand. Cohort studies are often impossible because of cost and time requirements and small numbers. If follow-up of a cohort defined years ago is feasible, the findings can be more reliable than cross-sectional study of prevalent cases. In the Danish follow-up study,[6] the group of probands and relatives was defined by Borberg in 1944. The results show the large influence of ascertainment bias on the mortality rate and frequency of cancer in neurofibromatosis.

A pressing question is what to tell the parents of a one-year-old with café-au-lait spots and axillary freckling or a person with neurofibromatosis who is considering a pregnancy. In general, information from a hospital or clinic series helps define the range of manifestations of neurofibromatosis, but 100 years of case reports have done that quite well. In short, most organ systems can have severe or mild symptoms, malignant or benign lesions, or none at all. The information that is needed for clinical management is lifetime mortality rates and true *natural* history (as opposed to *clinical* history).

Data Resources

The Borberg cohort is the oldest, large, defined group of patients. It has the further advantage of representing nearly complete nationwide ascertainment. Other groups that might be followed up are the Crowe, Schull, and Neel series in Michigan[7] or the Moscow series.[8] Each is more recent than the Borberg cohort, and neither achieves national coverage. Future consideration might be given to a truly population-based, household census study that would accurately sample the general population. Hereafter, it will not be sufficient to have patients come to any medical care setting at all if we want to know the true picture of neurofibromatosis.

The U.S. National Center for Health Statistics conducts periodic household surveys that, in the past, have incorporated dermatology examinations and, in the future, might enumerate individuals with signs of neurofibromatosis, even including results of split-lamp examination for Lisch nodules. Another data source of the National Center for Health Statistics is the multiple causes of death tapes for the years 1968 to 1980.[9,10] Usual mortality data are based only on the underlying cause of death determined by certain algorithms from the four lines allowed for medical events on most death certificates. The new multiple causes of death tapes list up to 20 medical

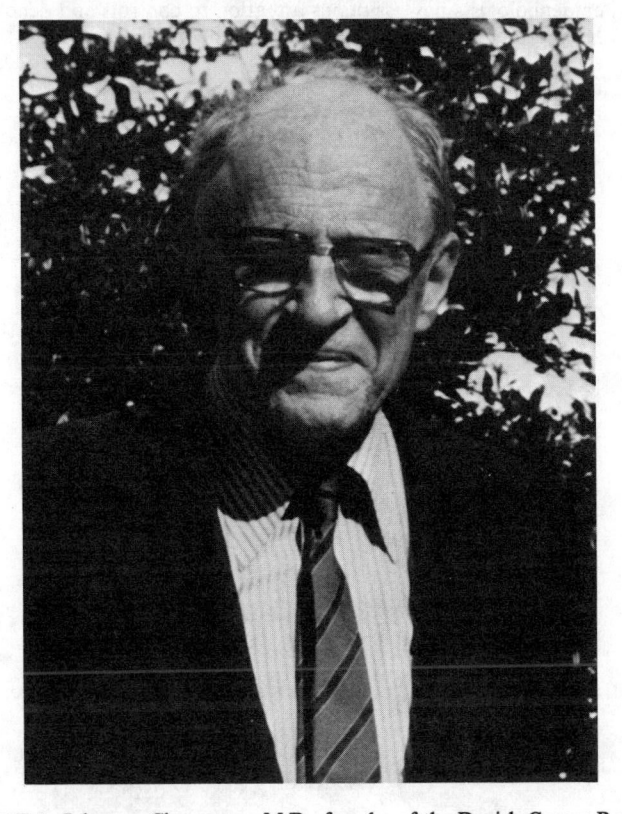

FIGURE 1. Johannes Clemmeson, M.D., founder of the Danish Cancer Registry.

events that a physician may have written on the death certificate. The 13 years of tapes costs only $9000 and can be expected to show associations of neurofibromatosis with other disorders that need to be quantified better than they have been in the past. The frequency of brain tumors and pheochromocytoma might be independently assessed. New associations might be revealed that have not been appreciated in clinic series.

Other potentially useful data sources are the Veterans' Follow-Up Agency (mostly male discharge records from all Veterans Administration hospitals)[11] and population-based surveillance of birth defects, as in metropolitan Atlanta, Georgia[12] and in

Hungary.[13] Bader has effectively used data collected by a cancer cooperative group, the Late Effects Study Group, to estimate that 1% of childhood cancer arises in individuals with neurofibromatosis.[14]

Denominators in Clinical Series

Finally, epidemiologists pay assiduous attention to controls and denominators. In estimating the prevalence of certain features of neurofibromatosis, it is obviously

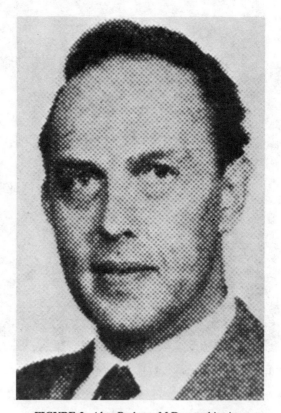

FIGURE 2. Alan Borberg, M.D., psychiatrist.

important to have the numerator as well defined and counted as possible. In general, the quality of numerators is excellent. What is lacking from most presentations is similar attention to the denominator. Rigorous epidemiologic studies have carefully defined comparison groups. In the Danish follow-up investigation,[6] the comparison was based on expectations calculated from vital records and cancer incidence rates that, like the cohort, were collected over the same years and throughout the nation.

In other studies, special control groups might have to be selected, sometimes at considerable but unavoidable expense.

By way of example, one may contrast the rates of cancer in neurofibromatosis reported by the Mayo Clinic[15] and the Memorial Sloan-Kettering Cancer Center, New York.[16] The frequencies were 3% and 28%. Apart from the problem of presenting just a percentage without regard to expected rates, it is obvious that the fraction of neurofibromatosis patients with cancer would be higher at a specialized cancer hospital than at a general medical facility. Similarly, when a neurology or an orthopedic center reports manifestations of neurofibromatosis, one must remember that the denominator is "all neurofibromatosis patients seen in a large referral center," and not "all persons with the neurofibromatosis gene."

CONCLUSIONS

Geneticists can teach epidemiologists that genes exist, that they cause disorders, like neurofibromatosis, and that there are environmental determinants in the expression of these genes that deserve epidemiologic study. Epidemiologists must teach geneticists that there are research techniques in neurofibromatosis that they have neglected, such as design of studies, development of data resources, and devotion to the denominator.

ACKNOWLEDGMENTS

I thank Drs. D. M. Parry and J. Byrne for critical comments on an early draft and Ms. L. E. Walton for manuscript preparation.

REFERENCES

1. MacMahon, B. & T. F. Pugh, Eds. 1970. Epidemiology: Principles and Methods. Little, Brown and Company. Boston, Mass.
2. Morton, N. E. & C. S. Chung, Eds. 1978. Genetic Epidemiology. Academic Press. New York, N.Y.
3. Miller, J. R., J. Clemmesen, E. Czeizel, H. J. Evans, E. B. Hook, J. D. Jansen, M. F. LeChat, E. Matsunaga, J. J. Mulvihill & P. Oftedal. 1983. A report to the International Commission for Protection against Environmental Mutagens and Carcinogens by Committee 5 (Epidemiology). Mutation epidemiology: review and recommendations. Mutat. Res. 123: 1-11.
4. Riccardi, V. M. & J. J. Mulvihill, Eds. 1981. Neurofibromatosis (von Recklinghausen's disease): genetics, cell biology, and biochemistry. Adv. Neurol. 29: 282.
5. Borberg, A. 1951. Clinical and genetic investigations into tuberous sclerosis and Recklinghausen's neurofibromatosis. Contributions to elucidation of interrelationship and eugenics of the syndromes. Acta Psychiatr. Neurol. 71(Suppl.): 1-239.
6. Sørensen, S. A., J. J. Mulvihill & A. Nielsen. 1986. Nation-wide follow-up of Recklinghausen's neurofibromatosis: survival and malignant neoplasms. N. Engl. J. Med. 314: 1010-1015.

7. CROWE, F. W., W. J. SCHULL & J. V. NEEL. 1965. A Clinical, Pathological and Genetic Study of Multiple Neurofibromatosis. Charles C. Thomas. Springfield, Ill.
8. SAVITSKY, V. A. & A. N. CHEREPANOV, Eds. 1972. Recklinghausen's Neurofibromatosis. Meditsina Press. Moscow, USSR.
9. National Center for Health Statistics. 1984. Multiple causes of death in the United States. Monthly Vital Statistics Report 32(10, Suppl. (2)). DHHS Publication No. (PHS) 84-1120. Public Health Service. Hyattsville, Md. (Feb. 14).
10. SCHOLL, T., Z. STEIN & H. HANSEN. 1982. Leukemia and other cancers, anomalies and infections as causes of death in Down's syndrome in the United States during 1976. Dev. Med. Child Neurol. 24: 817-829.
11. DEBAKEY, M. E. & G. W. BEEBE. 1962. Medical follow-up studies on veterans. J. Am. Med. Assoc. 182: 1103-1109.
12. Centers for Disease Control. 1980. Congenital malformations surveillance report January-December 1979. U.S. Department of Health, Education and Welfare. Atlanta, Ga.
13. CZIEZEL, A. & G. TUSNÁDY, Eds. 1984. Aetiological Studies of Isolated Common Congenital Abnormalities in Hungary. Akadémiai Kiadó. Budapest, Hungary.
14. BADER, J. L., A. T. MEADOWS, J. LEMERLE, P. A. VOUTE, P. MORRIS-JONES, W. A. NEWTON, A. BANFI & E. S. BAUM. 1980. Neurofibromatosis (NF) and other genetic defects associated with childhood cancer. (abstr.) Am. J. Hum. Genet. 32: 94.
15. D'AGOSTINO, A. N., E. H. SOULE & R. H. MILLER. 1963. Sarcomas of the peripheral nerves and somatic soft tissues associated with multiple neurofibromastosis (von Recklinghausen's disease). Cancer 16: 1015-1027.
16. BRASFIELD, R. D. & T. K. DAS GUPTA. 1972. Von Recklinghausen's disease: a clinicopathological study. Ann. Surg. 175: 86-104.

The Genetic Aspects of Neurofibromatosis[a]

JOHN C. CAREY,[b] BONNIE J. BATY,[b]
JOHN P. JOHNSON,[b] TRUDI MORRISON,[c]
MARK SKOLNICK,[c] AND JANE KIVLIN[d]

[b]Department of Pediatrics
[c]Department of Medical Biophysics and Computing
[d]Department of Ophthalmology
University of Utah School of Medicine
Salt Lake City, Utah 84132

Neurofibromatosis (NF) is one of the most common, potentially serious, autosomal dominant conditions in man. Crowe estimated the prevalence to be one in 2500 to 3300 and from this figure calculated a mutation rate of 1×10^{-4} per gamete per generation, long considered the highest in humans.[1] The phenotypic manifestations consist of cutaneous pigmentary changes and multiple benign neurofibromas; affected individuals are at risk for a diverse array of osseous, central nervous system, and neoplastic complications. There is marked variability in clinical involvement, making NF a prototypic condition for the study of the biologic mechanisms of variable expressivity in autosomal dominant disorders.[2] Because of the diversity of clinical manifestations, presentation can range from the child with a multiple congenital anomaly/dysplasia syndrome to the adult with a solid tumor malignancy. Various authors have labeled NF as a phacomatosis, a hamartomatous disorder, a neurocutaneous condition, and most recently a neurocristopathy.[3] Despite the recent increased interest in this genetic disorder, many unanswered questions about the clinical and biologic aspects of NF remain obvious and emphasize the need for this symposium.

Several comprehensive population studies in various parts of the world have established the mode of transmission of NF as autosomal dominant with high penetrance.[1,4–9] In particular, Riccardi's investigation in Houston consists of an ongoing longitudinal study of over 200 affected persons and continues to expand the growing knowledge base on the genetic aspects and natural history. On first glance, the number of series and their wide geographical distribution might suggest that further research into the classical genetics of NF is unnecessary. However, several basic genetic issues are still unresolved and the interpretation of the genetic data is often conflicting. These issues are of more than theoretical significance as the available genetic information is important for clinicians involved in the delivery of clinical genetic services.

The purpose of this paper is to review and document the unresolved issues regarding the hereditary aspects of the condition. We will summarize and reinterpret the recent available data on the genetics of NF. The presentation will overview the following

[a]This work was supported in part by National Institutes of Health Grant No. CA-28854, Genetic Epidemiology of Cancer in Utah Genealogies, and by March of Dimes Service Grant No. C-310.

areas: (1) NF and the classical principles of human genetics, (2) diagnostic criteria, (3) maternal effect on severity of NF, (4) heterogeneity, and (5) genetic counseling. In addition, some preliminary data on an investigation of 11 Utah kindreds will be introduced. These families were evaluated clinically as part of an ongoing study of linkage using restriction fragment length polymorphisms.

FORMAL GENETIC PRINCIPLES AND NF

As stated above, NF is considered to be an autosomal dominant condition with high penetrance and variable expressivity. The evidence to support the hypothesis that NF is due to an autosomal dominant gene comes from analysis of well-documented published pedigrees and from the calculation of classic segregation ratios in three major population studies.[1,4,5] Borberg reviewed the familial cases of NF, reported prior to 1950.[4] The findings included concordance of identical twins, several pedigrees of two-generation inheritance, 18 pedigrees of three-generation transmission, and at least 6 with four-generation transmission. Of course, the most well-known, early report of familial cases was in siblings by von Recklinghausen in 1882. Borberg's own data documented 9 families with three-generation transmission and 3 with transmission through four generations. Since several of these pedigrees showed male-to-male transmission, simple dominant inheritance is implied from a mere perusal of the pedigrees/case reports. Crowe's population study in Michigan adds 11 additional families with three generations and 2 with four-generation transmission. Prior to these two monographs, several authors had come to different conclusions, including irregular dominance and autosomal recessive inheritance.[4] However, the milder expression of the condition was not well documented until these reports and consanguinity was noted only once.[4] The results of the segregation ratios of frequency of affected offspring of affected adults in the three major population studies were consistent with dominant inheritance, as the frequencies were 0.51, 0.43, and 0.49 respectively.[1,4,5] Thus, the data from the recent studies are clearly consistent with simple autosomal dominant inheritance. No cases of apparent homozygosity have been documented.

Penetrance is the term that applies to a gene's ability to be expressed at all; it is an all or none situation and is contingent on the methods for studying genotype and phenotype. Although the gene for NF is frequently stated to have high penetrance, data on the direct estimation of penetrance are sparse. Using 6 informative, three-generation families and Crowe's pedigrees, Sergeyev directly estimated that the penetrance of NF cannot be under 80%.[5] This figure is based on a sample size of only 17 three-generation chains. The actual penetrance is likely much higher and close to 100%. The Utah kindreds that have been recently evaluated consist of 4 three-generation pedigrees and 1 four-generation family. The gene was 100% penetrant in these kindreds and when these data are added to Sergeyev's calculation, the sample size increases and, thus, the minimum penetrance estimation increases (data to be published later). It is also of note that the family reported by Carey as an example of incomplete penetrance probably has the central type of NF.[8] The segregation ratios stated above indirectly support the high penetrance.

The term *expressivity* refers to the variable manifestations of a given gene and is related to the degree of involvement. In regard to NF, the clinical significance of the genetic concept of expressivity relates to the natural history and the frequency of occurrence of the various manifestations. This issue is of obvious significance to families when a member is newly diagnosed to have NF. Because of the inherent bias in the hospital-ascertained population studies, data from the literature in counseling a family regarding a particular complication tend to emphasize the more severe aspects of NF.[8,10] Crowe and Borberg documented the occurrence of minimally affected individuals and labeled them as "forme fruste" cases. More recent authors have attempted to develop a clinical severity scale: two recent reports would suggest that about one-third of affected individuals have more severe manifestations, while the remainder have predominantly cutaneous expression.[6,8] This issue of the risk for the more serious and specific complications of NF is important for anticipatory guidance in families of NF. Future studies of natural history will ideally refine the limited figures on risk for the severe manifestations[8] and provide guidelines for routine health supervision of affected individuals.

The concept of *pleiotropy* refers to the fact that a single mutation can have many different consequences in a single individual. The clinical correlate of this basic genetic concept is encompassed in the term "syndrome." The many discussions about the pathogenesis of NF exemplify this genetic principle. Other presentations in this volume deal specifically with pathogenesis, and it is beyond the scope of this paper to review this literature.

One of the most commonly cited statements about the genetics of NF is that it is the most common autosomal dominant *mutation* in man. This statement has taken on an aura of conventional wisdom as it is present in the more widely used texts and most comprehensive reviews of NF.[7,11,12] However, the evidence to substantiate this conclusion is not clear-cut. The direct method for calculating a mutation rate is based on the prevalence of the condition and the frequency of sporadic (nonfamilial) cases among the total. The figure that is most commonly cited comes from Crowe[1] and was estimated as 1×10^{-4} or 100×10^{-6}. Review of Crowe's assumptions suggests that this estimation may be too high. The reasons for this comment are the following. (1) The estimation of prevalence in Crowe's study came from indirect information that involved a number of assumptions and a large error factor. Crowe estimates the prevalence of NF indirectly by examining the number of his ascertained cases in two other hospital settings. If he had found a second case in either of his two other sources, the prevalence figure would have been halved and this makes the prevalence estimate a very rough one. The figure of 1 in 2500-3300, however, is often stated as definite by most sources. (2) Sergeyev's estimation of prevalence is based on systematic examination of consecutive cases of 16-year-olds in Russia for military examination.[5] This figure of 1 in 7800 may also be an underestimation since the penetrance of NF may not be complete by the age of 16. Thus, while Crowe's prevalence figure of 1 in 2500-3300 may be high, Sergeyev's estimation is probably low. This still puts the mutation rate of NF as one of the highest in man, but close to those estimates of adult polycystic kidney disease, Duchenne muscular dystrophy, and hemophilia A.[5,11] It is important to be aware of the assumptions that go into the estimation of prevalence before one makes the strong statement of NF's excessively high mutation rate.

The other assumption that goes into the calculation of mutation rates is the frequency of sporadic cases among propositi. This figure has been derived in five separate studies. The frequency of sporadic cases ranges from 0.45 to 0.77, i.e., 45% to 77% of propositi represent nonfamilial probands.[1,4-6,8] As in the studies of expressivity, it is difficult to derive a very precise figure because of the varying ascertainment of cases and the different methods that the authors utilize in deriving the figure. In regard to ascertainment, for example, the San Francisco study was based on cases ascertained in a genetic counseling clinic and thus may be an overestimate of the frequency of familial probands.[8] On the other hand, the studies that ascertain their cases from hospital surveys vary in the thoroughness of examining parents and, thus, will affect the estimate of the sporadic cases. It is difficult to understand why the frequency of sporadic cases of 77% is so high in the Russian study compared to the other data bases.[5]

There is a body of evidence in the human genetics literature that would suggest that advanced paternal age is related to the occurrence of de novo mutations. This effect has been adequately documented for sporadic cases of achondroplasia, the Apert syndrome, and Marfan syndrome.[11] Data from three of the population studies of NF did not claim a paternal effect,[1,4,8] while Sergeyev's investigation did document such an effect.[5] Recently Riccardi et al. indicated that these conflicting results may be due to the large time span for birth years of the cases and to the problems in designating the proper control group for comparing paternal ages. Their approach to the situation led them to develop a methodology for controlling the general population, and these authors demonstrated a paternal age effect in NF.[13]

DIAGNOSTIC CRITERIA IN NF

Precision in diagnosis of any disorder is of obvious significance in discussing genetic aspects. Therefore, diagnostic criteria in NF will be reviewed. The two most consistent features used in the clinical diagnosis of NF are the cutaneous manifestations of café-au-lait spots and neurofibromas. However, the marked variability of expression, including these cutaneous ones, makes secure diagnosis or exclusion of NF sometimes difficult. Crowe documented that 79% of the 149 personally examined individuals had six or more café-au-lait spots of greater than 1.5 cm in diameter.[1] The "six spots" rule has become the established diagnostic criteria by many clinicians. However, it is important to note that the number six was chosen because an evaluation of 1000 normal individuals indicated that no one had more than five café-au-lait spots.[1] Crowe chose the 1.5 cm measurement arbitrarily to distinguish the café-au-lait spot from the common freckle. Thus, there is nothing magical about the stated number and if utilized in young children may lead to underdiagnosis. The actual frequency of multiple café-au-lait spots in the general population has not been studied in any extensive manner. Whitehouse's data from a well-baby clinic form the single well-documented frequency study and indicate that about 10% of otherwise normal children will have one or two café-au-lait spots of at least 0.5 cm. He suggests that the presence of more than five spots should raise the diagnosis.[14] In the populations studies, various authors have established their own criteria for the purposes of standardization. Riccardi's most recent criteria are helpful in research and consist of six or more café-au-lait spots accompanied by any one of the following three findings: axillary freckling, multiple neurofibromas, or family history.[15]

Recently, the presence of Lisch nodules of the iris has been emphasized as an important diagnostic feature in NF.[7] These nodules are iris hamartomata, probably of melanocytic origin.[16] Lewis has emphasized that Lisch nodules can be differentiated from the more common iris nevi and has documented the frequent occurrence and the age dependence of these iris hamartomata in individuals with NF. In their study, 92% of individuals over the age of 6 with NF exhibited the nodules.[15] In the evaluation of 11 Utah kindreds, 37 of 40 clearly affected persons over 6 years had Lisch nodules, substantiating Lewis' data and those of earlier reports.[15] This finding can be of importance in two common clinical situations in the genetics clinic: (1) the asymptomatic child who has five or more café-au-lait spots, and (2) the asymptomatic school-age child who is the offspring of an affected adult. Even though the frequency of Lisch nodules (as opposed to iris nevi) is not known in the general population, the presence of the nodules in these situations would point toward the individual having NF. Riccardi states that he knows of no disorder other than NF in which these iris hamartomata occur.[2] However, future studies are needed to confirm that Lisch nodules are not otherwise present in the general population. In addition, investigations where the ophthalmologist is blind to the status of the examined individual would be helpful in substantiating Lewis's statement that iris nevi and Lisch nodules are easily separable. During the evaluation of the Utah kindreds, two individuals at risk for NF (because of having an affected parent) exhibited Lisch nodules *without* diagnostic cutaneous manifestations. One of the individuals was an 8-year-old girl with one café-au-lait spot and the other was a 20-year-old man with two café-au-lait spots. Neither of these individuals had neurofibromas or any other distinctive manifestation of NF. It was concluded that these persons probably have the gene for NF with minimal expression; however, a secure conclusion would require the above information.

For genetic counseling purposes, an age of onset / penetrance curve would be helpful in evaluating NF families. Since café-au-lait spots and Lisch nodules both are age dependent, one could theoretically construct a curve of increasing number of affected individuals over time. If Lisch nodules turn out to be as useful a marker as is suggested above, the gene penetrance from the presence of iris nodules could be estimated as 90% by age 10. (Thirteen of 15 affected individuals in Lewis's study between the ages of 6 and 10 exhibited Lisch nodules.)[15] The same type of estimate could be applied to café-au-lait spots. With this approach in mind, Crowe's data on the frequency of café-au-lait spots according to age were reevaluated. Because of the rarity in the general population of four or more café-au-lait spots, the presence of this number of spots in a person at 50% risk for the gene (offspring of an affected parent) would suggest the diagnosis. From Crowe's data, there appears to be some age effect to the occurrence of café-au-lait spots as the mean number of spots from 0 to 4 is less than the mean number of spots in affected persons between 5 and 9. It is also of note that the mean number of café-au-lait spots in affected people between the ages of 5 and 9 is the same as the older 10-year age groups (10-19, 20-29, etc.). Thus, this would imply that the number of café-au-lait spots increases during these first five years of life; and then if one is going to develop café-au-lait spots, they are present between 5 and 9. Interestingly, the age grouping 6-10 overlaps in the peak development of both café-au-lait spots and iris nodules. The other age effect of café-au-lait spots of importance in Crowe's data is the fact that the mean number of café-au-lait spots in individuals over 50 is less than in the younger age groups. Although the numbers are smaller, this would suggest that there may be some fading of spots in older individuals. Crowe personally examined 149 affected individuals with NF in the study; these included 4 individuals with segmental form of NF, 3 with acoustic neuromas, and several who were at the extremes of age (i.e., younger than 5, older than 50). Twelve of the individuals who had less than four spots fell into these groups and made up almost 50% of those with less than four spots. If they are eliminated from the analysis, then 89.5% of affected individuals with classic NF between the ages of 5 and 50 have four or more café-au-lait spots. This makes the presence of this number of cutaneous nevi a consistent finding and would suggest that the expression of four café-au-lait spots is about 90% by age 10. The frequency of café-au-lait spots and Lisch nodules by the age of 10 can be used to develop an age-penetrance curve for NF and would help in estimating the probability of an at-risk person who has no signs, including Lisch nodules, of being affected. It appears that the age period of 5 to 10 is a crucial time in the expression of both of these manifestations. On the other hand, the absence of both of these findings after age 10 does not eliminate the possibility of the gene, since neurofibromas and other manifestations may appear in the second decade of life. These above estimates are based on several assumptions and are rough; prospective data on the development of these signs will be necessary for a more accurate estimation of an age of onset/penetrance curve for NF.

In addition to the more consistent diagnostic features of NF, there are a number of abnormalities that are suggestive of the diagnosis when one sees an individual with the particular finding. TABLE 1 lists the abnormalities in which greater than 50% of individuals with the finding will have NF. The Francois "syndrome" is certainly diagnostic of NF. Pseudoarthrosis of the tibia should always bring the condition to mind. Although the findings that are listed in the table are of low frequency in NF, they are distinctive enough that their presence in an individual with nondiagnostic cutaneous manifestations would support or suggest the diagnosis. There are many other manifestations of NF that are nonspecific and because of their commonness would not be as helpful or supportive; these would include seizures, short stature, scoliosis, macrocephaly, and mental retardation.

TABLE 2 presents a summary of the preliminary results of the clinical evaluation of the individuals in the 11 Utah kindreds. This study was initiated for the purpose of gathering familial cases for linkage analysis through restriction fragment length polymorphisms. The latter investigation is ongoing in the laboratory of Dr. Mark Skolnick. Thus far, 11 kindreds of at least two-generation transmission have been seen. The diagnosis of the affected individuals has been confirmed by history, physical examination, and ophthalmologic evaluation. Appropriate records have been gathered. As mentioned above, in these families the gene for NF has 100% penetrance. Thirty-seven out of 38 individuals between 5 and 50 years have four or more café-au-lait spots. The principle clinical finding of note is that 2 of the at-risk individuals exhibit more than three Lisch nodules in each iris and yet have nondiagnostic cutaneous manifestations.

TABLE 1. Summary of Distinguishing Features Associated with Neurofibromatosis

Greater than 50% of individuals with following abnormalities have NF
—presence strongly suggestive of NF:

  Pseudoarthrosis of tibia
  Francois "syndrome"
  Optic gliomas in infancy
  Thoracic meningoceles
  Sphenoid bone deficiency
  Lamboidal calvarial defect on x-ray

Less than 50% of individuals with the following abnormalities have NF
—presence of any of these findings should raise NF:

  Hemihypertrophy
  Macrodactyly
  Renal artery stenosis in childhood
  Diencephalic syndrome
  Meningiomas in childhood
  Precocious puberty

TABLE 2. Summary of Genetic and Clinical Data from Utah Families

---

Genetic
- 11 kindreds
  - 6 two-generation pedigrees
  - 4 three-generation pedigrees
  - 1 four-generation pedigree
- 54 affected individuals examined
- Age range: 7 months to 65 years
- 100% penetrance

Clinical
- 37/38 affected persons between 5-50 years have 4 or more café-au-lait spots
- 37/40 affected persons older than 6 years have Lisch nodules of iris
- All but 1 person over 20 have 1 or more cutaneous neurofibromas
- 2 at-risk family members have Lisch nodules and 1-2 café-au-lait spots

---

MATERNAL EFFECT ON SEVERITY OF NF

In 1978, Miller and Hall suggested that there may be a maternal effect in neu-rofibromatosis similar to the one documented in myotonic dystrophy.[17] Their cases who were offspring of affected mothers were more often severely involved and had an earlier age of onset. The authors suggested that one of the factors affecting the variation in expressivity of NF may be related to the intrauterine environment and humoral factors transmitted across the placenta. Subsequent reports that have inves-tigated this hypothesis have not substantiated the data either in general or examining more specific manifestations.[2,8,15]

HETEROGENEITY OF NF

Recent reports have indicated that an autosomal dominant disorder of bilateral acoustic neuromas with occasional peripheral signs of NF is a distinct genetic entity.[18] This particular condition has been designated as central neurofibromatosis or the acoustic neuroma form. The delineation of this disorder as an entity distinct from classical von Recklinghausen neurofibromatosis establishes the heterogeneity of NF. Heterogeneity for genetic conditions is clearly becoming one of the basic principles of genetic disease. Documentation of heterogeneity in the history of the delineation of many genetic disorders has helped sort out what was initially interpreted to be variability in clinical expression. Examples of this principle are typified in the clas-sification of osteogenesis imperfecta, Ehlers-Danlos, albinism, and many inborn errors of metabolism. Riccardi recently proposed a classification of the NF disorders.[19] Numerical designations from I to VII were applied to the various entities. However, this classification has not come into common usage, probably because clearly distinctive disorders are lumped with not-well-established entities. The so-called type III mixed form and the type IV variant form are not well defined by this classification and their usage is not clinically practical at this point. Certainly, the four established disorders would consist of (1) von Recklinghausen neurofibromatosis, (2) the central form with acoustic neuromas, (3) familial café-au-lait spots, and (4) segmental neurofibromatosis. Recently Hall *et al.* described four children with peripheral manifestations of NF accompanied by a phenotype similar to the Noonan syndrome.[20] We would feel that this also represents a distinguishable fifth entity. The late onset form of NF as described by Riccardi may be another presentation of the segmental form of NF.

In Crowe's original monograph, four of the affected individuals exhibited peripheral signs of NF localized to one segment of the body. Since that study, several cases of this presentation have been documented in the literature. Miller and Sparks reviewed the literature, reported two cases, and labeled this as segmental neurofibromatosis.[21] Since that time, four additional cases have been reported.[19,22,23] The Utah genetics clinic group has evaluated three individuals with segmental NF in the last six years. These cases will be briefly reported here:

Case 1. This eight-year-old female was referred for evaluation of multiple café-au-lait spots. Medical history was otherwise uncomplicated, and family history was noncontributory. On physical examination, the head circumference and height were between the 50th and 75th percentile. Physical examination was normal except for the examination of the skin. There were two café-au-lait spots of 1 cm in diameter in the right abdominal area. Several 1 to 2 mm freckles were present above these spots near the right costal margin. On the back, one pigmented café-au-lait spot and several freckles were present along the spine. The skin over the right flank and back area was slightly increased in pigment compared to the left side. No neurofibromas were present.

Case 2. This 18-year-old man was referred with the diagnosis of NF. Medical history had been uncomplicated until age 17, when an extensive plexiform neurofibroma was discovered along the ulnar nerve of the left arm. No other medical problems were present. Family history was noncontributory. On physical examination, the height was just above the mean. The only findings were limited to the left arm and left back area. The plexiform neurofibroma of the upper arm was palpable and tender. Café-au-lait spots of greater than 1 cm were present on the left hand and the left shoulder area. In addition, there were several 2-4 mm freckles along the distribution of the ulnar nerve from the wrist to the upper arm. There was no axillary freckling, and the remainder of the exam was normal. Slit lamp examination of the irises has not yet occurred.

Case 3. This 14-year-old girl was referred with NF. Medical history was uncomplicated except for the recent occurrence of a single seizure. Family history was noncontributory. Physical examination showed that the height and weight were at the 50th percentile where the head circumference was at the 90th percentile. Eye examination including slit lamp showed no Lisch nodules. The remainder of the examination was normal except for the skin. There was no axillary freckling. Multiple café-au-lait spots were noted on the anterior and posterior aspects of the right leg and lower abdominal area. There were five spots of greater than 1.5 cm in greatest diameter and five spots of 0.5 to 1.5 cm in diameter.

These cases make a total of 17 individuals in the literature with localized involvement of multiple café-au-lait spots and/or cutaneous neurofibromas. All of the cases thus far are sporadic. In only 4 cases have Lisch nodules been looked for and in 1 of these the hamartomata were found on the iris ipsilateral to the segmental involvement and in the others the nodules were absent. Because of the uniqueness of the localized involvement, these data would suggest that a segmental form is a distinctive entity. Whether or not these cases represent an actual somatic mutation cannot be stated with certainty. The hypothesis of somatic mutation and cryptic mosaicism has been discussed for retinoblastoma as well.[24] Some of the cases of later onset NF may represent this segmental disorder. If future studies using recombinant DNA analysis are productive, application of the analysis to different tissue sites in these cases will be important for examining the somatic mutation hypothesis.

The line between the principle of heterogeneity in genetic disorders and the conventional clinical approach to differential diagnosis would be difficult to draw. Besides the conditions mentioned above, other disorders with overlapping phenotypic features need to be considered when evaluating a person with NF. These include the McCune-Albright syndrome, Watson syndrome, autosomal dominant gastrointestinal neurofibromatosis, and the multiple mucosal neuroma syndrome (multiple endocrine adenomatosis III) (TABLE 3).

TABLE 3. NF: Heterogeneity and Differential Diagnosis

NF disorders:
    I Von Recklinghausen NF
    II central, acoustic neuroma NF
    Segmental NF
    Familial café-au-lait spots
    NF/Noonan phenotype

Other disorders with overlapping manifestations:
    McCune-Albright syndrome
    Watson syndrome
    Gastrointestinal neurofibromas
    Multiple mucosal neuroma syndrome (MEA III)

GENETIC COUNSELING

In 1975, an *ad hoc* committee of the American Society of Human Genetics defined genetic counseling as

> a communication process which deals with the human problems associated with the occurrence, or the risk of occurrence, of a genetic disorder in a family. This process involves an attempt by one or more appropriately trained persons to help the individual or family (1) comprehend the medical facts, including the diagnosis, the probable course of the disorder, and the available management; (2) appreciate the way heredity contributes to the disorder . . . ; (3) understand the options for dealing with the risk of recurrence; (4) choose the course of action which seems appropriate to them . . . ; and (5) make the best possible adjustment to the disorder . . . and/or the risk of recurrence of this disorder.[25]

The first task in counseling a family with NF relates to precision in the diagnostic process and discussion of the natural history. In reviewing the potential complications, the professional must balance the possibility of developing one of the more serious manifestations with the perspective that more than half of all people with NF live a normal life and have no serious manifestations. Provision of medical risk information to a family of an asymptomatic individual with NF is a common occurrence. The professional has the opportunity to provide anticipatory guidance by outlining guidelines for routine health supervision. Leaving the message that an index for suspicion for certain problems should increase with the NF diagnosis is important for the referring primary care physician. In addition, education of the family and the referring physician of the natural history should ideally increase the possibility of earlier detection of a potential complication. We would agree with Riccardi that a thorough and sensitive discussion of the natural history balanced with perspective helps to demystify the disorder rather than alarm the family.[7]

The second goal outlined above requires knowledge of autosomal dominant inheritance with variable expression. Even though the risk for an affected person to transmit the gene is 50-50, the risk for offspring to have NF with a serious complication is less, since over half of all affected individuals have only cutaneous signs. The third task deals with the options for dealing with the risk. In this regard prenatal diagnosis of NF is not possible at the present time.

The fourth task of genetic counseling implies a recognition of the family's own autonomy in reproductive decision making. Although it is sometimes stated that the only preventive measure in NF is genetic counseling, this premise contradicts a respect for a family's own right and opportunity to make a reproductive choice. Although used frequently, the term prevention is not appropriate in this genetic counseling model.

The fifth task involves the role of genetic counseling as a helping service. Assisting a family in their coping process is an ongoing task and can hardly be accomplished in a single one to two hour clinic visit. Uncertainty is a common theme in discussions with a family where NF is present. Distribution of appropriate reading material and referral to a local chapter of the National Neurofibromatosis Foundation are two practical suggestions in single-visit consultations. A review of the complex psychological dimensions of genetic counseling is beyond the scope of this paper. Recently established multidisciplinary NF clinics in several centers in the United States can potentially help in meeting this need.

SUMMARY

1. Although the genetic pattern in NF has been definitely established as autosomal dominant, more precise data regarding penetrance, natural history, prevalence, and heterogeneity are needed for the counseling of families.

2. NF is the prototypic disorder for the study of the biologic mechanisms of variable expressivity.

3. The widely cited prevalence figure of Crowe is probably too high; thus the mutation ratio estimation in NF is among the highest in man but close to other common Mendelian disorders.

4. With the existing data on frequency of Lisch nodules and with future prospective date on café-au-lait spot development, an age-of-onset penetrance curve for NF could be constructed for genetic counseling purposes.

5. The segmental form of NF is of interest as cases of this presentation may be helpful in studying the hypothesis of human somatic mutation when DNA analysis is available.

6. Guidelines for routine evaluation and ongoing health supervision of individuals with neurofibromatosis need to be developed; multidisciplinary NF clinics and collaborative study groups are appropriate settings for this undertaking.

7. Neurofibromatosis is an important disorder for the study of the psychodynamic processes that families experience in dealing with uncertainty.

ACKNOWLEDGMENTS

The authors wish to express their appreciation to Liz Stierman, M.S., Susan Demsey, M.S., and Janice Palumbos, M.S. for assistance in evaluating the families and to Kalene Neff, Susan Neff, and Jann Cox for help in preparing the manuscript.

REFERENCES

1. CROWE, F. W., J. SCHULL & J. V. NEEL. 1956. A Clinical, Pathological, and Genetic Study of Multiple Neurofibromatosis. Charles C. Thomas. Springfield, Ill.
2. RICCARDI, V. M. 1981. Neurofibromatosis: an overview in new directions in clinical investigations. Adv. Neurol. 21: 1-9.
3. BOLANDE, R. P. 1981. Neurofibromatosis—the quintessential neurocristopathy: pathogenic concepts and relationships. Adv. Neurol. 29: 67-75.
4. BORBERG, A. 1951. Clinical and genetic investigations into tuberous sclerosis and Recklinghausen's neurofibromatosis. Acta Psychiatr. Neurol. (Suppl.) 71: 1-239.
5. SERGEYEV, A. S. 1975. On the mutation rate of neurofibromatosis. Hum. Genet. 28: 129-138.
6. RICCARDI, V. M. & B. KLEINER. 1977. Neurofibromatosis: a neoplastic birth defect with two age peaks of severe problems. Birth Defects 13(3C): 131-138.
7. RICCARDI, V. M. 1981. Von Recklinghausen neurofibromatosis. N. Engl. J. Med. 305: 1617-1627.
8. CAREY, J. C., J. M. LAUB & B. D. HALL. 1979. Penetrance and variability in neurofibromatosis: a genetic study of 60 families. Birth Defects 15(5B): 271-281.
9. SAMUELSSON, B. 1981. Neurofibromatosis (von Recklinghausen's disease): a clinical psychiatric and genetic study. Doctoral Thesis. University of Goteborg, Sweden. (As cited in Riccardi, V. M. 1982. Am. J. Med. Genet. 13: 107-108.)
10. TUGWELL, P. X. 1981. How to read clinical journals: to learn the clinical course in prognosis of disease. Can. Med. Assoc. J. 124: 869-872.
11. VOGEL, F. & A. G. MOTULSKI. 1979. Human Genetics: Problems and Approaches. Springer-Verlag. Berlin, FRG.
12. THOMPSON, J. S. & M. W. THOMPSON. 1980. Genetics in Medicine. 3rd edit. W. B. Saunders. Philadelphia, Pa.
13. RICCARDI, V. M., C. E. DOBSON, R. CHAKRABORTY & C. BONTKE. 1984. The pathophysiology of neurofibromatosis: paternal age as a factor in the origin of new mutations. Am. J. Med. Genet. 18: 169-176.
14. WHITEHOUSE, D. 1966. Diagnostic value of the café-au-lait spot in children. Arch. Dis. Child. 41: 316.
15. LEWIS, R. A. & V. M. RICCARDI. 1981. Von Recklinghausen neurofibromatosis incidence of iris hamartoma. Ophthalmology 88: 348-354.
16. PERRY, H. & R. L. FONT. 1982. Iris nodules in von Recklinghausen's neurofibromatosis. Arch. Ophthalmol. 100: 1635-1640.

17. MILLER, M. & J. G. HALL. 1978. Possible maternal effect on severity of neurofibromatosis. Lancet 2: 1071-1073.
18. ELDRIDGE, R. 1981. Central neurofibromatosis with bilateral acoustic neuromy. Adv. Neurol. 29: 57-65.
19. RICCARDI, V. M. 1982. Neurofibromatosis. Curr. Probl. Cancer 7: 2-34.
20. HALL, J. G., J. E. ALLANSON & M. VAN ALLEN. 1983. Noonan phenotype associated with neurofibromatosis. Proc. Greenwood Genet. Clin. 2: 114-115.
21. MILLER, R. M & R. S. SPARKES. 1977. Segmental neurofibromatosis. Arch. Dermatol. 113: 837-838.
22. ZONANA, J. & R. G. WELEBER. 1984. Segmental neurofibromatosis and iris hamartoma. Proc. Greenwood Genet. Clin. 3: 140-141.
23. SAUL, R. A. & R. E. STEVENSON. 1984. Segmental neurofibromatosis: a distinctive type of neurofibromatosis? Proc. Greenwood Genet. Clin. 3: 3-6.
24. CARLSON, E. A. & R. J. DESNICK. 1979. Mutational mosaicism in genetic counseling in retinoblastoma. Am. J. Med. Genet. 4: 365-381.
25. 1975. Ad Hoc Committee on Genetic Counseling: report to the American Society of Human Genetics. Am. J. Hum. Genet. 27: 240-242.

Neurofibromatosis and Cancer

JUDITH L. BADER

Radiation Oncology Branch
National Cancer Institute
National Institutes of Health
9000 Rockville Pike
Building 10, Room B3B69
Bethesda, Maryland 20892

Cancer is among the most serious complications of the autosomal dominant genetic disorder neurofibromatosis (NF). This review will address 13 key questions relevant to the study of NF and cancer.

Before beginning, however, certain basic issues must be clarified. First, this paper will consider only peripheral NF, not central NF (bilateral hereditary acoustic neuroma). Second, the definition of cancer is operational. Optic glioma, meningioma, and other low-grade neural tumors that act like and are treated like cancer are herein considered malignant tumors, even though by strict pathologic appearance and nomenclature they may not be malignant. Neurofibromas, including plexiform neurofibromas, are not considered cancers in this discussion. Third, because there is as yet no biomarker, the diagnosis of NF is made on clinical grounds and may not always be straightforward. Young children may not yet have developed a sufficient number of NF stigmata and certain adults may have an equivocal number or array of stigmata when the diagnosis of cancer is made. In these individuals, linking NF to cancer cannot be done with certainty.

IS THE OVERALL RISK OF CANCER INCREASED WITH NF?

Several large institutions have reported their experience with cancer as a complication of NF (TABLE 1).[1-8] The usual interpretation of these data is that the overall risk of cancer is 14%. Clarification of how the information was collected suggests that no simple interpretation is possible. First, all the series are derived from hospital-based populations, which certainly biases ascertainment toward more complicated cases of NF (e.g., cases with cancer) than may occur in a randomly selected sample of NF patients in the nonhospitalized general population. In fact, Memorial Hospital (TABLE 1, series 7) is a highly specialized oncology center, which not surprisingly reported a cancer frequency of 48% in their NF patients. The Mayo Clinic (TABLE 1, series 5) reported a 3% frequency, counting only one form of cancer, neurofibrosarcoma. Second, these frequencies report cancer observed (numerator) at the time when the author collected the data by chart review; they do not represent lifetime risk of all cancer. Patients without cancer, counted in the denominator, were of various ages, had not lived out a lifetime, and might still go on to develop cancer at a later date. Third, no control population is compared to the NF patients to determine whether the cancer frequency or pattern by age, race, and sex is different from what would be expected by chance.

For the general population in the United States, the lifetime risk of cancer is about 25%. It is against this background that the NF data must be interpreted. If the cancer risk is only 3% with NF, the disorder might be thought to protect against cancer, clearly not the case. If the cancer risk is 48%, it might be thought to confer twice the risk, also not the case.

A series not listed in TABLE 1 addresses the issue of cancer and NF in children.[9] An international registry of nearly 5000 children with all forms of cancer was surveyed for a variety of genetic disorders. NF, identified in 48 children with 52 cancers, was the most frequent genetic disorder reported. By chance only about 1.6 NF cases were expected, given that the disorder is seen only about once in 3000 live births.[2]

Another series not listed in TABLE 1 studied cancer with NF outside the hospital setting.[10] One hundred forty-five member families of the National Neurofibromatosis Foundation responded to a mailed questionnaire survey, reporting 31 malignancies among 266 individuals with NF. The reported cancers were compared to expected numbers based on age- and sex-specific incidence rates from the Third National Cancer Survey. For all cancers, the observed to expected ratio was 2.5 in males and 4.1 in females, with the excess of cancers accounted for largely by cancers arising in brain, cranial, and peripheral nerves.

A conservative view of cancer frequency with NF, considering the limitation of the numerators, denominators, and methodology in published data, is that NF probably does increase the risk of cancer slightly due to an excess of only neural tumors. A precise figure cannot yet be determined, however.

WHICH CANCERS APPEAR TO OCCUR EXCESSIVELY WITH NF?

A summary of the cancers that appear to occur excessively with NF in adults and children is shown in TABLE 2. These data are derived from the major case series

TABLE 1. Cancer Frequency in Eight Large NF Case Series

Series	Date	Number of NF Patients	Number with Cancer (%)
1. Denmark[1]	1951	172	26 (15)
2. Michigan[2]	1956	223	23 (10)
3. Illinois VA Hospital[3]	1952	61	26 (43)
4. Cardiff, Wales[4]	1962	79	12 (15)
5. Mayo Clinic[5]	1963	678	21 (3)
6. Turin, Italy[6]	1968	179	33 (18)
7. Memorial Hospital[7]	1972	110	53 (48)
8. University of Pennsylvania[8]	1977	116	34 (29)
TOTAL		1618	228 (14)

TABLE 2. Tumors Occurring Excessively with Neurofibromatosis

Children	Adults
Gliomas/astrocytomas[a]	Gliomas/astrocytomas[a]
Ependymomas	Spinal cord tumors[a]
Spinal cord tumors[a]	Ependymomas
Meningiomas[a]	Neurofibrosarcomas[b]
Optic gliomas[a]	Spinal cord tumors[a]
Neurofibrosarcomas[b]	Pheochromocytomas[a]
Rhabdomyosarcomas[c]	
Nonlymphocytic leukemias[c]	

[a]Histology may be benign or malignant.
[b]Also called peripheral nerve sheath tumor or malignant schwannoma.
[c]Nonneural tumor.

already discussed and numerous case reports and smaller series which also support a disproportionate occurrence of cancers derived from neural crest tissue.

In children but not adults, two cancers not apparently derived from neural crest seem to occur excessively. Rare forms of childhood leukemia (juvenile chronic myelocytic and acute myelomonocytic leukemia) have been reported in over 45 patients, a surprising finding since together they account for less than 10% of all leukemia before 16 years of age.[11] Rhabdomyosarcoma, a soft tissue tumor of mesenchymal origin, has also been observed excessively.[12] An explanation for these associations is not yet clear.

One important point worth stressing is that the common adult forms of cancer, e.g., lung, breast, colon, and prostate, do *not* appear to occur with NF any more commonly than they do in the general population. NF neither predisposes to nor protects against the normal development of these cancers.

CAN THE NF PATIENT WHO WILL DEVELOP CANCER BE PREDICTED IN ADVANCE?

At present there is neither a biomarker to identify patients with NF nor one to predict susceptibility to cancer. One group has reported that skin fibroblasts from NF patients show enhanced sensitivity to transformation by the Kirsten murine sarcoma virus and suggests this as a laboratory assay to predict predisposition to cancer.[13] Further work is needed to verify the assay and its conclusions.

Other than in very rare case reports,[14] neither the location nor the number of café-au-lait spots or dermal neurofibromas has been shown to correlate with the development of cancer either locally or systemically. Other stigmata have not been correlated with cancer either. One report suggested that severity of NF was positively correlated with maternal transmission;[15] other reports have failed to confirm this observation.[16] The relationship between plexiform neurofibromas and cancer is considered in a later section.

DO SOME NF FAMILIES HAVE MORE CANCER THAN OTHERS AND CAN THEY BE PREDICTED?

It is clear from reviewing the National Neurofibromatosis Foundation question-naire data and from clinical reports that some families do indeed have a dispropor-tionate amount of NF-associated cancer. Neither clinical history nor pattern of disease manifestations appeared to correlate with appearance of cancer, however.

DO NF PATIENTS DEVELOP MULTIPLE PRIMARY MALIGNANCIES?

The literature reports numerous instances of NF patients with multiple primary malignancies. The true frequency of second cancers cannot be established from case reports, and it is not possible to predict which individuals will develop this compli-cation.

WHAT IS MALIGNANT DEGENERATION?

Malignant degeneration means the development of a neurofibrosarcoma at the site of a preexisting *plexiform* neurofibroma. This process rarely if ever develops in dermal neurofibromas. The term malignant degeneration with NF is commonly misused to mean either the occurrence of any cancer with NF or the occurrence of any neuro-fibrosarcoma with NF, not necessarily at the site of a preexisting plexiform neurofibroma.

WHAT IS THE RISK OF MALIGNANT DEGENERATION?

Because the term malignant degeneration has been used to mean various things in the literature, the reported risk varies from 3 to 48%, as discussed in an earlier section. To establish the precise estimate of the occurrence of neurofibrosarcoma within a plexiform neurofibroma, one would have to decide whether to count as the denom-inator either all plexiform neurofibroma lesions in the population or all individuals with NF who have at least one plexiform neurofibroma. Because many plexiform neurofibromas are clinically silent, neither denominator is ascertainable precisely.

Pathologists are supposed to report malignant degeneration when coexisting plexi-form neurofibroma is identified within the excised cancer. Unfortunately, however, the presence or absence of a benign precursor lesion, even if present, is not always mentioned in a pathology report. When only the report is reviewed in preparing a publication, underestimate of risk may result.

Given the vast number of plexiform neurofibromas occurring with NF, and the relative rarity of neurofibrosarcoma, one could conclude that the risk of true malignant degeneration is low, probably much lower than the 3% estimate cited in the report from the Mayo Clinic, a specialized referral center. Thus, for affected individuals who appear to have multiple plexiform neurofibromas, there is no reason to propose surgical excision to lessen the chance of cancer. Surgery might be considered, however, if the lesion grows rapidly or causes local problems with pain, function, or cosmesis.

ARE NF PATIENTS MORE SUSCEPTIBLE THAN OTHERS TO THE ENVIRONMENTAL CAUSES OF CANCER?

Clinical evidence suggests that dermal and plexiform neurofibromas may increase in size and number in response to the hormonal stimuli of puberty, pregnancy, and perhaps exogenous administration of hormones (such as birth control pills, although this is somewhat controversial). These observations suggest increased susceptibility of NF patients to hormonally mediated carcinogenesis, although data to support this notion are lacking. Investigation of steroid receptors, actions, and metabolism within neurofibromas and neurofibrosarcomas would be a worthwhile area for future study, however, perhaps leading to new therapeutic strategies.

The possibility of increased susceptibility to postirradiation second tumors, usually sarcomas, has also been suggested by recent publications.[17-19] The risk of inducing cancer after therapeutic irradiation is small but well documented and certainly occurs in the *absence* of NF.[20] The crucial question is whether NF patients are *more* susceptible than others to radiation carcinogenesis. As in other studies of cancer risk with NF, ascertainment bias in the numerator and definition of the denominator create problems with data interpretation.

A recent report from the Mayo Clinic suggests greater risk for radiation-induced neurofibrosarcoma among NF patients than unaffected persons.[18] Careful analysis of the data fails to support that suggestion, however. Between 1912 and 1981, 109 neurofibrosarcomas were identified at the Mayo Clinic, 65 in NF patients and 44 in non-NF patients. Seven of 65 NF patients (11%) and 5 of 44 non-NF patients (11%) had had prior irradiation for benign or malignant disease, clearly no excess for NF patients. Many had been treated with equipment, doses, and radiation techniques no longer used and some had had radiation for conditions no longer so treated. The paper concludes that NF patients should not receive "unnecessary" radiation. Actually, no one should receive "unnecessary" radiation. However, many of the neural tumors typically associated with NF are life threatening and are usually treated with surgery and/or radiation. To withhold x-ray treatment for a current life-threatening cancer seems unwise on the basis of either a low probability of subsequent cancer or an as yet *unproven* hypothesis of excess susceptibility to radiation carcinogenesis.

Recently, radiation sensitivity of NF cells *in vitro* has also been studied, with alterations found in some assay systems but not in others.[21-23] Additional work is needed to clarify these studies and determine whether there is any clinical correlation for the *in vitro* findings. Work has also begun on response to ultraviolet light, alkylating agents, growth factors, and viral transformation as well as oncogene expression and gene amplification within NF-related sarcomas.[24,25] Analysis of conflicting results among studies is difficult, however, because cell type, passage number, assay, end point, and adequacy of controls vary considerably.

DOES CANCER HAVE A WORSE PROGNOSIS WITH NF?

Conflicting reports have been published comparing survival following treatment for neurofibrosarcoma, optic glioma, and brain tumors with and without NF.[26-30] All are collected retrospective case series, however, with many patients treated prior to the era of modern combined modality cancer therapy. No studies have been done with appropriate methodology—rigorous staging, similar therapy for all patients, analysis of outcome with and without NF, controlling for important prognosis variables such as tumor stage, grade, location, performance status, age, etc. Until technically adequate study is made of prognosis, no firm conclusions can be drawn. Thus, NF patients with cancer should be treated aggressively for cure, and managed with the same clinical principles as patients without NF.

ARE THERE PARTICULAR PROBLEMS IN MANAGING THE NF PATIENT WITH CANCER?

Some NF patients have coexisting clinical problems which may complicate the clinical presentation and result in delay of diagnosis and presentation of disease at a late stage, e.g., patients with long-standing large plexiform neurofibromas which gradually start to grow, patients with preexisting neurologic conditions which mask the clinical signs of a growing intracranial mass. Initial cancer staging evaluation of NF patients may also be complicated by the presence of other nonmalignant lesions visualized on imaging scans or identified on physical exam.

Socioeconomic considerations may hinder optimal cancer management as well, with some families unable to afford care at cancer centers or lacking the sophistication to search beyond the initial local medical opinion that "nothing can be done."

WHAT IS THE ROLE OF SCREENING STUDIES FOR EARLY DETECTION OF CANCER WITH NF?

Use of *baseline* screening studies such as computerized axial tomography (CAT) or magnetic resonance imaging (MRI) scans of the head, orbits, torso, or extremities is controversial, recommended by some centers and not by others. A conservative view is that in the absence of any clinical suspicion, no baseline studies need be done for the otherwise well and asymptomatic child or adult, outside the bona fide approved protocol setting. Screening tests and health maintainance regimens recommended for the general population are recommended for NF patients as well, however.

As mentioned in an earlier section, *in vitro* tests to predict the development of cancer are as yet unproven and cannot be advised routinely.

WHAT CLINICAL OBSERVATIONS MIGHT BE RELEVANT TO CANCER DEVELOPMENT WITH NF?

The extremely high spontaneous mutation rate with NF is among the most unusual aspects of NF. If a molecular genetic explanation could be identified, it might help explain the apparent cancer predisposition as well as the extreme variability in the pattern and severity of noncancerous clinical manifestations.

The relationship of hormones to growth and development of benign and malignant tumors also bears further investigation, with potential for use in therapy.

WHAT CLINICAL AND LABORATORY AREAS MIGHT BE STUDIED NOW IN NF AND CANCER?

Many important clinical questions might be studied by investigators willing to use rigorous methodology instead of the traditional and less revealing retrospective clinical institutional case series: (1) What is the life expectancy of the "average" NF patient, one who is not identified in the secondary or tertiary care medical center? (2) What are the prime causes of death with NF, and how do they differ from those in the general population? (3) Are there any trends in cancer incidence, treatment, survival? Can etiologic clues be derived from analysis of cancer demographics? (4) Do the newer imaging techniques help differentiate between benign and malignant masses?

The most important laboratory project facing NF researchers today is the development of a biomarker for the NF gene. Pre- and postnatal diagnosis would be facilitated as would the recognition of equivocal cases, disorders with similar phenotype, and subgroups within peripheral NF, including segmental disease. If the biomarker identifies the responsible gene and thereby its gene product, relationship to cancer development would certainly be explored. Analysis of multigenerational NF pedigrees is already in progress to help with gene mapping and identification.[31] Since this work may take some time, currently available technology could be applied to look for known oncogenes, gene rearrangements and amplification, tumor markers, and growth factors. Biology of neural tumors associated with NF could be compared to the same tumors occurring without NF. Also, further work is needed on sensitivity of NF cell types to mutagens and carcinogens. Potential animal models for the disorder should also be pursued. Finally, evaluation of normal and abnormal neuron and Schwann cell biology may produce clues to NF etiology and treatment.

WHAT CAVEATS ARE IMPORTANT IN STUDYING NF AND CANCER?

Because cancer generates much concern among NF patients and physicians, care must be taken to avoid making sweeping general conclusions about the whole NF population based on small numbers of patient observations or few laboratory specimens. Conclusions based on observations from severely affected individuals, from highly specialized referral centers, may not apply to the majority of mildly or moderately affected individuals in the general NF population. This suggestion applies equally to studies about biology, etiology, screening, treatment, and prognosis. Use of the proper type and number of normal controls is essential both in clinical and laboratory studies. And finally, methodology is key in understanding the potential significance of any new report on cancer with NF: what specific methodology was used, what system was analyzed, what end point was chosen. With increasing interest in *in vitro* work with NF, assays are being performed on a variety of cell types: normal skin, plexiform and dermal neurofibromas, café-au-lait spots, lymphocytes, malignant tumors, cells from young and old, mild and severely affected individuals, cells from early and late passage, Schwann cells, neurons, fibroblasts. How to correlate and interpret often conflicting observations will be facilitated by rigorous attention to detail in reporting methodology and specimen accrual.

In conclusion, cancer with NF remains a grave clinical concern. Although considerable study has already been done,[32] opportunities still exist for the alert clinician and laboratory scientist to help understand this complex and important puzzle.

[**Note added in proof:** Since preparation of this manuscript, a population-based study of cancer incidence with NF in Denmark has been published.][33]

REFERENCES

1. BORBERG, A. 1951. Clinical and genetic investigations into tuberous sclerosis and Recklinghausen's neurofibromatosis. Acta Psychiatr. Neurol. **71**(Suppl.): 1-239.
2. CROWE, F. W., W. J. SCHULL & J. V. NEEL. 1956. A Clinical, Pathological and Genetic Study of Multiple Neurofibromatosis. Charles C. Thomas. Springfield, Ill.
3. PRESTON, F. W., W. S. WALSH & T. H. CLARKE. 1952. Cutaneous neurofibromatosis (von Recklinhausen's disease. Arch. Surg. **64**: 813-827.
4. HEARD, G. 1962. Nerve sheath tumours and von Recklinghausen's disease of the nervous system. Ann. R. Coll. Surg. Engl. **31**: 229-248.
5. D'AGOSTINO, A. N., E. H. SOULE & R. H. MILLER. 1963. Sarcomas of the peripheral nerves and somatic soft tissues associated with multiple neurofibromatosis (von Recklinghausen's disease). Cancer **16**: 1015-1027.
6. DALFORNO, S., M. RAMELLA GIGLIARDI & R. FARIELLO. 1968. Cancro **21**: 100-148.
7. BRASFIELD, R. D. & T. K. DAS GUPTA. 1972. Von Recklinghausen's disease: a clinicopathologic study. Ann. Surg. **174**: 86-104.
8. CASSELMAN, E. S., W. T. MILLER, S. R. LIN & G. A. MANDELL. 1977. Von Recklinghausen's disease: incidence of roentgenographic findings with a clinical review of the literature. CRC Crit. Rev. Diagn. Imaging **9**: 387-419.
9. BADER, J. L., A. T. MEADOWS, J. LEMERLE, P. A. VOUTE, P. MORRIS-JONES, A. BANFI, W. A. NEWTON & E. BAUM. 1980. Neurofibromatosis (NF) and other genetic defects associated with childhood cancer. Am. J. Hum. Genet. **32**(6): 97A.
10. BADER, J. L., A. F. KANTOR & A. E. RUBENSTEIN. 1981. Increased risk of cancer with neurofibromatosis. Proc. Am. Soc. Clin. Oncol. **20**: 339.
11. BADER, J. L. & R. W. MILLER. 1978. Neurofibromatosis and childhood leukemia. J. Pediatr. **92**: 925-929.
12. MCKEEN, E. A., J. BODURTHA, A. T. MEADOWS, E. C. DOUGLAS & J. J. MULVIHILL. 1978. Rhabdomyosarcoma complicating multiple neurofibromatosis. J. Pediatr. **93**: 992-993.
13. BIDOT-LOPEZ, P. & J. W. FRANKEL. 1983. Enhanced viral transformation of skin fibroblasts from neurofibromatosis patients. Ann. Clin. Lab. Sci. **13**: 27-32.

14. PERKINSON, N. G. 1957. Melanoma arising in a cafe au lait spot of neurofibromatosis. Am. J. Surg. **93:** 1018-1021.
15. MILLER, M. & J. G. HALL. 1978. Possible maternal effect on severity of neurofibromatosis. Lancet **2:** 1071-1073.
16. BADER, J. L. & R. W. MILLER. 1979. No maternal effect in childhood leukemia with neurofibromatosis. Lancet **1:** 503.
17. CORKILL, A. G. L. & C. F. ROSS. 1969. A case of neurofibromatosis complicated by medullublastoma, neurogenic sarcoma, and radiation-induced carcinoma of the thyroid. J. Neurol. Neurosurg. Psychiatry **32:** 43-47.
18. DUCATMAN, B. S. & B. W. SCHEITHAUER. 1983. Postirradiation neurofibrosarcoma. Cancer **51:** 1028-1033.
19. FOLEY, F. M., J. M. WOODRUFF, F. T. ELLIS & J. B. POSNER. 1980. Radiation-induced malignant and atypical nerve sheath tumors. Ann. Neurol. **7:** 311-318.
20. BOICE, J. D. 1981. Cancer following medical irradiation. Cancer **47**(Suppl.): 1081-1090.
21. SCHWENN, M. R., R. R. WEICHSELBAUM & J. B. LITTLE. 1985. Investigation of the cytytoxic effects of DNA damaging agents on neurofibromatosis cells. Mutat. Res. **142**(1-2): 55-58.
22. HAFEZ, M., L. SHARAF, S. EL-NABI & G. EL-WEHEDY. 1985. Evidence of chromosomal instability in neurofibromatosis. Cancer **55:** 2434-2436.
23. WOODS, W. G., B. A. MCKENZIE & T. D. BYRNE. 1985. Sensitivity of cultured skin fibroblasts from patients with neurofibromatosis to DNA damaging agents. (Submitted for publication.)
24. SCHWENN, M. R., P. C. BILLINGS & J. B. LITTLE. 1985. N-myc amplification and expression in a malignant schwannoma from a patient with neurofibromatosis. (Abstr.) Proc. Am. Assoc. Cancer Res. **26:** 65.
25. ROWLEY, P. T., B. KOSCIOLEK & J. L. BADER. Oncogene expression in neurofibromatosis. Ann. N.Y. Acad. Sci. (This volume.)
26. STORM, F. M., F. R. EILBER, J. MIRRA & D. L. MORTON. 1979. Neurofibrosarcoma. Cancer **45:** 126-129.
27. SORDILLO, P. R., L. HELSON, S. I. HAJDU, G. B. MAGILL, C. KOSLOFF, R. B. GOLBEY & E. J. BEATTIE. 1981. Malignant schwannoma—clinical characteristics, survival, and response to therapy. Cancer **47:** 2503-2509.
28. WRIGHT, J. E., W. E. MCDONALD & N. B. CALL. 1980. Management of optic gliomas. Br. J. Ophthalmol. **64:** 545-552.
29. KLUG, G. L. 1982. Gliomas of the optic nerve and chiasm in children. Neuro-ophthalmology **2:** 217-223.
30. DANOFF, B. F., S. KRAMER & N. THOMPSON. 1980. The radiotherapeutic management of optic nerve gliomas in children. Int. J. Radiat. Oncol. Biol. Phys. **6:** 45-50.
31. SPENCE, M. A., D. M. PARRY, J. L. BADER, M. L. MARAZITA, M. BOCIAN, S. J. FUNDERBURK, J. J. MULVIHILL & R. S. SPARKES. Genetic linkage analysis of neurofibromatosis. Ann. N.Y. Acad. Sci. (This volume.)
32. HOPE, D. G. & J. J. MULVIHILL. 1981. Malignancy in neurofibromatosis. Adv. Neurol. **29:** 33-56.
33. SORENSON, S. A., J. J. MULVIHILL & A. NIELSON. 1986. Long-term follow-up of von Recklinghausen neurofibromatosis. N. Engl. J. Med. **314:** 1010-1015.

Investigations on the Neural Crest[a]

Methodological Aspects and Recent Advances

NICOLE M. LE DOUARIN

Institute of Embryology of the CNRS and of the College of France
49bis, Avenue de la Belle-Gabrielle
94130 Nogent-sur-Marne, France

The neural crest, a transient structure of the vertebrate embryo, arises from the lateral ridges of the neural primordium (the neural plate) as they join mediodorsally to form the neural tube. The central nervous system (CNS) subsequently differentiates from the neural tube while the neural crest cells lose their initial epithelial arrangement and move away from their source. They migrate along preformed migration pathways and become distributed all over the body within a variety of microenvironments where they develop into a large number of cell types (TABLE 1).

Because of its pluripotentiality and the striking migratory behavior of its component cells, the neural crest has attracted the interest of many developmental biologists. In a monograph, Horstadius reported the pioneering work carried out essentially in the amphibian embryo during the first half of this century;[1] another monograph appeared later on this subject and was mainly based on experiments performed on the avian embryo.[2] Information on the mammalian neural crest is still very scarce due to the difficulty of gaining access to the embryo at the time of organogenesis. It is likely, however, that most of the knowledge acquired from birds is also valid for mammals.

The first techniques used to decipher the complex migratory behavior of crest cells and to demonstrate the multiplicity of their fates consisted in the removal of the neural folds from definite regions of the embryo and the subsequent analysis of the deficiencies resulting from the extirpation. This method, classical in experimental embryology, yielded interesting, but imprecise, results due to the partial replacement of the removed embryonic regions by "rescuing" neighboring cells. Marking the presumed migratory cells is a much more accurate way to follow them throughout their developmental history. This was first achieved for the neural crest by using various natural markers, such as differences in the size and staining properties of cells of various amphibian species experimentally combined for this purpose (see Reference 1, for references). These markers, however, were not conspicuous and stable enough to fulfill the requirements for a precise analysis of neural crest ontogeny. Radioisotopic labeling of the nucleus by tritiated thymidine (^{3}H-TdR) represented significant progress in this field.[3–8] More stable and easier to use, the quail-chick marker system was subsequently introduced.[9–11] It allowed the normal fate of the avian neural crest to be

[a]This work was supported by the Centre National de la Recherche Scientifique, the Institut National de la Santé et de la Recherche Médicale, the Fondation pour la Recherche Médicale Française, and the Ligue contre le Cancer and aided by Basic Research Grant No. 1-866 from the March of Dimes Birth Defect Foundation.

TABLE 1. The Derivatives of the Neural Crest

PERIPHERAL NERVOUS SYSTEM
   I. SENSORY GANGLIA:

SENSORY NEURONS
in:

Spinal Ganglia
Trigeminal nerve (V) root ganglion: *Trigeminal ganglion* (partly)
Facial nerve (VII) *root ganglion*
Glossopharyngeal nerve (IX) root ganglion: *Superior ganglion*
Vagal nerve (X) root ganglion: *Jugular ganglion*
Cells of Rohon-Béard (Amphibians)

SATELLITE CELLS

In all sensory ganglia including geniculate (nerve VII); otic (nerve VIII); petrosum (nerve IX); and nodose (nerve X).

   II. AUTONOMIC NERVOUS SYSTEM:
Sympathetic ganglia and plexuses: neurons and satellite cells.
Parasympathetic ganglia and plexuses: neurons and satellite cells.

   III. SCHWANN CELLS OF THE PERIPHERAL NERVES

ENDOCRINE AND PARAENDOCRINE CELLS
Carotid body type I cells;
Calcitonin-producing (C-cells);
Adrenalmedulla.

PIGMENT CELLS

MESECTODERMAL DERIVATIVES:

CEPHALIC CREST
Skeleton

Nasal and orbitary
Palate and maxillary
Trabeculae (partly)
Sphenoid complex (small contribution)
Cranial vault (squamosal and small contribution to frontal)
Otic capsule (partly)
Visceral skeleton

Connective tissue

Dermis, smooth muscles and *adipose tissue* of the *skin* in the face and ventral part of the neck
Ciliary muscles
Small contribution to striated muscle cells of the face and neck
Connective and *muscular* tissues of the *wall* of the *large arteries* derived from the *aortic arches* (except endothelial cells)
Tooth papillae (except endothelium of blood vessels)
Cornea: corneal "endothelium" and stromal fibroblasts
Meninges: in prosencephalon and partly in mesencephalon
Connective component of the pituitary, lacrymal, salivary, thyroid, parathyroid glands and of the thymus

TRUNK CREST

Dorsal fin mesenchyme (lower vertebrates)

unraveled, and various problems accessible to the *in vivo* approach of experimental embryological techniques to be investigated, e.g., questions concerning the real potentialities carried by neural crest cells in various parts of the body and the interplay of genetic determination and epigenetic factors in their differentiation (see References 2 and 12-14).

Many of the problems posed by neural crest cell development can also be approached through *in vitro* culture research, and during the last 10 years a number of interesting findings have resulted from experiments carried out in culture (see References 2 and 14-17).

Recently, monoclonal antibody technology has been applied to neural crest cell ontogeny and important developments are to be expected from the multifocal approach directed now to exploiting this model system.

CELL MARKERS IN NEURAL CREST RESEARCH

Acetylcholinesterase (AChE) activity, first observed in neural crest cells by Drews and co-workers (see Reference 18), was the subject of a detailed study by Cochard and Coltey[19] and Miki *et al.*[20]

Since about 90% of crest cells express this enzyme throughout the migratory phase while the other tissues of the embryo do not, AChE activity, a character easily detectable by cytochemistry, can be used as a cell marker. However, the enzyme remains a permanent feature of certain crest derivatives only, and therefore does not allow most of the neural crest cells to be followed during their entire developmental history. In spite of these limitations, AChE provides a clear-cut vision of the moving crest cell strands in the normal embryo during the early migratory phases.

Monoclonal antibodies (Mabs) recognizing crest cell surface antigens have been obtained by immunizing mice with peripheral ganglia from quail embryos.

NC1 was raised against crude extracts of 8-day quail embryo ciliary ganglia[21-22] and GlN2 against 15-day quail nodose ganglia.[23] Although the antigens recognized are slightly different in their cellular distribution at later developmental stages, both Mabs decorate most neural crest cells soon after the onset of their migration to their final sites of arrest (FIGURE 1). Subsequently, the antigens recognized are found on certain cells belonging to the peripheral nervous system (PNS) but not on the ectomesenchymal derivatives of the cephalic crest or on the melanocytic lineage. During the second half of incubation, the CNS also exhibits NC1 and GlN2 immunostaining. However, since their binding properties are restricted to neural crest cells during their migratory phase, these Mabs are useful for following them along their various pathways in intact quail or chick embryos.

Using the quail-chick marker system involves the graft of the neural primordium at stages preceding the onset of the migratory process (FIGURE 2). The procedures for the isotopic and isochronic grafting of the neural tube associated with the neural folds, or of the neural fold exclusively, have been described elsewhere (e.g., Reference 2). The former type of graft (replacement of fragments of the chick neural tube + neural crest, by their quail counterpart) has recently given rise to quail-chick spinal cord chimeras that can reach the stage of hatching and exhibit completely normal behavior after birth.[24]

This shows that the neuronal connections between the host and graft cells are correctly established and substantiates the reliability of the information yielded by

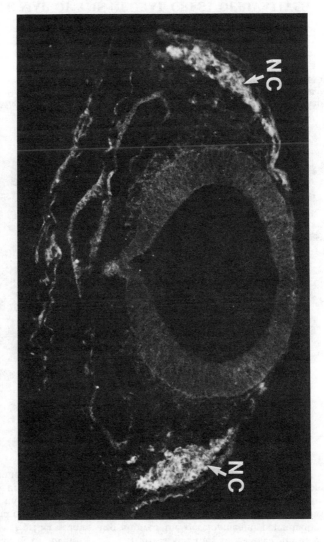

FIGURE 1. Transverse section in the midbrain of a seven-somite quail embryo showing the neural crest (NC). Magnification: ×500.

this developmental model during embryogenesis. Its validity is further supported by the complete identity of the conclusions reached about the pattern of neural crest migration pathways from experiments using the markers applied to intact embryos (AChE and Mabs) and those based on the quail-chick neural chimeras.[25] Moreover, the stability of the quail nuclear marker makes it a unique tool to investigate the long-term evolution of the neural crest derivatives and thus to establish the fate map of this structure. Further studies also allowed the developmental potentialities of the crest cells and of their progeny contained in peripheral ganglia to be examined. They revealed the unexpected presence, in the ganglia, of progenitor cells able to yield a variety of neuronal and nonneuronal cell types if provided with an appropriate microenvironment.

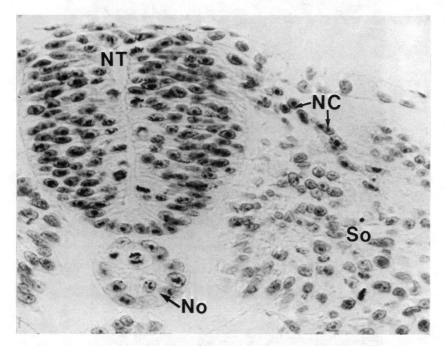

FIGURE 2. Migration of neural crest cells (NC) visualized by the quail nuclear marker, in a three-day (E3) chick embryo into which a quail neural primordium (neural tube + neural folds) was grafted at the level of somites 23 to 28 at the 28-somite stage. The embryo was observed 18 hours after surgery; No, notochord; NT, neural tube; So, somite.

FATE MAP OF THE NEURAL CREST DERIVATIVES

Fate maps of the neural crest and of the placodal ectoderm participating in the formation of the PNS were constructed on the basis of isochronic and isotopic substitutions of parts of the neural primordium between quail and chick embryos.[2,26] This led to the identification of certain previously unrecognized neural crest derivatives (see TABLE 1) and to the delimitation of the territories from which the various neural crest—and placode—derived PNS precursors arise in normal development (FIGURE 3).

This being established, one can raise the question as to whether, in the different areas defined, the developmental potentials of crest cells are already strictly limited. Several experimental designs have been devised to study this problem. One has consisted in heterotopically transplanting fragments of the entire neural primordium,[27] or of the neural fold alone, from quail embryos into chick recipients.[28-29] The migratory behavior and developmental potential of a given region of the neural crest subjected to a different embryonic environment could then be investigated.

The cephalic and vagal neural crest, when transplanted at the level of somites 18-24 ("adrenomedullary" level of the crest), yielded adrenergic cells that colonized the host sympathetic ganglia and suprarenal glands. Conversely, cells from the cervicotruncal neural crest, which normally do not penetrate the mesentery and gut, did so when the neural tube was transplanted prior to crest cell migration in the vagal area of the neuraxis.[27] These truncal crest cells migrating into the gut become distributed into myenteric and submucosal plexuses and fail to express the adrenergic phenotype that is characteristic of their normal fate. Instead, they differentiate, like the vagal crest, into cholinergic[30] and peptidergic[31] neurons.

The latter finding was confirmed in a different experimental system. Pieces of hindgut, taken before they received their supply of neural crest cells, were transplanted on the chick chorioallantoic membrane. After 7 to 10 days, the transplanted gut was found to display normal muscular development except for a total absence of enteric ganglia.[32] However, enteric plexuses developed if neural crest was transplanted in association with aneural hindgut, irrespective of whether the crest cells would normally have given rise to enteric ganglia, to sympathoblasts, or adrenomedullary cells. The cholinergic nature of the ganglia formed in the culture was revealed by the presence of choline acetyltransferase activity and high levels of AChE, while neither tyrosine hydroxylase, the key enzyme for catecholamine (CA) synthesis, nor formaldehyde-induced fluorescence of CA could be detected.

Initial pluripotentiality of premigratory neural crest cell populations was also shown by Noden through heterotopic transplantation of different regions of the cranial neural crest.[33] When the forebrain crest, which normally does not yield neural elements, was grafted at the mesencephalic/metencephalic region, crest cells emigrated from their new position and formed normal ciliary and trigeminal ganglia. These ganglia were absent when the reverse transplantation (i.e., replacement of diencephalic by mid/hindbrain crest) was performed, showing that some regional heterogeneity of the head neural crest is established early.

Quail neural crest, removed surgically from various levels of the neuraxis before the onset of migration, can also be inserted into a slit made between somites and neural tube in a normal chick embryo. The fate of this supernumerary population of crest cells can be identified several days later in the host. In this experimental system as well, the implanted crest cells develop according to their position in the host rather than to their normal fate in the donor. Forebrain crest, for example, which normally does not yield PNS derivatives, contributes significantly to PNS ganglia if transplanted to the 18-24-somite area producing not only Schwann cells and glia but also sensory dorsal root ganglion (DRG) neurons, sympathetic cells, and adrenomedullary cells.[29]

Therefore, at each axial level, the neural crest can be considered as potentially able to give rise to the various cell types of the PNS. However, this does not necessarily imply that all regions of the neural crest are exactly equivalent. In fact, certain differences exist between the different populations of crest cells. For example, cephalic

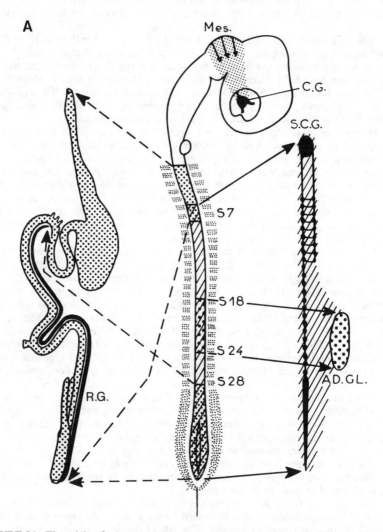

FIGURE 3A. The origin of adrenomedullary and autonomic ganglion cells. The spinal neural crest caudal to the level of the fifth somite gives rise to the ganglia of the sympathetic chains. The adrenomedullary cells originate from the spinal neural crest between the level of somites 18 and 24. The vagal neural crest (somites 1-7) gives rise to the parasympathetic enteric ganglia of the preumbilical region, the ganglia of the postumbilical gut originating both from the vagal and lumbosacral neural crest. The ganglion of Remak (R.G.) is derived from the lumbosacral neural crest (posterior to the level of somite 28). The ciliary ganglion (C.G.) is derived from the mesencephalic crest (Mes). AD.GL, adrenal gland; S.C.G., superior cervical ganglion. (From Reference 2 with permission.)

B

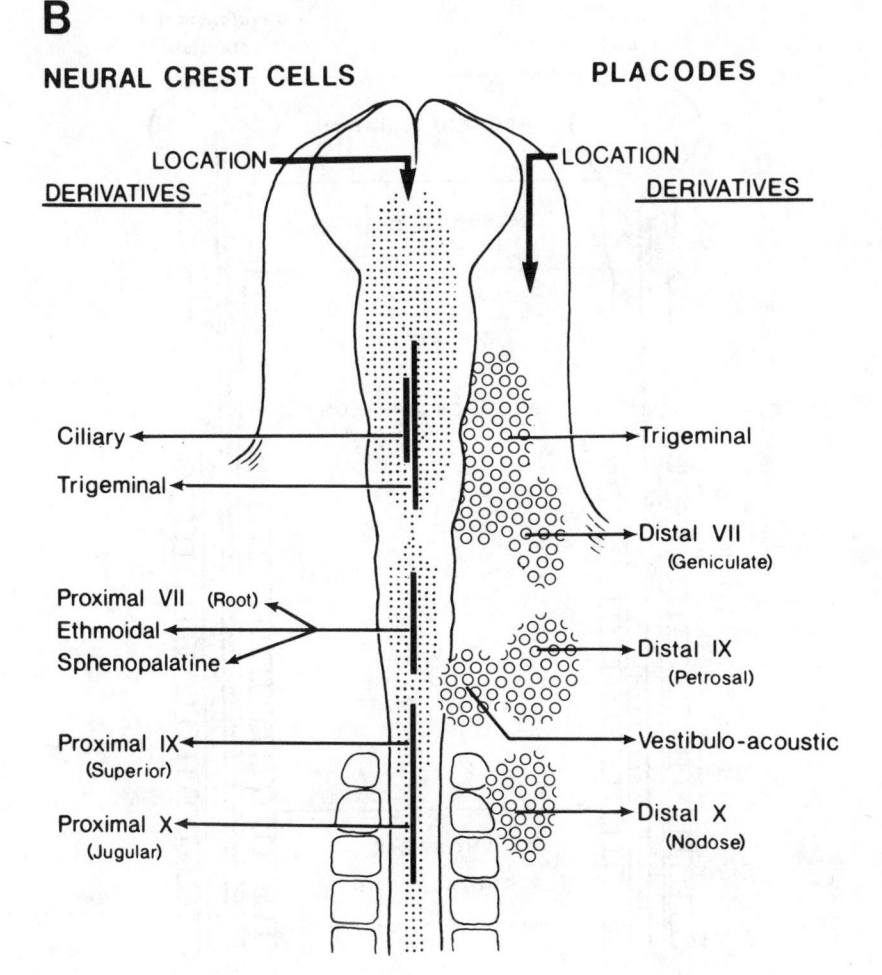

FIGURE 3B. Schematic drawing of a stage 9.5 chick embryo (about 10 somites) indicating positions of neural crest and placodal anlagen for cranial sensory and autonomic ganglia. (From Reference 26 with permission.)

crest grafted at the level of somites 24-28 migrated into the dorsal mesentery and colonized the gut, whereas normal truncal crest migration is restricted to the dorsal trunk structures.[27] Furthermore, trunk neural crest grafted in place of mesencephalic crest did not result in development of a normal trigeminal ganglion.[33]

As far as the PNS is concerned, the fate map of the neural crest differs strikingly from the distribution of crest cell developmental potentials along the neuraxis (FIGURE 4). Since each axial level of the body is provided with a specific set of PNS structures, a decisive role must be attributed to the various embryonic microenvironments, not only in gangliogenesis, but also in choosing within the large array of differentiation capacities that characterize neural crest cell populations at the different levels. It is

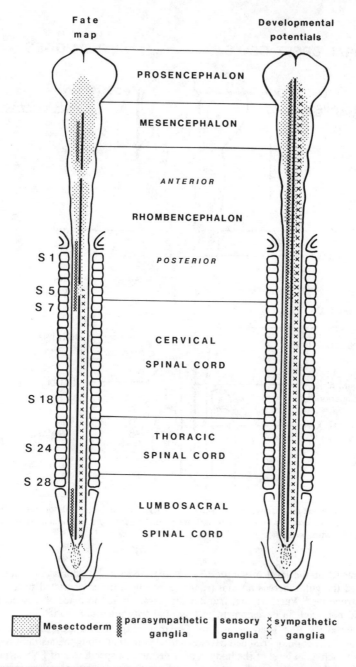

FIGURE 4. Diagram showing, on the left ("Fate map"), the distribution along the neural crest of the presumptive territories yielding the mesectoderm, the sensory, parasympathetic, and sympathetic ganglia in normal development. On the right ("Developmental potentials"), distri-

evidently through this selection that environmental cues control the development of the PNS. Moreover, it has to be underlined that the capacity of neural crest cells to yield mesectodermal derivatives is restricted to the cephalic region of the neuraxis down to the level of the 5th somite in the two avian species investigated in this respect.[34]

The nature of the environmental factors directing neural crest cell differentiation, the timing of their action, and the state of determination of the reacting cells at different stages of embryogenesis are the subjects of further investigations carried out essentially on the neural derivatives of the crest.

RESTING UNDIFFERENTIATED CELLS IN DEVELOPING PERIPHERAL GANGLIA

Certain of these investigations have led to the demonstration that resting undifferentiated cells remain in the nonneuronal cell population of quail PNS ganglia at least until hatching, i.e., after all the neurons of these ganglia have withdrawn from the cell cycle (no relevant experiments have been performed on postnatal ganglia).

The potentialities of these undifferentiated cells are restricted to the autonomic cell lineage, including sympathetic, chromaffin, and enteric ganglion cells. Such progenitor cells exist in all types of ganglia, be they sensory (DRG and cranial nerve sensory ganglia) or autonomic (ciliary and sympathetic ganglia).

In the sensory ganglia, however, cycling precursors of sensory neurons that can survive and differentiate after grafting are present during the early stages of PNS ontogeny before all the sensory neurons of the ganglia have reached the postmitotic state.

These conclusions were drawn from experiments in which fragments of embryonic quail peripheral ganglia were implanted into the neural crest migratory pathway of younger chick hosts, as described in FIGURE 5.

Soon after the graft, the solid piece of ganglion loses cohesiveness and its histological structure becomes disrupted while the component cells become dispersed in the host somitic structures. Twenty-four hours after grafting, quail cells can be seen, singly or in small groups, among the host dorsal mesenchymal cells. After 48 hours, this dispersion is followed by homing of the progeny of the grafted cells into the host's neural crest-derived structures.

The phase of homing revealed interesting cell-cell recognition mechanisms through which the graft-derived cells recognized the host's crest elements with which they agglomerated and formed chimeric ganglia. Moreover, it was only when young sensory ganglia were grafted that quail cells (i.e., quail neurons) were found in the host's DRG. In all the other cases, the progeny of implanted ganglion cells colonized peripheral nerves (as Schwann cells), autonomic ganglia (sympathetic, enteric), and paraganglia (adrenal-medulla).[29,30,35-38]

---

bution of the developmental potentials for the same cell types is indicated. In fact, if neural crest cells from any level of the neural axis are implanted into the appropriate site of a host embryo, they can give rise practically to all the cell types forming the various kinds of PNS ganglia. This shows that the target tissue of crest cell migration, rather than their origin on the neural axis, determines their fate. This is not true, however, for the ectomesenchymal cells (also called mesectoderm) whose precursors are confined to the cephalic area of the crest down to the level of somite 5.

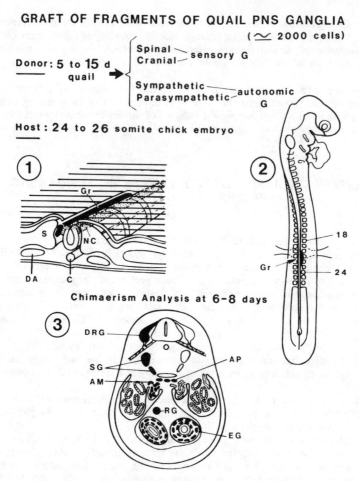

FIGURE 5. Diagram showing the experimental procedure followed in the back transplantation of quail PNS ganglia into the chick neural crest migration pathway: 1 and 2 show the positioning of the graft; 3 shows the various host crest derivatives in which quail cells are found in the 6-8 day chick host. AM, adrenal medulla; AP, aortic plexus; C, notochord; DA, dorsal aorta; DRG, dorsal root ganglion; EG, enteric ganglia; Gr, graft; NC, neural crest; RG, ganglion of Remak; S, somite; SG, sympathetic ganglia.

THE DUAL CELL LINE SEGREGATION MODEL

These results suggested an early heterogeneity of the neural crest, in which at least certain neuronal precursors are already committed to a particular differentiation pathway at the time of migration. These are the precursors that give rise, respectively, to sensory (type "S" progenitors) and autonomic (type "A" progenitors) neurons. Developmental potentials of the two postulated progenitor cells are already restricted to the autonomic and sensory pathways, either in the migrating crest or in the very young ganglia, even though choices concerning their terminal differentiation can still take place under the influence of environmental cues, as demonstrated with sympathetic nerve cells of the newborn rat (see Reference 39 for a review) even at the single cell level.[40-41]

Autonomic and sensory potentialities both exist in the emigrating flow of crest cells (FIGURE 6). The fact that in the back-transplantation experiments, no sensory neurons can be obtained, from either distal sensory or autonomic ganglion grafts, while autonomic derivatives arise from all types of grafted peripheral embryonic ganglia, could reflect different survival requirements for the two types of precursor. Sensory precursors may be able to survive and differentiate only in ganglia situated

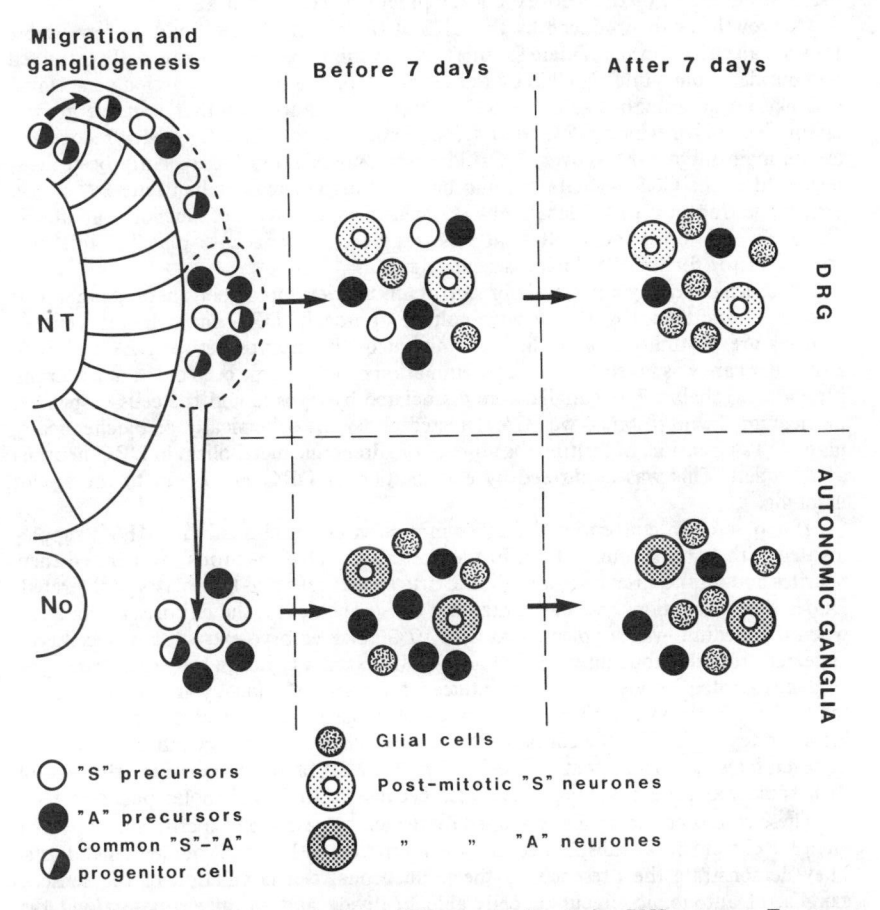

FIGURE 6. Hypothesis accounting for cell line segregation during PNS ontogeny. Two types of precursors, sensory ("S") and autonomic ("A"), arise from a common progenitor during neural crest cell individualization and/or migration and in the early steps of gangliogenesis.

in close proximity to the CNS, while autonomic precursors remain alive in all types of PNS ganglia, at least until hatching. Sensory neuronal precursors either become postmitotic neurons or disappear from the DRG after E7 in quail embryos, while autonomic precursors remain present in large excess in all types of peripheral ganglia. Proliferation and differentiation of the latter can be triggered by the microenvironment of a younger host in the back transplantation experimental system.

In support of this view is the fact that all the sensory ganglia whose neurons originate from the neural crest develop in contact with the CNS. This is true not only for the DRG but also for the proximal part of the trigeminal ganglion (situated on cranial nerve V) and for the superior-jugular complex corresponding to the root ganglia of nerves IX and X. Furthermore, as soon as they withdraw from the cell cycle, sensory neurons readily extend neurites toward the CNS, as can be seen on sections treated with antibodies directed against neurofilament proteins.[42] It can be proposed that the CNS exerts a short-range positive effect on the survival, and perhaps also the differentiation, of the sensory lineage precursor cells (FIGURE 7).

A growth factor produced by the CNS at these early stages could be responsible for such an effect. One candidate for this function might be the factor recently extracted and purified from adult pig CNS by Barde et al.,[43] on the basis of its action on survival and neurite outgrowth of chick DRG neurons in culture. Another is nerve growth factor (NGF), for which DRG (and sympathetic neurons) have long been recognized as the main targets. Moreover, NGF-like immunoreactivity has recently been demonstrated in the CNS (spinal cord and brain) of certain mammalian fetuses,[44] as has retrograde transport of ^{125}I-labeled NGF from the spinal cord of newborn rats to the DRG via the dorsal roots. NGF at this stage seems, in fact, to play the role of a trophic factor for the developing sensory neurons.

Presence of resting autonomic precursors in the developing peripheral ganglia was further substantiated by the in vitro culture approach. DRG in which all sensory neurons are postmitotic were dissected out of quail embryos between E9 and E15. Particular care was taken to avoid contamination by adrenergic cells of the neighboring sympathetic chains. The ganglia were dissociated by trypsin, and the cells suspended in medium. In no instance was CA detected either histochemically or biochemically in the cell suspension, indicating the absence of adrenergic metabolism in DRG neurons of the quail. This was confirmed by examination of DRG in situ up to the age of hatching.

If explanted in conventional Eagle's minimum essential medium (MEM) supplemented with horse serum and NGF, the postmitotic DRG neurons regenerated their neurites and, in the absence of antimitotic drugs, glial cells and fibroblasts proliferated. Under these conditions, no CA-containing cells appeared in the culture. In contrast, when the medium was supplemented with 10% chick embryo extract, a new cell type appeared from day four onward. These cells displayed a typical adrenergic phenotype as demonstrated by glyoxylic acid-induced fluorescence[45] and by immunoreactivity for tyrosine hydroxylase (TH) (FIGURE 8). A large proportion of TH-positive cells incorporated ^{3}H-TdR in the course of the culture. Their morphology differed strikingly in several respects from that of the sensory neurons of the DRG since the size of their soma was generally smaller and also because of their multipolar phenotype.[21,46]

These results confirm those obtained by the above-described experiments, in which quail DRG were back transplanted into the migration pathway of younger chick hosts. They demonstrate the presence, in the nonneuronal cell population of the sensory ganglia, of autonomic precursor cells able to divide and to differentiate along the adrenergic pathway under the influence of one or more factors contained in chick embryo extract.

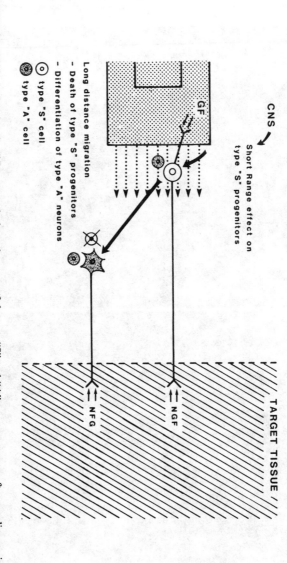

FIGURE 7. Diagram showing the different survival requirements of the type "S" and "A" precursors soon after gangliogenesis (see text for explanation).

CNS

Short Range effect on
type "S" progenitors

GF

Long distance migration
— Death of type "S" progenitors
— Differentiation of type "A" neurons

⊙ type "S" cell
⊛ type "A" cell

NFG

NGF

TARGET TISSUE

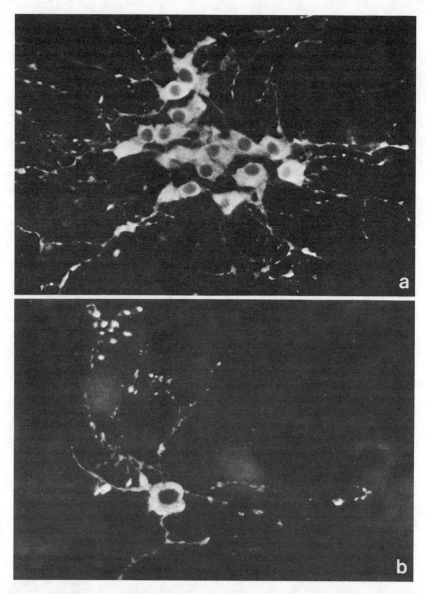

FIGURE 8. Culture of dissociated cells from 10-day embryonic quail DRG in a medium supplemented with serum and chick embryo extract. Numerous cells with tyrosine hydroxylase immunoreactivity differentiate in the culture (a). Many of them incorporate ³H-TdR as in (b), where the nucleus of a TH-positive cell shows dense silver grains in the nucleus. Magnification: (a) × 555; (b) × 530 (figure reduced to 85%).

Studies on the Dual Cell Line Segregation Model Carried Out In Vitro

If heterogeneity is established early in the neural crest cell population, this might be apparent in tissue culture, where environmental conditions can be modified to trigger selectively the expression of developmental potentialities. This is why a series of studies have been undertaken in several laboratories with a view to addressing this question.

The Various Techniques of Crest Cell Explantation

Differentiation of neural crest cells into neurons or paraganglionic type cells in culture has been documented by the work of several laboratories. One of the first successful attempts in this direction was due to Cohen and Konigsberg,[47] who isolated the neural primordium (comprising the neural tube + the neural folds) from quail embryos at E2 and observed, within 12 to 24 hours, the emigration of the neural crest cells around the tube explant. Removal of the tube thereafter eliminated most of the cells belonging to the CNS, with the exception, however, of those that had migrated from the tube itself. This technique, particularly easy to handle, has been widely used.

In order to avoid contamination by cells of the neural tube, other methods were devised involving surgical removal of the crest, either when still in the folds or when migrating. This latter instance, which is the "safest" if neural tube cell contamination is to be avoided, is particularly appropriate for the mesencephalic neural crest which, as mentioned before, migrates, as a multisheet of cells, underneath the superficial ectoderm (FIGURE 1).

Whether the crest cells are explanted along with the tube or selectively removed microsurgically, it was found that their differentiation into various phenotypes could be modulated by monitoring the composition of the culture medium and substrate.

Modulation of Neural Crest Cell Development by the Culture Conditions

When cultured *in vitro* in serum-containing medium (DMEM + 15% fetal calf or horse serum), isolated mesencephalic or trunk neural crest cells grew rapidly but did not exhibit a morphologically identifiable neuronal phenotype (FIGURE 9a). However, acetylcholine (ACh) synthetic activity was significantly higher in these cultures than in the freshly removed crest.[48] Moreover, CA synthesis became detectable and a modulatory effect of serum was observed with horse serum generally favoring ACh synthesis and fetal calf serum preferentially stimulating CA production.[49] None of the neuronal markers tested, such as tetanus toxin or neurofilament protein immunoreactivity, revealed any neuronal phenotypic expression in the culture or in the crest prior to cultivation. The intermediate filament protein, vimentin, was present in virtually 100% of crest cells prior to and during culture.[50]

Crest cultures evolve differently in a fully defined medium, totally devoid of serum but provided instead with hormones, growth factors, and transferrin, the "basic Brazeau medium" (BBM).[50-51] In a few hours, a subpopulation of crest cells, both from trunk and mesencephalic regions, readily differentiated into neurons without dividing

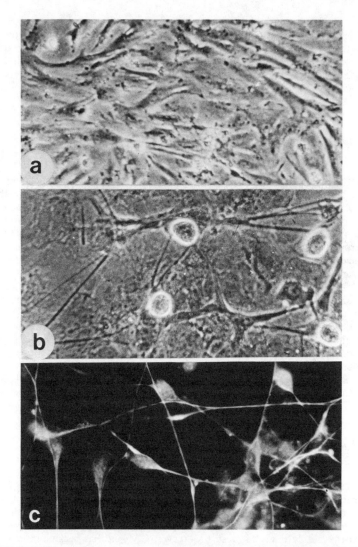

FIGURE 9. Culture of E2 quail mesencephalic neural crest cells in DMEM + 10% fetal calf serum (FCS) (a) and in the defined medium of Brazeau (BBM)[49] (b, c). In (a), examination of the culture by phase contrast at 14 days, shows cells with fibroblastic morphology; no differentiated neurons are visible. In (b), E2 quail mesencephalic crest cells have been cultured in BBM for 30 days. Neuronal somas and bundles of nerve fibers are visible on top of a sheet of flat cells. In (c), 200 KD neurofilament protein antibody has been applied to a 2-day culture of mesencephalic crest in BBM. Both fibers and cell bodies of the neuronlike cells are immunoreactive. Magnification: (a) × 360; (b) × 360; (c) × 435.

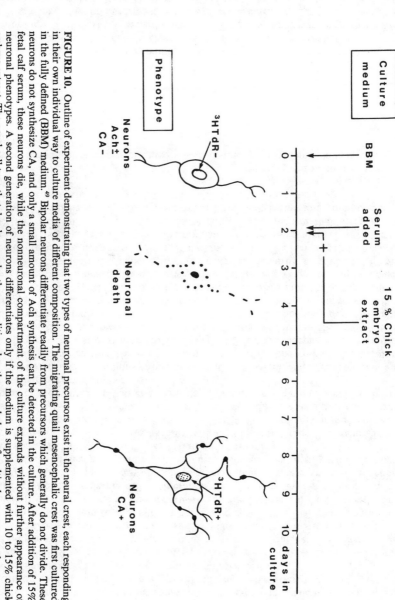

FIGURE 10. Outline of experiment demonstrating that two types of neuronal precursors exist in the neural crest, each responding in their own individual way to culture media of different composition. The migrating quail mesencephalic crest was first cultured in the fully defined (BBM) medium.[49] Bipolar neurons differentiate readily from precursors which generally do not divide. These neurons do not synthesize CA, and only a small amount of Ach synthesis can be detected in the culture. After addition of 15% fetal calf serum, these neurons die, while the nonneuronal compartment of the culture expands without further appearance of neuronal phenotypes. A second generation of neurons differentiates only if the medium is supplemented with 10 to 15% chick embryo extract. The novel cell type that develops under these conditions has the morphology of multipolar neurons and possesses manifest adrenergic traits (TH immunoreactivity and CA-specific fluorescence). This cell type arises from cycling precursors.

(FIGURE 9b). Expression of tetanus toxin binding sites and neurofilament protein synthesis could be detected very early in these cells, which extended neuronal outgrowths. Application of a pulse of depolarizing current to the cells with typical neurite outgrowths revealed their aptitude to generate action potentials from day four in culture,[52] thus confirming their neuronal nature. Coexpression of neurofilament protein (FIGURE 9C) and vimentin was a general rule in the neurons, while only vimentin was detectable in the still cycling, nonneuronal, flat cells.

Biochemical or histochemical analysis failed to reveal CA synthesis and storage and only low levels of ACh synthesis could be detected in the neurons differentiating in serum-free medium. The neurotransmitter they produce is as yet unknown.

Addition of serum to the cultures had a strong inhibitory effect on neurite outgrowth from the neuronal precursors thus revealed in the crest, and it appeared clearly that conditions stimulating cell proliferation were incompatible with the promotion of neuronal phenotypic expression. It became plain that culture in serum-free medium stops proliferation and triggers neurite extension in cells that, *in vivo,* would normally have gone through several divisions before differentiating.

Culture of neural crest cells with or without the neural tube (Reference 53 and our own unpublished observations) can, however, yield neurons even in the presence of serum if 10 to 15% of chick embryo extract is added to the medium. The neurons appear in the culture only after several days, and at least some of them exhibit the catecholaminergic phenotype.

Moreover, two generations of neurons can be successively obtained from the same explanted neural crest if the conditions are modified in the course of the culture according to the pattern indicated in FIGURE 10. In mesencephalic crest cultures initiated in BBM, the bipolar neurons readily differentiate within the first 24 hours and disappear rapidly if serum is added at 48 hours; the nonneuronal cells divide actively, but no morphologically recognizable neurons develop. In contrast, if chick embryo extract prepared from E9 chicks is added to BBM along with the serum, a novel generation of neuronlike cells arises from about day six onward. Glyoxylic acid fluorescence[45] reveals CA content in these cells, the majority of which arise from cycling precursors, as shown by ^{3}H-TdR incorporation.[54] The fact that the adrenergic phenotype develops in culture when their precursors are allowed to divide is consistent with the observation by Kahn and Sieber-Blum,[55] who showed that in crest cells explanted with the neural tube in the presence of both serum and embryo extract, appearance of CA-containing cells is inhibited by antimitotic agents such as cytosine arabinoside.

These results support the contention that the developing neural crest contains at least two types of neuronal precursors with distinct behavior and differentiation requirements.

CONCLUDING REMARKS

As seen before, several data point to the notion that a certain degree of commitment already exists at least in certain crest cells when they migrate away from the neural primordium. This view was recently further supported when it was found that a Mab (GlN1), prepared by immunizing a mouse with crude extract of quail nodose ganglion, recognizes a surface antigen on about 10% of the migrating neural crest and, subsequently, on all glial (satellite and Schwann) cells but only on a small number of neurons.[23]

The nature of the antigen recognized and its relationship with the phenotypes of the differentiated cells in which it is expressed at later stages are now under investigation. It is hoped that this approach will open new avenues in neural crest research, namely, in the recognition of the cell line segregation occurring during the course of its ontogeny.

REFERENCES

1. HÖRSTADIUS, S. 1950. The Neural Crest: Its Properties and Derivatives in the Light of Experimental Research. Oxford University Press. London, England.
2. LE DOUARIN, N. M. 1982. The Neural Crest. Cambridge University Press. Cambridge, England.
3. WESTON, J. A. 1963. Dev. Biol. 6: 279-310.
4. WESTON, J. A. 1970. Adv. Morphog. 8: 41-114.
5. CHIBON, P. 1964. C. R. Acad. Sci. Paris 259: 3624-3627.
6. CHIBON, P. 1966. Mem. Soc. Zool. Fr. 36: 1-107.
7. JOHNSTON, M. C. 1966. Anat. Rec. 156: 143-156.
8. NODEN, D. M. 1975. Dev. Biol. 42: 106-130.
9. LE DOUARIN, N. M. 1969. Bull. Biol. Fr. Belg. 103: 435-452.
10. LE DOUARIN, N. M. 1973. Exp. Cell Res. 77: 459-468.
11. LE DOUARIN, N. M. 1973. Dev. Biol. 30: 217-222.
12. LE DOUARIN, N. M. 1980. Curr. Top. Dev. Biol. 16: 31-85.
13. LE DOUARIN, N. M., M. A. TEILLET & J. FONTAINE-PERUS. 1984. In Chimaeras in Developmental Biology. N. M. Le Douarin & A. Mc Laren, Eds.: 313-352. Academic Press. London, England.
14. LE DOUARIN, N. M. 1985. In Handbook of Physiology, Development of the Nervous System. Max Cowan, Ed. American Physiological Society. (In press.)
15. WESTON, J. A. 1982. In Cell Behaviour. R. Bellairs, A. Curtis & G. Dunn, Eds.: 429-470. Cambridge University Press. Cambridge, England.
16. WESTON, J. A. 1983. In Cell Interactions and Development: Molecular Mechanisms. K. M. Yamada, Ed.: 153-184. John Wiley and Sons. Chichester, England.
17. WESTON, J. A., J. GIRDLESTONE & G. CIMENT. 1983. In Cellular and Molecular Biology of Neuronal Development. I. Black, Ed.: 51-62. Plenum Publishing Corporation. New York, N.Y.
18. DREWS, V. 1975. Prog. Histochem. Cytochem. 7: 1-52.
19. COCHARD, P. & P. COLTEY. 1983. Dev. Biol. 98: 221-238.
20. MIKI, A., E. FUGIMOTO & H. MIZOGUTI. 1983. Histochemistry 78: 81-93.
21. VINCENT, M., J.-L. DUBAND & J. P. THIERY. 1983. Dev. Brain Res. 9: 235-238.
22. VINCENT, M. & J.-P. THIERY. 1984. Dev. Biol. 103: 468-481.
23. BARBU, M., C. ZILLER, P. M. RONG & N. M. LE DOUARIN. J. Neurosci. (In press.)
24. KINUTANI, M. & N. M. LE DOUARIN. 1985. Dev. Biol. 111: 243-255.
25. LE DOUARIN, N. M., P. COCHARD, M. VINCENT, J.-L. DUBAND, G. C. TUCKER, M.-A. TEILLET & J. P. THIERY. 1984. In The Role of Extracellular Matrix in Development: 373-398. Alan R. Liss, Inc. New York, N.Y.
26. D'AMICO-MARTEL, A. & D. M. NODEN. 1983 Am. J. Anat. 166: 445-468.
27. LE DOUARIN, N. M. & M.-A. TEILLET. 1974. Dev. Biol. 41: 162-184.
28. NODEN, D. M. 1976. J. Gen. Physiol. 68: 13a.
29. SCHWEIZER, G., C. AYER-LE LIÈVRE & N. M. LE DOUARIN. 1983. Cell Differ. 13: 191-200.
30. LE DOUARIN, N. M., D. RENAUD, M.-A. TEILLET & G. LE DOUARIN. 1975. Proc. Nat. Acad. Sci. USA 72: 728-732.
31. FONTAINE-PERUS, J., M. CHANCONIE & N. M. LE DOUARIN. 1982. Cell Differ. 11: 183-193.
32. SMITH, J., P. COCHARD & N. M. LE DOUARIN. 1977. Cell Differ. 6: 199-216.
33. NODEN, D. M. 1978. Dev. Biol. 67: 313-329.

34. LE LIÈVRE, C. & N. M. LE DOUARIN. 1975. J. Embryol. Exp. Morphol. **34:** 125-154.
35. LE DOUARIN, N. M., C. S. LE LIÈVRE, G. SCHWEIZER & C. M. ZILLER. 1979. *In* Cell Lineage, Stem Cells and Cell Determination. N. M. Le Douarin Ed.: 353-365. Elsevier North Holland Publishing Company. Amsterdam, Holland.
36. LE LIÈVRE, C. S., G. G. SCHWEIZER, C. M. ZILLER & N. M. LE DOUARIN. 1980. Dev. Biol. **77:** 362-378.
37. AYER-LE LIÈVRE, C. S. & N. M. LE DOUARIN. 1982. Dev. Biol. **94:** 291-310.
38. DUPIN, E. 1984. Dev. Biol. **105:** 288-299.
39. PATTERSON, P. H. 1978. Annu. Rev. Neurosci. **1:** 1-17.
40. FURSHPAN, E. J., P. R. MAC LEISH, P. H. O'LAGUE & D. D. POTTER. 1976. Proc. Nat. Acad. Sci. USA **73:** 4225-4229.
41. LANDIS, S. C. 1976. Proc. Nat. Acad. Sci. USA **73:** 4220-4224.
42. COCHARD, P. & D. PAULIN. 1984. J. Neurosci. **4:** 2080-2094.
43. BARDE, Y. A., D. EDGAR & H. THOENEN. 1982. EMBO J. **1:** 549-553.
44. AYER-LE LIÈVRE, C. S., T. EBENDAL, L. OLSON & A. SIEGER. 1983. Med. Biol. **61:** 296-304.
45. KÖNIG, R. 1979. Histochemistry **61:** 301-305.
46. XUE, Z. G., J. SMITH & N. M. LE DOUARIN. 1985. C. R. Acad. Sci. Paris **300:** 483-488.
47. COHEN, A. M. & I. R. KONIGSBERG. 1975. Dev. Biol. **46:** 262-280.
48. SMITH, J., M. FAUQUET, C. ZILLER & N. M. LE DOUARIN. 1979. Nature **282:** 853-855.
49. FAUQUET, M., J. SMITH, C. ZILLER & N. M. LE DOUARIN. 1981. J. Neurosci. **1:** 478-492.
50. ZILLER, C., E. DUPIN, P. BRAZEAU, D. PAULIN & N. M. LE DOUARIN. 1983. Cell **32:** 627-638.
51. ZILLER, C., N. M. LE DOUARIN & P. BRAZEAU. 1981. C. R. Acad. Sci. Paris **292:** 1215-1219.
52. BADER, C. R., D. BERTRAND, E. DUPIN & A. C. KATO. 1983. Nature **305:** 808-810.
53. COHEN, A. M. 1977. Proc. Nat. Acad. Sci. USA **74:** 2899-2903.
54. ZILLER, C., M. FAUQUET, J. SMITH & N. M. LE DOUARIN. Dev. Biol. (In press.)
55. KAHN, C. R. & M. SIEBER-BLUM. 1983. Dev. Biol. **95:** 232-238.

Sympathetic Neuronal Density and Cell Membrane Contact Regulate Phenotypic Expression in Culture[a]

IRA B. BLACK AND JOSHUA E. ADLER

Department of Neurology
Division of Developmental Neurology
Cornell Medical College
515 East 71st Street
New York, New York 10021

INTRODUCTION

Neuronal development consists of apparently discrete, reproducible processes including cellular migration, aggregation, transmitter phenotypic expression, and synaptogenesis. A number of these processes have been defined in some detail. However, potential mechanistic relationships among the processes are unclear. While it is well recognized, for example, that aggregation generates the stable formation of nuclei in the brain and ganglia in the periphery, the relationship of aggregation to transmitter expression is undefined.

One hint concerning interrelationships may derive from observations in the embryonic rat *in vivo*: initial expression of the catecholamine (CA) enzymes tyrosine hydroxylase (TH) and dopamine-β-hydroxylase (DBH) and of CAs coincides with cellular aggregation to form the primordial sympathetic ganglia.[1] The temporal association of cellular aggregation and transmitter expression suggests that these processes may be causally related. This possibility has gained indirect support from the observations that growth of bovine adrenal chromaffin cells[2] or PC12 rat pheochromocytoma cells[3] in high-density cell culture selectively increases TH specific activity.

We have examined the relationship of cell aggregation and transmitter phenotypic expression by growing virtually pure neonatal rat sympathetic neurons in fully defined, serum-free medium at varying cell densities.[4] We have found that increasing cell density, with consequent neuronal aggregation, differentially affects TH, choline acetyltransferase (CAT), a cholinergic enzyme, and substance P (SP), a putative peptide transmitter, in these neurons. The differential effects appear to be mediated by cell aggregation and contact, and not through elaboration of diffusible factors.

[a] This work was supported by National Institutes of Health Grants NS 10259 and HD 12108 and was aided by a grant from the March of Dimes Birth Defects Foundation.

METHODS

Experimental Animals and Culture Techniques

Sprague-Dawley rat pups, less than 24 hours old, were used. Methods of dissociation and culture have been described elsewhere.[5] Ganglion dissociates were plated at varying concentrations of 7000-35,000 neurons per 35-mm dish in Ham's nutrient mixture F12 supplemented with transferrin, putrescine, insulin, selenium, and progesterone.[6] After 24 and 72 hours in culture, cytosine arabinofuranoside (10^{-5} M, ARA-C) was added to destroy the dividing nonneuronal cells. Medium was replaced 24 hours after each addition of ARA-C. Efficacy was confirmed by phase microscopic examination.

Cell Counts

Cultures were rinsed with calcium/magnesium-free Puck's saline G (Sal G) and then incubated at 37°C for 30 minutes in 1 ml of 1 mM EGTA and trypsin (0.25%) in calcium/magnesium-free Sal G. Neurons were gently triturated from the dish bottom, and duplicate counts were performed in a hemocytometer.

Extraction and Radioimmunoassay of Substance P

SP was extracted and assayed as described elsewhere.[7]

Assay of Tyrosine Hydroxylase Activity

Cultures were rinsed with ice-cold Sal G, following which 200 μl of potassium phosphate buffer (20 mM) pH 7.6 with 0.2% Triton X-100 was added. Dishes were then scraped as for SP extraction. A 10 μl aliquot of extract was assayed for activity as previously described.[8,9]

Assay of Choline Acetyltransferase Activity

Enzyme was extracted similarly to tyrosine hydroxylase except that 100 μl of EDTA (10mM) pH 7.4 with 0.5% Triton X-100 was used. A 2 μl aliquot of extract was assayed for activity according to the method of Fonnum.[10]

Statistics

Data were analyzed with a one-way analysis of variance and the Newman-Keuls test.

RESULTS AND DISCUSSION

Differential Effects of Neuronal Density on Phenotypic Expression

Under normal circumstances, sympathetic neurons of the rat superior cervical ganglion (SCG) express both TH and SP.[11,12] To define the effect of increasing neuronal density on these different phenotypic characters, virtually pure dissociated ganglion neuron cultures were grown at varying densities. At relatively low densities of 7000-8000 neurons/dish, moderate levels of TH were detectable (728 pm/dish × hour) after one week (FIGURE 1). Increasing cell density yielded a linear rise in TH activity to a maximum of 2200 pm/dish × hour for 25,000 neurons/dish (FIGURE 1). Consequently, TH per neuron remained constant over a broad range of cell densities.

In contrast, cell density had a profound, nonlinear effect on SP content. Low-density cultures contained 20 pg SP (FIGURE 1). A 2-fold increase in cell density increased SP 3-fold, whereas a 4-fold increase in density yielded a striking *30-fold* rise in the peptide (FIGURE 1).

We also examined the effect of cell density on cholinergic expression by assaying the activity of CAT, the enzyme that synthesizes acetylcholine. While CAT activity is predominantly localized to presynaptic terminals of the SCG *in vivo*,[13,14] nonneuronal factors in culture elicit cholinergic expression in postsynaptic ganglion neurons.[15] To determine whether increased neuronal density can also elicit cholinergic expression, CAT activity was examined. At low cell densities CAT activity was undetectable (FIGURE 2). However, CAT activity appeared *de novo* at an intermediate density of 15,000 neurons/dish, and increased sixfold when cell density was doubled (FIGURE 2).

To definitively evaluate the effects of cell density, the specific content (or activity) of each transmitter character was expressed per neuron for the entire range of neuron densities examined. TH activity per neuron remained constant (FIGURE 3). In contrast, CAT activity per neuron increased fourfold and SP content per neuron increased sevenfold at high neuronal densities, suggesting that cell density affected different traits differently.

The observations indicate that neuronal density differently regulates distinct transmitter traits. While we have not localized these traits to specific individual neurons in these particular cultures, previous work has indicated that cholinergic, noradrenergic, and peptidergic characters are, in fact, present in the same sympathetic neurons under a variety of conditions.[12,16] Our observations confirm the general contention that phenotypic traits for different transmitters may be differentially regulated in the same neuronal populations,[11,15-21] and, more specifically, indicate that cell density is one condition evoking differential effects. Moreover, the fact that SP and CAT activity increased per neuron while TH remained constant suggests that there is no *obligatory* reciprocal relationship between CAT and SP on the one hand and TH on the other.

Our observations may also be relevant to the general problem of conditions necessary for cholinergic and peptidergic expression in classical noradrenergic sympathetic

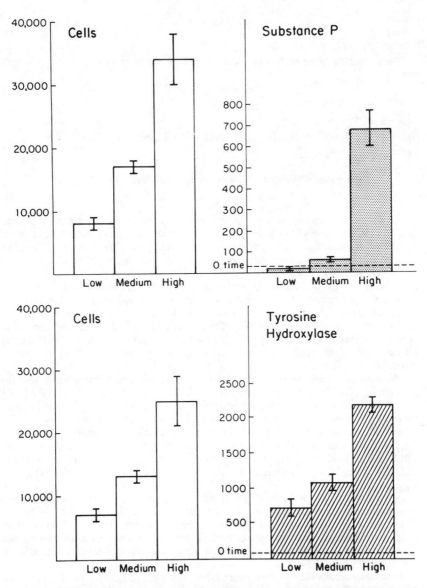

FIGURE 1. Effects of neuronal density on tyrosine hydroxylase activity and substance P content. Cell dissociates were plated at low, medium, and high densities. After one week, neuronal number (six dishes) and tyrosine hydroxylase activity (six dishes; bottom panel) were determined in sister cultures at all densities. Neuronal number is expressed as mean cells per dish ± standard error of the mean; tyrosine hydroxylase activity is expressed as pmol product per dish × hour (± SEM). Dashed line represents mean tyrosine hydroxylase activity for high cell densities six hours after plating. Substance P content (top panel) is expressed as pg per dish (± SEM). Dashed line represents mean substance content for high cell densities six hours after plating. (Data from Reference 4.)

neurons. Previous studies suggested that expression and increases of peptidergic and cholinergic traits required the presence of nonneuronal cells or factors elaborated therefrom.[15,16,19–23] The present studies, performed in the virtual absence of nonneuronal cells, in fully defined serum-free medium, indicated that sympathetic neurons may express cholinergic and peptidergic characters in the absence of nonneuronal elements. In this context, high neuronal density elicited the same effects as the presence of nonneuronal cells. Consistent with this contention, only TH demonstrated a time-dependent increase in low-density cultures in our studies.

To begin examining mechanisms underlying the apparent neuron-neuron interactions, a number of different approaches were employed. We initially examined the effects of medium conditioned by high-density cultures.

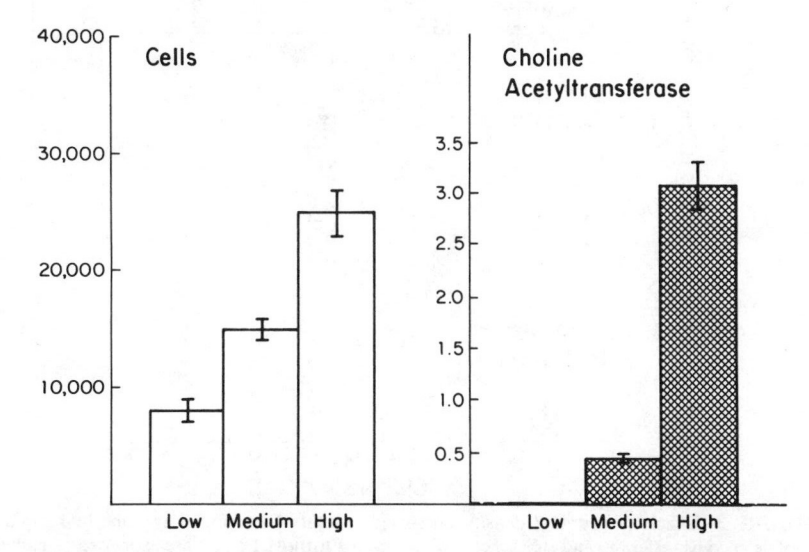

FIGURE 2. Effects of neuronal density on choline acetyltransferase activity. Cell dissociates were plated as in FIGURE 1. After one week, neuronal number (six dishes) and choline acetyltransferase activity (six dishes) were determined in sister cultures at all densities. Neuronal number is expressed as mean cells per dish (± SEM); choline acetyltransferase activity is expressed as nmol product per dish × hour (± SEM). Dashed line represents mean choline acetyltransferase activity for high cell densities six hours after plating. (Data from Reference 4.)

Conditioned Medium and Transmitter Expression

To determine whether the effects of increased density were mediated by diffusible neuronal factors, low-density cultures were exposed to culture medium conditioned by one-week-old, high-density cultures. High-density cultures prepared from the same dissociates served as controls. Conditioned medium did not elicit any increase in either CAT activity or SP, whereas high-density *control* cultures exhibited marked, nonlinear increases in both characters, as expected (FIGURE 4). These results suggested that diffusible factors elaborated by high-density neurons were not regulating differential transmitter expression. Consequently, we examined the possibility that cell contact itself might be critical.

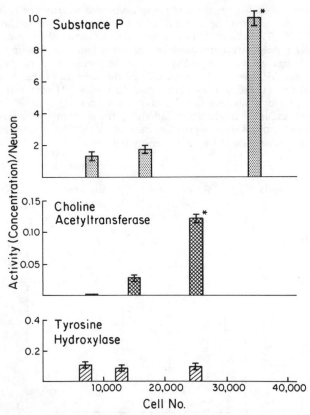

FIGURE 3. Effects of neuronal density on specific activity (content) of tyrosine hydroxylase, choline acetyltransferase, and substance P. Data from FIGURES 1 and 2 are expressed as activity or content per neuron for tyrosine hydroxylase (pmol product per neuron $\times$ hour), choline acetyltransferase (pmol product per neuron $\times$ hour), and substance P (fg per neuron) $\pm$ SEM. *Differs from all other groups at $p < 0.01$. (Data from Reference 4.)

Culture Density and Neuronal Aggregation

To determine whether increased density actually increased neuronal aggregation over the range examined, cultures derived from the same dissociate were examined by phase microscopy. Twenty-four and 48 hours after plating, cells in the high- and low-density cultures exhibited the same low incidence of aggregation. However, by one week, high-density cultures contained multiple cellular aggregates, whereas few, if any, were observed in low-density culture. To define the dynamics of high-density aggregation in greater detail, culture dishes were marked and time-lapse phase microscopy was performed over the course of one week. No detectable differences in aggregation between high- and low-density cultures were apparent at 24 hours, when perikaryal diameter was increasing. However, between 48 and 96 hours in high-density cultures only, perikarya appeared to migrate toward one another, eventually forming large multicellular aggregates. Thereafter, little further aggregation occurred. Aggregation was not observed at any time in low-density cultures.

Inhibition of Perikaryal Aggregation

To examine the potential causal relationship between perikaryal aggregation and phenotypic expression, aggregation was inhibited with methylcellulose, an agent that increases medium viscosity. Addition of the agent to medium inhibited perikaryal aggregation and simultaneously inhibited the rises in CAT and SP without affecting neuronal survival. Moreover, inhibition of aggregation with tunicamycin, an agent that blocks lipid-dependent glycosylation and cell membrane interactions, reproduced the effects of methylcellulose.[24]

These observations suggest that cell membrane interactions per se are critical in the regulation of transmitter phenotypic expression.

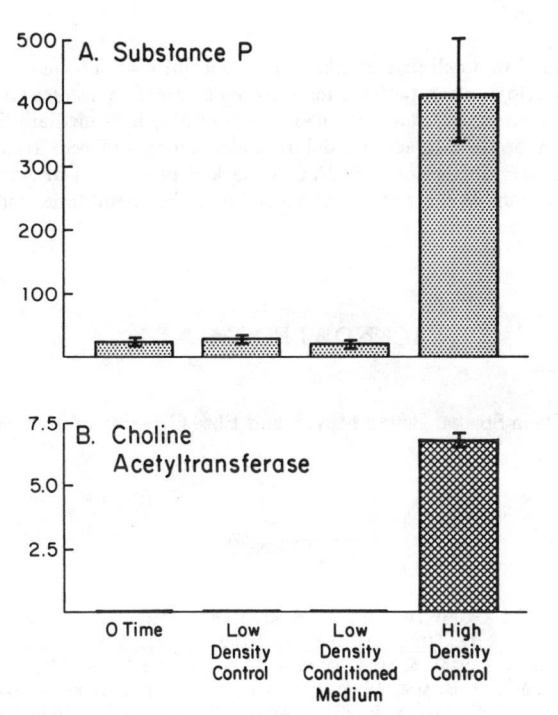

FIGURE 4. Effects of conditioned medium on substance P content and choline acetyltransferase activity. Cell suspensions were plated at low and high densities. Low-density control (six dishes) and high-density control (six dishes) cultures were fed with fresh medium. Low-density conditioned-medium cultures (six dishes) were fed with medium conditioned by previously plated high-density cultures. All cultures were grown for one week. Substance P is expressed as pg per dish ($\pm$ SEM); choline acetyltransferase activity is expressed as nmol product per dish $\times$ hour ($\pm$ SEM).

The Effects of Cell Membranes

To determine whether cell membrane interactions do, in fact, regulate phenotypic expression, low-density cultures were exposed to whole ganglion membrane preparations for three days. Crude membrane preparations derived from a 30,000 $\times$ g pellet of whole ganglia were used. Membranes elicited the *de novo* appearance of CAT activity, strongly suggesting that interactions of cell membrane components regulate phenotypic expression in aggregating neurons.[24] We are presently defining the characteristics of the membrane factors involved. The present system offers the opportunity to define the intercellular molecular interactions regulating transmitter expression and increases. In this manner it may be possible to define causal relationships among the apparently distinct ontogenetic processes of cellular migration, aggregation, and phenotypic expression.

CONCLUSIONS

We have found that cell density plays an important role in transmitter phenotypic expression in developing sympathetic neurons in culture. Our studies strongly suggest, moreover, that neuronal contact and membrane interactions mediate this effect. The influence of membrane interactions differentially affects different transmitter traits, eliciting the *de novo* appearance of CAT, a marked increase in SP/neuron, but not altering TH/neuron. We are presently analyzing the membrane components and mechanisms involved.

ACKNOWLEDGMENTS

We thank Dana Straka, Bettye Mayer, and Elise Grossman for excellent technical assistance.

REFERENCES

1. COCHARD, P., M. GOLDSTEIN & I. B. BLACK. 1979. Dev. Biol. **71:** 100-114.
2. ACHESON, A. L. & H. THOENEN. 1983. Cell Biol. **97:** 925-928.
3. LUCAS, C. A., D. EDGAR & H. THOENEN. 1979. Exp. Cell. Res. **121:** 79-86.
4. ADLER, J. E. & I. B. BLACK. 1985. Proc. Nat. Acad. Sci. USA **82:** 4296-4300.
5. KESSLER, J. A., J. E. ADLER & I. B. BLACK. 1983. Science **221:** 1059-1061.
6. BOTTENSTEIN, J. & G. SATO. 1979. Proc. Nat. Acad. Sci. USA **76:** 514-517.
7. ADLER, J. E., J. A. KESSLER & I. B. BLACK. 1984. Dev. Biol. **102:** 417-425.
8. BLACK, I. B., A. HENDRY & L. L. IVERSEN. 1971. Brain Res. **34:** 229-240.
9. BLACK, I. B., F. E. BLOOM, I. A. HENDRY & L. L. IVERSEN. 1971. J. Physiol. London **215:** 24-25P.
10. FONNUM, F. 1975. Neurochemistry **24:** 407-409.
11. KESSLER, J. A., J. E. ADLER, M. C. BOHN & I. B. BLACK. 1981. Science **214:** 335-336.

12. BOHN, M. C., J. A. KESSLER, J. E. ADLER, K. MARKEY, M. GOLDSTEIN & I. B. BLACK. 1984. Brain Res. **298:** 378-381.
13. HEBB, C. O. & G. M. H. WAITES. 1956. J. Physiol. London **132:** 667-671.
14. HEBB, C. O. 1956. J. Physiol. London **133:** 566-570.
15. PATTERSON, P. H. & L. L. Y. CHUN. 1977. Dev. Biol. **56:** 263-280.
16. FURSHPAN, E. J., P. R. MACLEISH, P. H. O'LAGUE & D. D. POTTER. 1976. Proc. Nat. Acad. Sci. USA **73:** 4225-4229.
17. KESSLER, J. A., J. E. ADLER, W. O. BELL & I. B. BLACK. 1983. Neuroscience **9:** 309-318.
18. PATTERSON, P. H. 1978. Annu. Rev. Neurosci. **1:** 1-17.
19. O'LAGUE, P. H., K. OBATA, P. CLAUDE, E. J. FURSHPAN & D. D. POTTER. 1974. Proc. Nat. Acad. Sci. USA **71:** 3602-3606.
20. LANDIS, S. C. 1976. Proc. Nat. Acad. Sci. USA **73:** 4220-4224.
21. JOHNSON, M., D. ROSS, M. MEYERS, R. REES, R. BUNGE, E. WAKSHULL & H. BURTON. 1976. Nature **262:** 308-310.
22. PATTERSON, P. H. & L. L. Y. CHUN. 1974. Proc. Nat. Acad. Sci. USA **71:** 3607-3610.
23. KESSLER, J. A., J. E. ADLER, G. M. JONAKAIT & I. B. BLACK. 1984. Dev. Biol. **103:** 71-79.
24. ADLER, J. E. & I. B. BLACK. 1985. Soc. Neurosci. Abstr. **2:** 947.

Molecular and Immunocytochemical Studies of Neurofibromas and Related Cell Types[a]

JOHN E. PINTAR,[b] KENNETH H. SONNENFELD,[c]
JOHN FISHER,[b] ROBYN S. KLEIN,[b] AND
BARBARA KREIDER[d]

[b]Department of Anatomy and Cell Biology
Columbia University College of Physicians and Surgeons
630 West 168th Street
New York, New York 10032

[c]Department of Neurology
Mount Sinai School of Medicine
1 Gustav Levy Place
New York, New York 10029

[d]Department of Neurology
Children's Hospital of Philadelphia
34th Street and Civic Center Boulevard
Philadelphia, Pennsylvania 19017

INTRODUCTION

Abnormal proliferation of cell types normally associated with peripheral neurons is a central feature of neurofibromatosis. Although the molecular basis underlying the localized development of dermal neurofibromas is not known, it is conceivable that abnormal expression of growth factor genes or oncogenes directs this proliferation. At present nerve growth factor (NGF), which has well-defined effects on specific populations of embryonic and adult cells (see References 1-4 for reviews), has been the most extensively studied growth factor. Despite extensive biochemical character-ization of this molecule and molecular studies of its effects on NGF-responsive cells, relatively little is known about its relevance to specific disease states. Although linkage analysis has strongly suggested that a structurally altered β-NGF gene is not correlated with neurofibromatosis[5] (but see Reference 6), the possibility remains that altered regulation or processing of β-NGF in neurofibroma tissue may be related to the development of this condition.

Recent, but indirect, evidence has offered some support for this possibility. Some sympathetic nerve endings exhibit hypertrophy and fail to innervate appropriate target organs following development of dermal neurofibromas.[7] Although it is not known

[a]This work was supported in part by grants from the Neurofibromatosis Foundation (to JP and KHS) and from the National Institutes of Health (NS-21970 to JP).

how early this disruption occurs, it might alter the proliferation of cell types normally associated with neurons, such as perineural fibroblasts and peripheral Schwann cells, that are possible synthetic sites for NGF-like peptides. It is possible that NGF, if synthesized in these tumors, accumulates because aberrant connections prevent its removal, which may permit autoregulatory effects on Schwann cells in neurofibromas that express NGF receptors.[8] Since dermal neurofibromas transplanted to the anterior chamber of the rat eye can elicit sympathetic fiber outgrowth from the host iris into the tumors[9] and since extracts of dermal neurofibromas contain NGF-like bioactivity in standard sensory ganglia and PC12 bioassays,[10] it is tempting to speculate that this effect on fiber outgrowth is NGF mediated; however, NGF radioimmunoreactivity in these tissues has not yet been demonstrated. In view of the potential false positives often given by immunochemical procedures for NGF analysis, it is clear that a more refined analysis of NGF presence in neurofibroma tissue and any relationship between NGF and the development of neurofibromas requires more direct methods for detecting and localizing NGF gene expression.

The availability of recombinant DNA probes for all subunits of the NGF molecule[11-15] makes it possible to study the structure of NGF genes in inherited disease, to determine whether expression of these genes is altered, and to identify cell types containing specific mRNA using *in situ* hybridization. One of the most important applications of recombinant DNA technology uses DNA probes as histochemical tools.[16-18] Radiolabeled single-stranded DNA or RNA probes incubated with sections of fixed tissue can form stable, double-stranded hybrids with complementary mRNA molecules under appropriate conditions. The distribution of radiolabeled probe can be visualized following autoradiography of the hybridized section, and the distribution of specific mRNA thus determined at the single-cell level. It is likely that both the ability to determine whether differences exist in NGF (or other growth factor or oncogene) mRNA content between normal skin and neurofibromas and the ability to localize specific mRNA-containing cells with *in situ* hybridization will be required to accurately assess the role of NGF (or other relevant growth factor or oncogene) expression in the development of neurofibromatosis. *In situ* hybridization may be especially informative when specific mRNA is concentrated in relatively few cells and in any case will be required to identify specific cell types responsible for synthesis of specific RNA detected in extracts.

In this paper, we demonstrate the localization of cells in mouse submaxillary gland tissue sections containing β-NGF mRNA by *in situ* hybridization. In addition, we present a method for assessing specificity of *in situ* hybridization signals by hybridization of nonhomologous fragments to adjacent tissue sections. Further, we demonstrate the presence of β-NGF mRNA in a rat Schwann cell-schwannoma hybrid cell line that shares characteristics with neurofibroma cells. Finally, we have used antibodies to the NGF receptor[19] and to monoamine oxidase B (MAO-B),[20,21] the primary degradative enzyme for catecholamines, to characterize other biochemical properties of neurofibroma cells.

MATERIALS AND METHODS

DNA Probes

Recombinant pBR322 plasmids containing a 760 base-pair mouse NGF cDNA insert (pBR322-NGF-2C11)[11] were propagated in *E. coli* HB101, amplified, and isolated by standard procedures. The mouse NGF plasmid has been used to isolate human genomic clones[11] and cross-hybridizes in all species examined. A recombinant pBR322 plasmid containing a 550 base-pair cDNA insert of the proopiomelanocortin (POMC) gene was obtained from Dr. James Roberts. For *in situ* hybridization experiments, nonhomologous NGF cDNA fragments were obtained by digestion of NGF plasmid DNA with Pst and Rsa (see Results).

Northern Blot Analysis

Several rat hybrid cell lines derived from fusion of primary Schwann cells and a rat schwannoma cell line (RN-22) were provided by Dr. David Pleasure. One line, RNS5, which showed greatest binding capacity for ^{125}I-NGF, was examined for expression of the NGF gene. Total RNA was isolated from these cells using the guanidine-isothiocyanate LiCl procedure, and poly A+ RNA isolated by oligo-dT chromatography. Poly A+ RNAs were separated by agarose gel electrophoresis, transferred to Gene-Screen (New England Nuclear), hybridized with ^{32}P-labeled NGF cRNA (synthesized after a Pst fragment from the NGF cDNA clone originally obtained from Axel Ullrich was subcloned into Sp64), and washed to a final stringency of 0.05X SSC at 68°C (SSC is 0.15 M sodium chloride and 0.015 M sodium citrate).

Immunocytochemistry

The immunocytochemical localization of MAO-B in neurofibroma tissue sections and in cultured cells derived from neurofibromas was performed using an antiserum raised in rabbits against bovine MAO-B.[20,21] This antiserum does not show detectable cross-reactivity with rat or human MAO-A by immunoprecipitation or immunoblotting procedures. Freshly excised neurofibromas were fixed by immersion in 4% paraformaldehyde in 0.1 M sodium borate buffer, pH 11 for 3-24 hours at 4°C, while cells cultured from dermal neurofibromas enriched in Schwann cells were fixed for 15-60 minutes at room temperature. Following fixation, neurofibroma tissues were prepared for cryostat sectioning by immersion for 24 hours at 4°C in 10% sucrose followed by 20% sucrose in 0.1 M sodium phosphate buffer, pH 7.0. Serial 10-μm sections were collected on gelatin-chrome alum coated slides.

For immunofluorescence, sections were hydrated in 0.1 M sodium phosphate, 0.5 M sodium chloride containing 0.3% Triton X-100 (high salt buffer, HSB). Slides were incubated for 5 minutes in a 1% sodium borohydride solution to reduce aldehyde groups and thus minimize background staining. Sections were then incubated overnight at room temperature in a 1:100 dilution of rabbit MAO-B antiserum containing 5% normal swine serum (Accurate Scientific). Alternate sections or coverslips incubated with rabbit preimmune serum served as controls. After washing in HSB, sections were incubated for 1 hour in a 1:25 dilution of rhodamine-conjugated swine anti-rabbit immunoglobulin G (IgG) (Dako Brand, Accurate Scientific) containing 5% normal swine serum.

Following visualization of MAO-B distribution, coverslips were removed and cells or slides incubated with mouse anti-human NGF receptor antibodies.[19] Ascites fluid from hybridoma-injected mice was incubated with sections or coverslips at a dilution of 1/1000 overnite; bound antibody was visualized following incubation with biotinylated anti-mouse antibody and avidin-biotin horseradish peroxidase.

In Situ *Hybridization*

Adult male and female mouse submaxillary glands were immersion fixed for 2 hours at room temperature in freshly prepared 4% paraformaldehyde-phosphate buffered saline (PBS) (pH 7.0), equilibrated overnight in 20% sucrose, and embedded in OCT. Cryostat sections containing both male and female tissue (8 μm) were hydrated and treated with 0.2 N HCl for 10 minutes. Section were then prehybridized at 24°C for 1 hour with prehybridization buffer containing 50% formamide, 4X SSC, 20 mM tris (pH 7.5), yeast total RNA (0.1 mg/ml), yeast transfer RNA (0.05 mg/ml), herring sperm DNA (0.1 mg/ml), 1 mM EDTA, 0.02 percent ficoll, 0.02% polyvinylpyrrolidone-20, and bovine serum albumin (0.2 mg/ml). Prehybridization buffer was removed and replaced with hybridization buffer containing the above components plus 10% dextran sulfate and ^{32}P- or ^{3}H-labeled NGF, I-13 or pBR322 DNA (specific activity, 10^7 cpm/μg; 2×10^4 cpm per section). The probe was heat denatured at 100°C for 10 minutes before it was applied to the tissue section. Incubation of tissue sections with hybridization mix continued overnight at 24°C. Sections were washed for 1 hour each time in two changes of 2X SSC containing 0.1% sodium dodecyl sulfate (SDS) at room temperature and for 5 hours in 0.2X SSC at 37°C. Sections were air dried and coated with emulsion (Kodak NTB-2) which had been diluted 1:1 with 0.6 M ammonium acetate. Sections were then exposed at 4°C for 6 weeks, developed with D-19, and counterstained with hematoxylin and eosin. ^{32}P- and ^{3}H-NGF were prepared by nick translation isolated inserts or insert fragments. The specific activity of ^{3}H-DNA probes used for *in situ* hybridization approached 10^7 cpm/μg. DNAase concentration during nick translations was adjusted to give radiolabeled probe fragments of 40-100 base-pairs which enhance probe penetration into the section but which allow stable DNA-RNA hybrids to be formed and maintained under the hybridization conditions used.

RESULTS AND DISCUSSION

The β-NGF Gene Is Expressed in a Rat Schwann Cell-Schwannoma Hybrid Cell Line

Northern blot analysis (FIGURE 1) demonstrated the presence of a radiolabeled band of 1.3 kilobases (kb), the size of NGF mRNA, in poly A+ extracts of a rat Schwann cell-schwannoma hybrid (RNS5) that expresses the NGF receptor and can bind axolemma. This observation is consistent with the possibility that the NGF gene may be expressed in cells with similar phenotype found in human neurofibromas and further raises the question of whether these hybrid cells can respond to exogenous NGF, and/or whether axolemma can alter NGF expression by these cells.

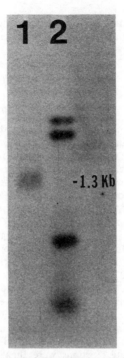

FIGURE 1. Northern blot analysis of RNA-5 poly-A+ RNA. 10 μg poly A+ RNA was separated on a 0.8% formaldehyde agarose gel, blotted, and hybridized with ^{32}P-NGF cRNA. A hybridizing species of about 1.3 kb (the size of NGF mRNA) is observed in lane 1; standards in lane 2 are 2.3, 2.0, 0.5, and 0.1 kb in length.

Distinct Populations of Neurofibroma Cells Can Be Visualized with MAO-B and NGF Receptor Antibodies

Previous use of MAO-B antisera has identified rodent and human central nervous system astrocytes as MAO-B positive[20,21] (and Levitt and Pintar, unpublished observations). Both tissue sections of dermal neurofibromas and cultures of cells derived from dermal neurofibromas contain cells with MAO-B immunoreactivity. Two morphologically distinct cell types are MAO-B positive. One type is ovoid, while the second is elongate and Schwann-like in appearance. The elongated MAO-B cells predominate both in tissue sections (FIGURE 2) and in vitro (FIGURE 3B). Following visualization of MAO-B immunoreactivity, subsequent incubation of cultured cells with anti-human NGF receptor antibodies demonstrated a distinct population of Schwann-like NGF receptor positive cells that are MAO-B negative.

Thus MAO-B and NGF receptor antibodies recognize distinct cell types within neurofibromas. As in situ hybridization begins to localize specific cells expressing growth factor genes or oncogenes within these tumors, the ability to couple immunocytochemical detection of MAO-B and NGF receptor containing cells with in situ hybridization[22] should prove useful.

Localization of NGF mRNA in Mouse Submaxillary Gland and Specificity of In Situ Hybridization

NGF cDNA probes have successfully been used for *in situ* hybridization of the mouse submaxillary gland. *In situ* hybridization of male and female submaxillary glands with radiolabeled NGF cDNA or cRNA reflects the difference in NGF mRNA content that is characteristic of this sexually dimorphic structure and demonstrates specific cell populations containing NGF mRNA.

We initially hybridized ^{32}P-labeled NGF to sections containing both male and female submaxillary glands, which can easily be distinguished histologically. Following the exposure of hybridized slides to x-ray film, film exposure (after 24 hours) was much greater over areas of the section containing male tissue (FIGURE 4). This difference between male and female submaxillary gland was not seen if sections were hybridized with radiolabeled plasmid or POMC DNA. These controls provide strong evidence that the differences seen reflect the known differences in NGF mRNA content of these tissues.

Further, we have hybridized submaxillary glands with ^{3}H-labeled NGF cDNA probes to obtain precise single cell localization following emulsion autoradiography. Following a four-week exposure, silver grains were concentrated in the male (FIGURE 5) and female secretory tubules and were essentially absent in the acini; this cellular

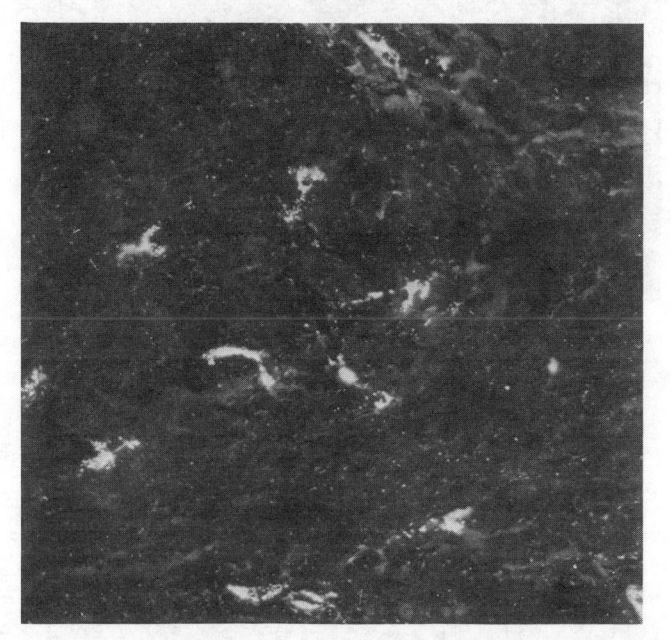

FIGURE 2. Demonstration of MAO-B immunoreactivity in dermal neurofibromas. Dermal neurofibromas were fixed for 2 hours in 4% paraformaldehyde-PBS, equilibrated with 20% sucrose, and sectioned on a cryostat after OCT embedding. Sections were stained with rabbit anti-bovine MAO-B antibodies that have previously been shown to recognize human MAO-B but not human MAO-A. Sites of anti-MAO-B binding were visualized with a rhodamine-labeled sheep anti-rabbit second antibody. MAO-B positive cells in this field have stellate appearance.

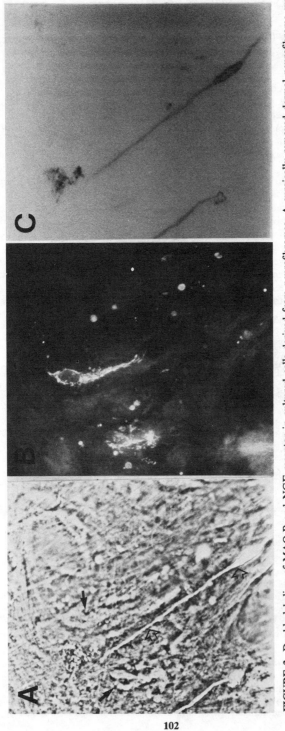

FIGURE 3. Double labeling of MAO-B and NGF receptor in cultured cells derived from neurofibromas. A surgically removed dermal neurofibroma was dispersed with dispase and cells plated on plastic coverslips, grown for five days, fixed, and sequentially treated with anti-MAO-B and anti-NGF receptor antisera. (A) Phase micrograph showing elongated Schwann-like cells sitting on a bed of fibroblasts; MAO-B positive cells and NGF receptor positive cells are denoted by arrows and arrowheads, respectively. (B) MAO-B immunostaining. (C) NGF receptor immunostaining; note that immunoreactive MAO-B and NGF receptor positive cells are distinct.

distribution of grains corresponds to the site of NGF storage in the submaxillary gland as demonstrated by immunocytochemistry. These results show that there are specific cellular locations of β-NGF mRNA in tissue sections using ^{3}H-labeled NGF probes and provide direct evidence that NGF is synthesized in secretory tubules. Strong hybridization signals are obtained following a four-week exposure. Since an "average" eukaryotic cell contains approximately 2×10^5 mRNA molecules/cell, and since the abundance of male submaxillary gland NGF mRNA is 0.1%,[11] 200 copies of NGF mRNA are readily detected using double-stranded probes.

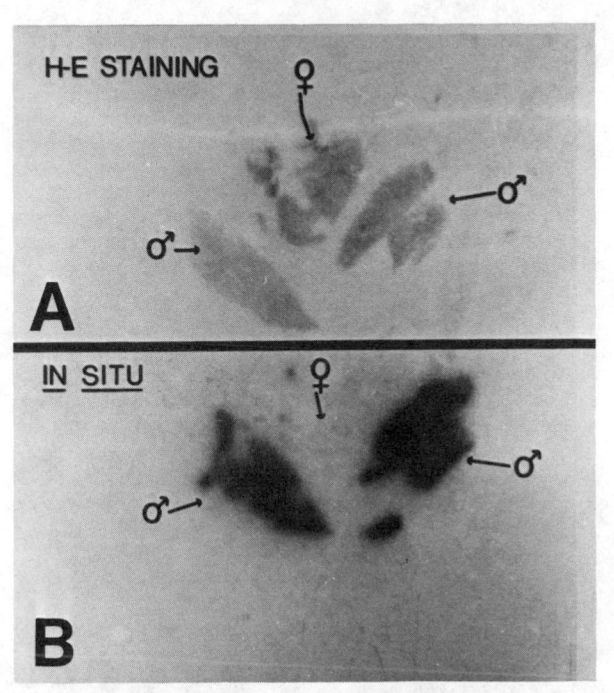

FIGURE 4. *In situ* hybridization of submaxillary gland with ^{32}P-NGF DNA. Adult male and female submaxillary glands were fixed for 2 hours in 4% formaldehyde-PBS, equilibrated with sucrose-PBS, and embedded in OCT. Eight-micrometer sections were rinsed in 95% ethanol for 10 minutes in 0.2 N HCl. Sections were prehybridized and hybridized as described in Methods. The hybridization buffer contained 50 K cpm ^{32}P-labeled NGF DNA. After washing, sections were exposed to x-ray film for one day at room temperature. Following autoradiography male and female tissues were identified histologically. A stained section containing both male and female tissue is shown in low power in FIGURE 4A; the corresponding x-ray film of the same section is shown in FIGURE 4B. The much greater hybridization of radiolabeled NGF DNA to areas of the section containing male tissue is apparent (FIGURE 4B).

Identical procedures have yet to identify NGF mRNA containing cells in neurofibroma tissue sections or in neurofibroma-derived cell cultures enriched in Schwann cells. Thus, although our present results appear to exclude high levels of NGF gene expression in specific neurofibroma cells, lower levels of NGF expression remain possible. It is likely that the use of single-stranded cRNA for *in situ* hybridization[23] will be necessary to detect cells expressing low levels of growth factor or oncogene mRNA unless a relatively low number of specific cells in a specific tissue contain this mRNA. Strong hybridization signals to mouse submaxillary gland secretory tubules are obtained within a week using ^{3}H-labeled cRNA β-NGF as a hybridization probe.[18]

Previous applications of *in situ* hybridization have relied on other information about the cellular location of peptides of interest as a major criterion for specificity

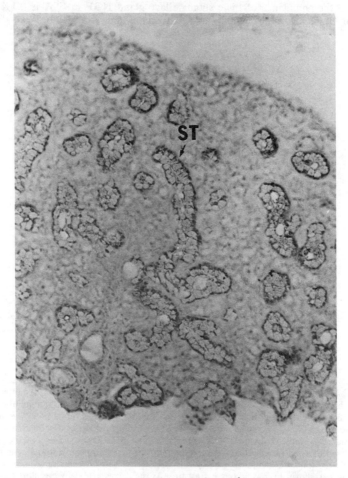

FIGURE 5. Hybridization of male submaxillary gland with ^{3}H-NGF DNA. NGF cDNA was radiolabeled with ^{3}H-nucleotides and hybridized to sections containing male mouse submaxillary gland. Following hybridization and washing, sections were coated with emulsion and exposed for 4 weeks at 4°C. Heavy labeling of the secretory tubules is apparent.

of the hybridization procedure. For example, in the demonstration that proopiomelanocortin mRNA was present in specific hypothalamic cells, adjacent sections were examined by immunocytochemistry and by *in situ* hybridization, and identical cells contained both immunoreactive endorphin and silver grains following binding of the POMC probe.[17] However, alternative methods to ensure specificity of *in situ* hybridization procedures when immunocytochemical procedures have proven elusive or controversial must be developed. In the procedure we use to ensure specificity, one nonspecific and two specific, but nonhomologous, DNA or RNA probes are hybridized to three adjacent tissue sections. If similar grain distributions are seen in sections hybridized with the two different, but gene-specific, probes that are not mimicked in the section containing nonspecific DNA, then the hybridization is considered specific. Digestion of NGF cDNA with Pst and Rsa produces such fragments that produce the same pattern of secretory tubule labeling as shown in FIGURE 5 when hybridized to mouse submaxillary glands.[18] Ultimately the greatest combination of sensitivity and assured specificity should result from hybridization of adjacent sections with non-homologous, but gene-specific, cRNA probes.

SUMMARY AND PROSPECTUS

We have demonstrated expression of the β-NGF gene in a rat Schwann cell-schwannoma hybrid cell line that possesses many characteristics of normal Schwann cells. This observation suggests that an investigation of NGF expression in neurofibromas of different growth states is warranted. Since Schwann cells from neurofibromas possess NGF receptors, possible autoregulation of Schwann cell function by NGF is conceivable. Distinct populations of cells expressing the NGF receptor and MAO-B should provide useful markers for further characterization of cells shown to express specific genes by *in situ* hybridization.

ACKNOWLEDGMENTS

The authors thank Axel Ullrich for providing the β-NGF cDNA plasmid used for initial *in situ* hybridization experiments and Alonzo Ross for providing ascites fluid containing monoclonal antibodies to the human NGF receptor. The authors are also pleased to thank Andy Stover for expert technical assistance and Ruth Carpino for preparation of the manuscript.

REFERENCES

1. GREENE, L. A. & E. M. SHOOTER. 1980. The nerve factor: biochemistry, synthesis, and mechanism of action. Annu. Rev. Neurosci. **3:** 353-402.
2. THOENEN, H. & Y.-A. BARDE. 1980. Physiology of nerve growth factor. Physiol. Rev. **60:** 1284-1335.
3. BRADSHAW, R. A. & N. V. COSTRINI. 1983. The structure and function of nerve growth factor. *In* Growth and Maturation Factors. G. Guroff, Ed. **1:** 1-31. John Wiley and Sons. New York, N.Y.
4. PINTAR, J. E. Structure and expression of the NGF genes. *In* Growth and Maturation Factors. G. Guroff, Ed. John Wiley and Sons. New York, N.Y. (In press.)

5. DARBY, J. K., J. FEDER, M. SELBY, V. RICCARDI, R. FERRELL, D. SIAO, K. GOSLIN, W. RUTTER, E. M. SHOOTER & L. L. CAVALLI-SFORZA. 1985. A discordant sibship analysis between β-NGF and neurofibromatosis. Am. J. Hum. Genet. 37: 52-59.
6. SPENCE, M. A., J. L. BADER, D. M. PARRY, et al. 1983. Linkage analysis of neurofibromatosis. J. Med. Genet. 20: 334-337.
7. RUBENSTEIN, A. E., C. MYTILINEOU, M. D. YAHR, J. PEARSON & M. GOLDSTEIN. 1981. Neurotransmitter analysis of dermal neurofibromas: implications for the pathogenesis and treatment of neurofibromatosis. Neurology 31: 1184-1188.
8. SONNENFELD, K. H., P. BERND, G. SOBUE, M. LEBWOHL & A. E. RUBENSTEIN. 1986. Nerve growth factor receptors on dissociated neurofibroma Schwann-like cells. Cancer Res. 46: 1446-1452.
9. RUBENSTEIN, A. E., C. MYTILINEOU & R. LADMAN. 1982. Neurofibromas transplanted to the anterior chamber of the eye: an animal model for axon-sheath cell trophic interactions in neurofibromatosis. Neurology 32: A158.
10. RUBENSTEIN, A. E., R. HADMAN, C. MYTILINEOU, A. M. ARON, S. WALLACE & S. SILLMAN. 1983. Nerve growth factor in neural tumors in disseminated neurofibromatosis. Neurology 33: 79.
11. ULLRICH, A., A. GRAY, C. BERMAN & T. J. DULL. 1983. Human β-nerve growth factor gene sequence highly homologous to that of mouse. Nature 303: 821-825.
12. SCOTT, J., M. SELBY, M. URDEA, M. QUIROGA, G. I. BELL & W. J. RUTTER. 1983. Isolation and nucleotide sequence of a cDNA encoding the precursor of mouse nerve growth factor. Nature 302: 538-540.
13. ULLRICH, A., A. GRAY, W. I. WOOD, J. HAYFLICK & P. H. SEEBURG. 1984. Isolation of the cDNA clone coding from the g-subunit of mouse nerve growth factor using a high-stringency selection procedure. DNA 3: 387-392.
14. ISACKSON, P. J., A. ULLRICH & R. A. BRADSHAW. 1984. Mouse 7S nerve growth factor: complete sequence of a cDNA coding for the a-subunit precursor and its relationship to serine proteases. Biochemistry 23: 5997-6002.
15. HOWLES, P. H., D. P. DICKINSON, L. L. DiCAPRIO, M. WOODWORTH-GUTAI & K. W. GROSS. 1984. Use of a cDNA recombinant for the g-subunit of mouse nerve growth factor to localize members of this multigene family near the TAM-1 locus on chromosome 7. Nucleic Acids Res. 12: 2791-2805.
16. BRAHIC, M. & A. T. HAASE. 1978. Detection of viral sequences of low reiteration frequence by in situ hybridization. Proc. Nat. Acad. Sci. USA 75: 6125-6129.
17. GEE, C., C-L. C. CHEN, J. L. ROBERTS, R. THOMPSON & S. J. WATSON. 1983. Identification of POMC neurons in the rat hypothalamus by in situ hybridization. Nature 306: 374-376.
18. PINTAR, J. E. & D. I. LUGO. Localization of peptide hormone gene expression in adult and embryonic tissues. In In Situ Hybridization: Applications of Neurobiology. K. Valentino, J. Eberwine & J. D. Barchas, Eds. Oxford University Press. Oxford, England. (In press.)
19. ROSS, A. H., P. GROB, M. BOTHWELL, D. E. ELDER, C. S. ERNST, N. MARANO, B. F. GHRIST, C. C. SLEMP, M. HERLYN & B. ATKINSON. 1984. Characterization of nerve growth receptor in neural crest tumors using monoclonal antibodies. Proc. Nat. Acad. Sci. USA 81: 6681-6685.
20. LEVITT, P., J. E. PINTAR & X. O. BREAKEFIELD. 1982. Immunocytochemical demonstration of monoamine oxidase-B in brain astrocytes and serotonergic neurons. Proc. Nat. Acad. Sci. USA 79: 6385-6389.
21. PINTAR, J. E., P. LEVITT, J. I. SALACH, W. WEYLER, M. B. ROSENBERG & X. O. BREAKEFIELD. 1983. Specificity of antisera prepared against pure bovine MAO-B. Brain Res. 276: 127-139.
22. SHIVERS, B. D., R. E. HARLAN, D. W. PFAFF & B. S. SCHACHTER. 1986. Combination of immunocytochemistry and in situ hybridization in the same tissue section of rat pituitary. J. Histochem. Cytochem. 34: 39-43.
23. COX, K., D. DELEON, L. ANGERER & R. ANGERER. 1984. Detection of mRNAs in sea urchin embryos by in situ hybridization using assymetric RNA probes. Dev. Biol. 101: 485-502.

Nerve Growth Factor Binding to Cells Derived from Neurofibromas[a]

KENNETH H. SONNENFELD,[b] PAULETTE BERND,[c]
ALLAN E. RUBENSTEIN,[b] AND GEN SOBUE[d]

[b]Department of Neurology
[c]Department of Anatomy
Mount Sinai School of Medicine
1 Gustave Levy Place
New York, New York 10029

[d]Department of Neurology
Aichi Medical University
Nagoya, Japan

INTRODUCTION

Neurofibromatosis (NF) is a disorder in which the proliferation of cellular components of neural sheaths to form either dermal or plexiform neurofibromas is one of the most frequent and characteristic features. Light and electron microscopic observations of neurofibromas have led investigators to postulate that the perineural fibroblast[1-4] or the Schwann cell[5-9] is the principal proliferating cell type comprising neurofibromas.

The origin in the neural crest of cells contributing to neurofibroma growth has prompted several investigators to postulate that effectors of neural crest differentiation such as nerve growth factor, a polypeptide required for normal development and function of sympathetic and sensory neurons, may be involved in neurofibroma growth.[10-14] Although studies have focused on identifying alterations in the amount and activity or structure of nerve growth factor (NGF) present in individuals with NF, few have focused on identifying cells in neurofibromas that might be targets for NGF action. In this communication, we describe a method for the complete dissociation of neurofibromas into individual cells, and the results of experiments directed at identifying binding sites for ^{125}I-NGF on cells from neurofibromas.

PREPARATION OF NEUROFIBROMA CULTURES

Cultures of dissociated neurofibromas were initiated from patients with neurofibromatosis treated at the neurofibroma clinic of the Mount Sinai Hospital in New York City. Following the removal of overlying skin, neurofibromas are minced into

[a]Supported by a National Neurofibromatosis Foundation Grant and Public Health Service Postdoctoral Training Grant NS07245 to K.H.S., and National Institutes of Health Grant HD17262 and a Familial Dysautonomia Award to P.B.

107

small pieces (approximately 1 mm³) while immersed in complete growth medium (CGM; RPMI 1640 with fetal calf serum, 15%). Minced tissue is washed once in CGM, centrifuged (500 × g for five minutes), and resuspended in digesting solution. A digesting solution we have found to be most efficient for dissociating neurofibromas contains Dispase (Boehringer-Mannheim, 1.25 U/ml), collagenase (Sigma, 0.05%), hyaluronidase (Sigma, 0.1%), CaCl₂ (5 mm), MgCl₂ (0.5 mm), and Hepes (25 mm) in RPMI 1640 with fetal calf serum (4%). Tissue is digested at 37°C either in a sterile spinner flask or a 15 ml plastic culture tube containing a magnetic stir bar. Incubations are continued until all the tissue is dissociated, and in several cases this lasted for approximately 18 to 24 hours. Cells dissociated with Dispase and kept in its presence during prolonged digestion remain viable and need not be continuously separated from digesting tissue as is necessary when trypsin is used. Enzyme solution is removed from cells by aspirating the supernatant following centrifugation of cells for five minutes at 1000 × g. Cells are resuspended in CGM and plated in 24 well cluster tissue culture dishes or 25 cm² tissue culture flasks.

This procedure resulted in cell dissociates containing long spindle-shaped cells with an elongated nucleus and round cells (FIGURE 1). Within 24 to 48 hours after plating, two distinctive morphologies were present in cultures of dissociated neurofibromas. Long, spindle, Schwann-like cells (SLC) comprised one population. The other, fibroblast-like population (fibroblast-like cells, FLC) contained cells that had a round nucleus and broad flat expanses of membrane. Proliferation of FLC appeared more rapid than SLC, and FLC were the predominant cell type within one week of plating.

RADIOAUTOGRAPHIC IDENTIFICATION OF ¹²⁵I-NGF BINDING SITES ON NEUROFIBROMA SLC

To determine whether cells from neurofibromas possess NGF binding sites and whether such sites would be distributed among all neurofibroma cell types or limited to a particular subpopulation, we used radioautography to detect binding of ¹²⁵I-NGF to cultured cells of dissociated neurofibromas. The beta subunit of NGF was isolated from male mouse saliva[15,16] and iodinated with lactoperoxidase.[17,18] Binding of ¹²⁵I-NGF to neurofibroma cultures and subsequent radioautographic localization were accomplished using a modification of the techniques described by Bernd and Greene.[19] Dissociated cells which had been grown on glass coverslips were rinsed with fresh CGM followed by incubation for one hour at 37°C in CGM containing ¹²⁵I-NGF (5 ng/ml = 0.2 nM). Nonspecific binding was determined by including in the incubation medium of parallel cultures unlabeled NGF (5 or 10 μg/ml). After the incubation period, coverslips with cells were rapidly washed six times (1 ml/wash) with phosphate-buffered saline (PBS, 4°C, pH 7.4) and fixed in glutaraldehyde (2.5% in phosphate buffer 0.1 M, pH 7.4). Coverslips mounted on slides were then washed in distilled water, dried, and dipped in photographic emulsion. Development of emulsion after about one week revealed grains over ¹²⁵I-NGF labeled cells.

Evidence of cell-specific ¹²⁵I-NGF binding is shown in the photomicrograph of cultured cells from a dissociated neurofibroma (FIGURE 2a and b). The localization of grains over SLC and not FLC indicates that NGF binding sites are present on

Schwann-like cells. The lack of ^{125}I-NGF binding to FLC and the inability of binding to be displaced by insulin, bovine serum albumin, and cytochrome C (data not shown) suggest that ^{125}I-NGF binding to SLC is specific. Displacement of ^{125}I-NGF by excess unlabeled NGF (FIGURE 4 a and b) indicates that NGF binding to SLC is saturable.

Two types of NGF binding sites, which can be distinguished from one another by their dissociation characteristics, have been described.[17,20] NGF dissociation from high-affinity sites (also referred to as slow or type I) occurs at 37°C with a $t_{1/2}$ of about 10 to 30 minutes depending on the cell type studied,[17,20,22] but occurs extremely slowly, if at all, when dissociation is attempted at 0°C. NGF dissociation from the low-affinity

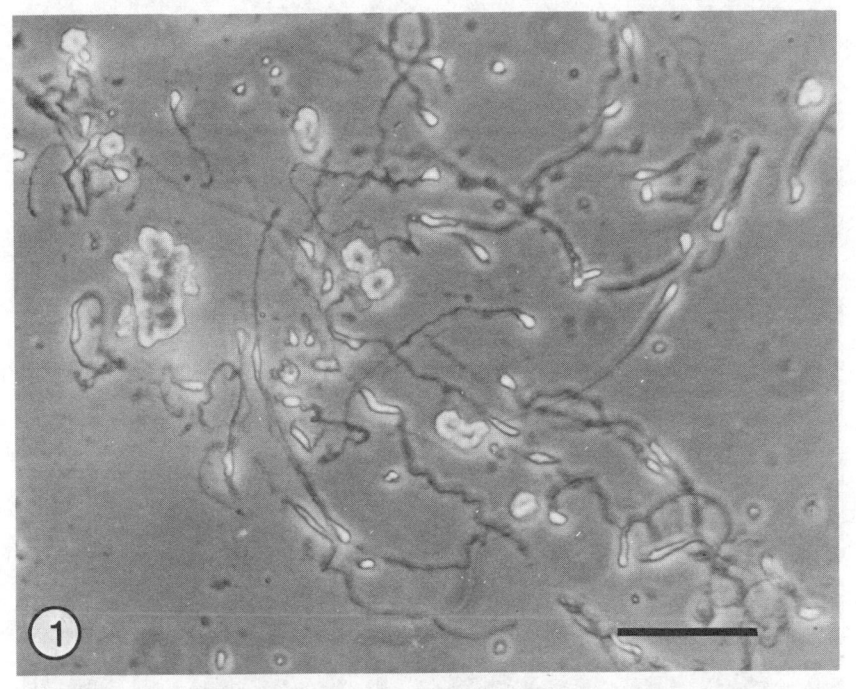

FIGURE 1. Photomicrograph of cells in suspension following dissociation of a dermal neuro-fibroma. Both round and elongated spindle-shaped cells are apparent. The scale bar equals 100 microns.

site (fast or type II) occurs within a few seconds[17,20,21] at both 37° and 0°C. Although the function of the fast (low-affinity) site is unclear, the slow (high-affinity) site appears to mediate NGF regulation of neurite outgrowth,[17,18,22] increased protein synthesis,[18] and enhanced survival.[17,21] To determine whether the ^{125}I-NGF binding to SLC was characteristic of fast or slow site binding, coverslips that had been incubated with ^{125}I-NGF at 37°C were transferred to CGM at 0°C containing ^{125}I-NGF and unlabeled NGF (10 μg/ml). After 15 minutes, cells were washed and processed for radioautography. The absence of an accumulation of grains over SLC (FIGURE 3 a and b) under these conditions supports the hypothesis that the majority of NGF binding sites on SLC are the fast type.

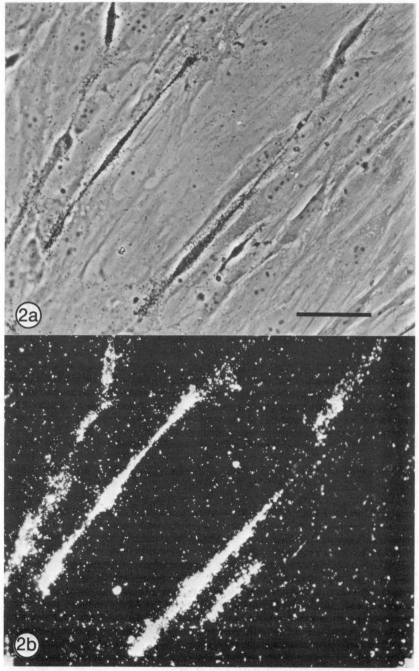

FIGURE 2. Radioautograph of cells from a dissociated neurofibroma incubated with ¹²⁵I-NGF (5 ng/ml) in CGM for one hour at 37°C. After one hour cultures were washed six times in phosphate-buffered saline and fixed in glutaraldehyde (2.5%). Cultures were then processed for radioautography by dipping coverslips with cells in photographic emulsion and exposing them for approximately one week. Following development, cultures were photographed on a Leitz microscope. Cells were photographed using both phase (a) and dark field (b) optics. Scale bar equals 50 microns.

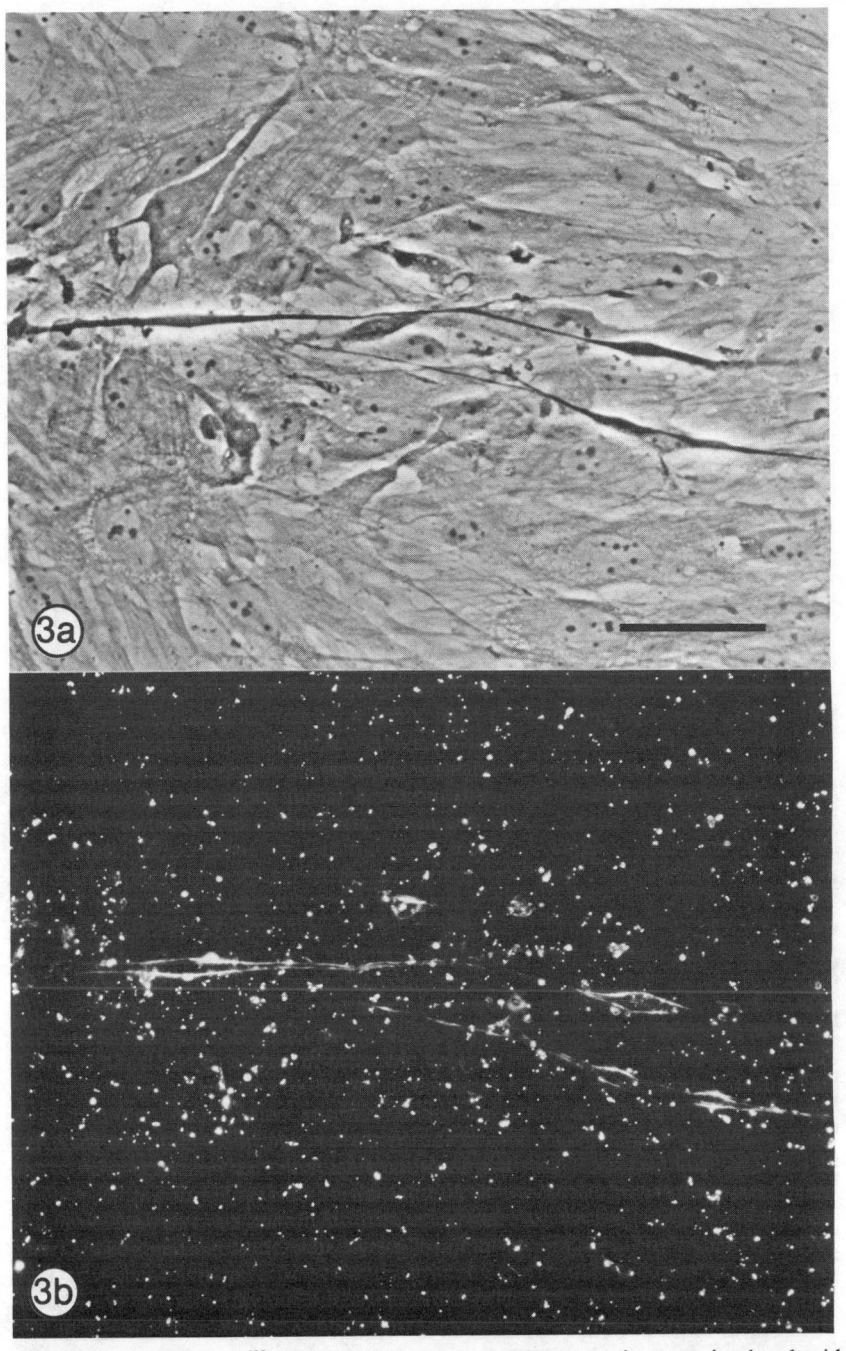

FIGURE 3. Absence of ^{125}I-NGF binding from neurofibroma cultures preincubated with ^{125}I-NGF (5 ng/ml) in CGM for one hour at 37°C, followed by transfer to fresh CGM at 0°C containing ^{125}I-NGF (5 ng/ml) and unlabeled NGF (10 μg/ml). After 15 minutes cells were washed and processed for radioautography. The absence of grains over Schwann-like cells is consistent with the NGF binding site being the fast type. Scale bar equals 50 microns.

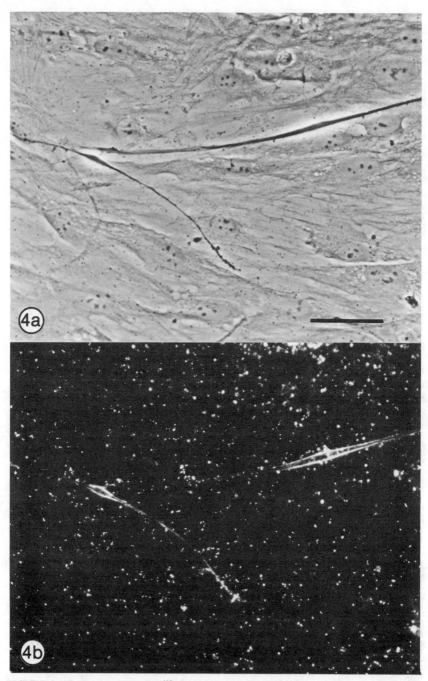

FIGURE 4. Nonspecifically bound ^{125}I-NGF. Parallel cultures to those used in FIGURES 2 and 3 were incubated with ^{125}I-NGF (5 ng/ml) and unlabeled NGF (10 μg/ml) for one hour at 37°C. Both Schwann-like and fibroblast-like cells are present (as seen with phase optics, a). As seen with dark field optics (b), displacement of ^{125}I-NGF from saturable sites is indicated by the lack of increased grain densities over Schwann-like cells.

CONCLUSIONS

Our results describe NGF binding sites, identified with ^{125}I-NGF on cells from dissociated neurofibromas. Radioautographic and biochemical[23] data suggest that the NGF binding site on neurofibroma SLC are the fast type. The binding by neurofibroma SLC of a monoclonal antibody raised against melanoma cells that appears to bind to the fast NGF receptor[24] is consistent with the ^{125}I-NGF binding experiments. Because cells present in histologic sections of neurofibromas bind the NGF-receptor monoclonal antibody,[24] it is likely that the NGF binding sites identified in culture are present *in vivo* and are not a culture artifact.

It is unclear what function is mediated by the presence of fast binding sites on neurofibroma SLC. NGF binding sites with similar characteristics have been described on Schwann cells from chick sensory ganglia[25,26] and RN6 schwannoma cells,[26] therefore making the observation of NGF binding sites on neurofibroma not unique. It has been suggested that NGF receptors on Schwann cells may modulate neuron-Schwann cell interaction.[26] Further investigation will be necessary to determine whether or not such a function exists and is important to the pathology associated with neurofibromatosis.

ACKNOWLEDGMENTS

The comments of Drs. Tibor Barka, David Pleasure, and Alonzo Ross are greatly appreciated.

REFERENCES

1. MALORY, F. B. 1920. The type cell of the so-called dural endothelioma. J. Med. Res. **41:** 349-346.
2. PENFIELD, W. 1927. The encapsulated tumor of the nervous system. Meningeal fibroblastoma, perineural fibroblastoma and neurofibromata of von Recklinghausen. Surg. Gynecol. Obstet. **45:** 178-188.
3. TARLOV, I. M. 1940. Origin of the perineural fibroblastomas. Am. J. Pathol. **16:** 33-40.
4. RAIMONDI, A. & F. BECKMAN. 1967. Perineural fibroblastomas: their fine structure and biology. Acta Neuropathol. **8:** 1-23.
5. VEROCAY, J. 1910. Zur Kenntnis der Neurofibrome. Beitr. Pathol. Anat. **48:** 1-68.
6. MASSON, P. 1923. Experimental and spontaneous schwannomas (peripheral gliomas). Am. J. Pathol. **8:** 367-416.
7. MURRAY, M. R. & A. P. STOUT. 1940. Schwann cell versus fibroblast as the origin of the specific nerve sheaths tumor. Observations of normal nerve sheaths and neurilemomas in vitro. Am. J. Pathol. **16:** 41-60.
8. RIO HORTEGA, DEL P. 1943. Estudio citologico de los neurofibromas de Recklinghausen (lemociomas). Arch. Histol. (BaAs) **1:** 373-414.
9. PINEDA, A. 1966. Electron microscopy of the lemmocyte in peripheral nerve tumors (neurolemmomas). J. Neurosurg. **25:** 35-55.
10. SCHENKEIN, I., E. D. BUEDKER, L. HELSON, F. AXELROD & J. DANCIS. 1974. Increased nerve growth factor stimulating activity in disseminated neurofibromatosis. N. Engl. J. Med. **390:** 613-614.

11. SIGGERS, D. C., S. H. BOYER & R. ELDRIDGE. 1975. Nerve growth factor in disseminated neurofibromatosis. N. Engl. J. Med. **292:** 1134.
12. FABRICANT, R. N. & G. J. TODARO. 1981. Increased serum levels of nerve growth factor in von Recklinghausen's disease. Arch. Neurol. **38:** 401-405.
13. RUBENSTEIN, A. E., R. HADMAN, C. MYTILINEOU, A. M. ARON, S. WALLACE & S. SILLMAN. 1983. Nerve growth factor in neural tumors in disseminated neurofibromatosis. Neurology **33:** 79.
14. RIOPELLE, R. J., V. M. RICCARDI, S. FAULKNER & M. C. MARTIN. 1984. Serum neuronal growth factor levels in von Recklinghausen's neurofibromatosis. Ann. Neurol. **16:** 54-59.
15. BURTON, L. E., W. H. WILSON & E. M. SHOOTER. 1978. Nerve growth factor in mouse saliva. Rapid isolation procedures for and characterization of 7S nerve growth factor. J. Biol. Chem. **253:** 7807-7812.
16. VARON, S., J. NOMURA & E. M. SHOOTER. 1968. Reversible dissociation of mouse nerve growth factor protein into different subunits. Biochemistry **7:** 1296-1303.
17. SUTTER, A., R. J. RIOPELLE, R. M. HARRIS-WARRICK & E. M. SHOOTER. 1979. Nerve growth factor receptors: characterization of two distinct classes of binding sites on chick embryo sensory ganglia cells. J. Biol. Chem. **254:** 5972-5982.
18. SONNENFELD, K. H. & D. N. ISHII. 1982. Nerve growth factor effects and receptors in cultured human neuroblastoma cell lines. J. Neurosci. Res. **8:** 375-391.
19. BERND, P. & L. A. GREENE. 1983. Electron microscopic radioautographic localization of iodinated nerve growth factor bound to and internalized by PC12 cells. J. Neurosci. **3:** 631-643.
20. SCHECHTER, A. L. & M. A. BOTHWELL. 1981. Nerve growth factor receptors in PC12 cells: evidence for two classes with differing cytoskeletal association. Cell **24:** 867-874.
21. SONNENFELD, K. H. & D. N. ISHII. 1985. Fast and slow nerve growth factor binding sites in human neuroblastoma and rat pheochromocytoma cell lines: relationship of sites to each other and to neurite outgrowth. J. Neurosci. **5:** 1717-1728.
22. ZIMMERMANN, A., A. SUTTER & E. M. SHOOTER. 1981. Monoclonal antibodies against beta-nerve growth factor and their effects of receptor binding and biological activity. Proc. Nat. Acad. Sci. USA. **78:** 4611-4615.
23. SONNENFELD, K. H., P. BERND, G. SOBUE, M. LEBWOHL & A. E. RUBENSTEIN. 1986. Nerve growth factor receptors on dissociated neurofibroma Schwann-like cells. Cancer Res. **46:** 1446-1452.
24. ROSS, A. H., P. GROB, M. BOTHWELL, D. E. ELDER, C. S. ERNST, N. MARANO, B. F. D. GHRIST, C. C. SLEMP, M. HERLYN & B. ATKINSON. 1984. Characterization of nerve growth-factor receptor in neural crest tumors using monoclonal-antibodies. Proc. Nat. Acad. Sci. USA **81:** 6681-6685.
25. CARBONETTO, S. & R. W. STACH. 1982. Localization of nerve growth factor bound to neurons growing nerve fibers in culture. Dev. Brain Res. **3:** 463-473.
26. ZIMMERMANN, A. & A. SUTTER. 1983. Beta nerve growth factor (beta NGF) receptors on glial cells. Cell-cell interaction between neurones and Schwann cells in culture of chick sensory ganglia. EMBO J. **2:** 879-885.

The Nerve Growth Factor Receptor in Normal and Transformed Neural Crest Cells[a]

ALONZO H. ROSS, MEENHARD HERLYN,
GERD G. MAUL, HILARY KOPROWSKI,
MARK BOTHWELL,[b] MOSES CHAO,[c]
DAVID PLEASURE,[d] AND
KENNETH H. SONNENFELD[e]

The Wistar Institute of Anatomy and Biology
3601 Spruce Street
Philadelphia, Pennsylvania 19104

INTRODUCTION

Nerve growth factor (NGF) is a peptide hormone essential for the development and maintenance of sympathetic and sensory neurons.[1] This dependence is readily demonstrated by injecting rodent embryos with anti-NGF antibodies. The resulting pups lack a functional sympathetic nervous system.[2,3] NGF is probably synthesized and released by the innervated tissues serving to guide the axons to the correct sites and acting as a survival factor for the neurons once the synapses are formed.[4] NGF can also act as a differentiation factor for embryonic adrenal and pheochromocytoma cells causing neurite extension.[5] For a subclone of a rat pheochromocytoma cell line PC12, NGF is mitogenic.[6]

The initial event for all of these responses is binding of NGF to specific receptors on the cell surface. A number of investigators have identified 90,000- and 200,000-dalton proteins as NGF receptors,[7,8] and there have been a few reports of an additional 140,000-dalton receptor.[9] To allow a more definitive molecular weight assignment of the NGF receptor, we prepared anti-NGF receptor monoclonal antibody (MAb)[10]

[a] This work was supported in part by Grants CA-25874, NS-08075, CA-10815, NS-21716, and NS-17551 from the United States Public Health Service and by grants from the National Neurofibromatosis Foundation and the Multiple Sclerosis Society.

[b] Department of Biochemistry, Princeton University, Princeton, N.J. 08544.

[c] Department of Cell Biology and Anatomy, Cornell University Medical School, New York, N.Y. 10021.

[d] Department of Neurology, Children's Hospital of Philadelphia, Philadelphia, Pa. 19104.

[e] Department of Neurology, Mount Sinai School of Medicine, 1 Gustave Levy Place, New York, N.Y. 10029.

and identified the human melanoma NGF receptor as a 75,000-dalton glycoprotein, which in some cell lines appears as a 180,000-dalton aggregate.[11] In this article we review the preparation of the MAb and the applications of these antibodies in characterizing the NGF receptor and its distribution.

IDENTIFICATION OF ANTIMELANOMA MAbs
AS ANTI-NGF RECEPTOR

Based on reports of Fabricant and co-workers that the NGF receptor is expressed on human melanoma cells,[12] we screened our collection of antimelanoma MAbs for an anti-NGF receptor MAb. The antimelanoma MAbs were prepared as part of an ongoing program studying tumor progression.[13] Most of these antibodies were generated by immunizing mice with live melanoma cells and fusing the primed splenocytes with myeloma cells. The resulting antibodies were then screened for reactivity with melanoma cells and for a relative lack of reactivity with normal cells.

The antimelanoma MAbs were further screened by comparing antibody binding to human melanoma cell line A875, which is unusually rich in NGF receptors, and to another human melanoma cell line, SK MEL 37, which has far fewer NGF receptors (TABLE 1). Only MAbs ME82-11 and ME20.4 preferentially bound to A875 cells. The identification of these antibodies as anti-NGF receptor was confirmed in two experiments. Both MAbs inhibited binding of ^{125}I-NGF to A875 cells even though normal mouse immunoglobulin had no effect. Both antibodies also immunoprecipitated the NGF receptor cross-linked to ^{125}I-NGF.[10]

Since we had prepared only two independent anti-NGF receptor MAbs from approximately 300 fusions using splenocytes immunized with whole melanoma cells, we sought a more efficient procedure to generate additional anti-NGF receptor MAbs.

TABLE 1. Expression of Melanoma-Associated Antigens and NGF Receptors by Human Melanoma Cell Lines[a]

	Bound Counts per Minute to:		
Ligand	SK MEL 37	A875	Receptor
NGF	444[b]	8,731[c]	NGF receptor
ME77-71	1,950	0	None identified
ME20.11	3,224	0	Protein (28)[d]
ME31.3	2,932	804	Chondroitin sulfate proteoglycan
ME82-11	912	11,592	Protein (75)[c]
ME20.4	1,288	12,872	Protein (75)[c]
ME311	1,626	0	Ganglioside
ME061	9,837	1,210	Protein (97)[c]
ME37-7	17,427	11,267	HLA-DR

[a] Reproduced from Reference 10 with permission.
[b] Determined by indirect radioimmunoassay.
[c] Determined by direct binding of ^{125}I-NGF.
[d] Number in parenthesis is the $M_r \times 10^{-3}$, as determined by SDS-gel electrophoresis.

TABLE 2. Properties of Anti–NGF Receptor MAbS

					Binding to:	
MAb	Isotypes	Immunogen	Inhibition of ^{125}I-NGF Binding to A875 Cells	Western Blotting	Frozen Tissue Sections	Fixed Paraffin-Embedded Tissue Sections
ME82-11	IgG$_1$	WM115 melanoma cells	+	−	±	−
ME20.4	IgG$_1$	WM245 melanoma cells	+	±[a]	+	±
NGF-R3	IgG$_1$	A875 melanoma cells + pure NGF receptor	+	+[b]	+	±

[a] Reactive with nonreduced samples but not reduced.
[b] Reactive with both reduced and nonreduced samples.

Mice were immunized with A875 cells and boosted with purified NGF receptor (Marano *et al.*, unpublished). The resulting hybridoma culture supernatants were screened using purified NGF receptor. Five MAbs were generated from a single fusion. The properties of the original MAbs and one of the new ones are summarized in TABLE 2. All of the antibodies react with the extracellular segment of the molecule and inhibit binding of ^{125}I-NGF. One MAb reacts with the receptor in Western blots, and two react with the receptor in frozen tissue sections. None of the MAbs consistently react with paraffin-embedded fixed tissue sections. The MAbs bind to species-specific epitope(s) since none of the MAbs react with PC12, the rat pheochromocytoma cell line.

MOLECULAR CHARACTERIZATION OF THE NGF RECEPTOR

The molecular nature of the human melanoma NGF receptor has been considerably clarified as a result of the anti-NGF receptor MAbs. A 75,000-dalton protein with an isoelectric point of 4.9-5.2 was immunoprecipitated from metabolically labeled melanoma A875 cells (FIGURE 1). However, the receptor from A875 cells without reduction of disulfide bonds migrates in sodium dodecyl sulfate-polyacrylamide gel electrophoresis (SDS-PAGE) as a mix of 75,000-dalton and 180,000-dalton proteins.[11,14] The latter form of the receptor appears to be a dimer of the 75,000-dalton form. Similar unreduced immunoprecipitates derived from metabolically labeled HS294 melanoma cells included no 180,000-dalton protein.

The NGF receptor undergoes several posttranslational processing steps including glycosylation probably on both N- and O-linked sites.[11] It is phosphorylated on at least one serine residue. Addition of NGF had no obvious effect on phosphorylation, and no phosphorylation activity was found associated with the receptor. The proposed structure of the human melanoma NGF receptor is shown in FIGURE 2.

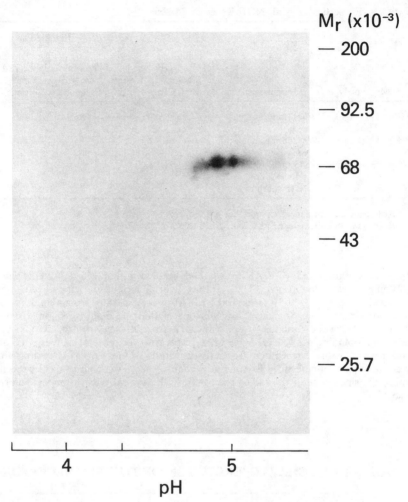

FIGURE 1. Charge heterogeneity of NGF receptor. A875 cells were labeled with [^{35}S]cysteine, extracted with detergent, and clarified by ultracentrifugation. Immunoprecipitates were prepared using either ME20.4 or P3X63Ag8 (control) immunoglobulin G (IgG) and analyzed by two-dimensional gel electrophoresis. An autoradiogram of the ME20.4 gel is shown. There were no evident spots on the P3X63Ag8 autoradiogram (not shown). (Reproduced from Reference 11 with permission.)

EXPRESSION OF THE NGF RECEPTOR BY TRANSFECTANT CELL LINES

Transfectant cell lines expressing the NGF receptor have been isolated using anti-NGF receptor MAbs.[15] Human DNA was co-precipitated with a cloned thymidine kinase gene using Ca^{++} and added to a thymidine kinase-minus variant of the murine fibroblastic L-cell line. The cells were then placed in hypoxanthine-aminopterin-thymidine (HAT) medium, and the resulting colonies were screened by rosetting assay for expression of the NGF receptor. Since our anti-NGF receptor MAbs react only with human receptor and not murine receptor, the assay would not detect any aberrant cells expressing the murine NGF receptor. The positive colonies (1 in 6000) were cloned and grown up for further study. The resulting cell lines bind NGF and bear a cell surface NGF receptor that appears to be identical to the melanoma receptor. We are presently evaluating the biological responsiveness of these cells to NGF.

IMMUNOLOCALIZATION OF NGF RECEPTOR USING MAbS

Anti-NGF receptor MAb ME20.4 was used to stain both frozen and fixed tissue sections in an effort to better define the distribution of the NGF receptor (TABLE 3).[10] There was no evident staining of normal melanocytes, but nevi—the benign melanocytic lesion—and melanomas were positive. Recent studies of melanocytic cells in culture mirrored these results (TABLE 4). Cultured melanocytes expressed barely detectable amounts of NGF receptor, nevi expressed larger amounts, and melanomas still larger amounts. Hence, in the melanocytic system there is a correlation between tumor progression and expression of NGF receptor. Neurofibromas, pheochromocytomas, and the perineuria of peripheral nerves were also NGF receptor positive, consistent with the accepted association between neural crest embryonic origin and expression of NGF receptor. Other tissues reported to bear NGF receptors or to be NGF responsive are now being screened.

The NGF receptor in a variety of immunoperoxidase-stained human melanoma tissue sections appeared to be present both in the cytoplasm and the plasma membrane, but for A875 human melanoma cells the receptor was mostly confined to the plasma membrane (TABLE 3).[10] This result was further investigated using A875 cells fixed and permeabilized with alcohol. The distribution of the NGF receptor was determined using MAb ME20.4 and a fluorescent second antibody (FIGURE 3). The antigen was most clearly detected in the plasma membrane and seemed to be associated with microvilli, similar to the distribution reported for the insulin receptor.[16] There was no detectable fluorescence associated with the nucleus.

The cell surface distribution of the NGF receptor was further investigated using intact melanoma cells lightly fixed with paraformaldehyde. Receptor was localized

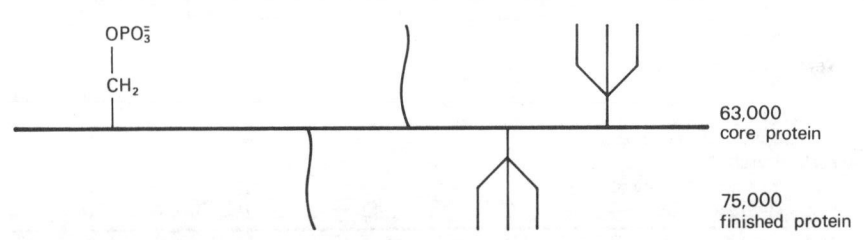

FIGURE 2. Proposed structure of the human melanoma NGF receptor. The receptor consists of an ~63,000-dalton core protein which, after posttranslational processing, has an apparent molecular weight of 75,000. The modifications include phosphorylation of serine residue(s), glycosylation of O-linked sites (wavy lines), and glycosylation of N-linked sites (branched lines).

TABLE 3. Summary of Immunoperoxidase Staining of Frozen and Fixed Tissue Sections with MAb ME20.4[a]

Tissue	Fixation	Ratio of Positive/Total[b]	Site of Staining
Melanocytes	Frozen	0/11	—
	Fixed	0/5	—
Nevi	Frozen	5/5	Cytoplasmic[c]
	Fixed	0/3	—
Melanomas	Frozen	6/9	Cytoplasmic
	Fixed	0/3	—
A875 melanoma cell line	Frozen	1/1	Plasma membrane
	Fixed	1/1	Plasma membrane
Peripheral dermal nerves	Frozen	8/8	Neural sheath
	Fixed	5/5	Neural sheath
Neurofibromas	Fixed	2/4	Cytoplasmic
Pheochromocytomas	Frozen	1/1	Cytoplasmic
Pancreas	Frozen	0/1	—
Adrenal gland	Fixed	0/1	—

[a] Reproduced from Reference 10 with permission.
[b] Ratio of positive samples to the total number of samples examined.
[c] Distributed throughout the cell not excluding the plasma membrane.

using MAb ME20.4 and then with a fluorescent MAb or with a second antibody coupled to colloidal gold. All incubations were carried out at 4°C to prevent redistribution of the antigen. Judging by immunofluorescence, the receptor on the cell surface was preferentially associated with microvilli, a pattern that was unaffected by the addition of NGF. Electron microscopy of sections of the melanoma cells showed the gold label over the entire cell membrane (FIGURE 3a) but again preferentially localized on microvilli (FIGURE 3b and c).

TABLE 4. Binding of Anti–NGF Receptor MAb to Cultured Melanocytic Cells

Source of Melanocytic Cells	Number of Cultures Tested	Number Positive for MAb ME82-11 Binding[a]				
		++++	+++	++	+	−
Newborn normal skin[b]	15	0	2	4	7	2
Nevi	26	1	11	1	3	10
Radial growth phase primary melanoma	2	2	0	0	0	0
Vertical growth phase primary melanoma	11	9	1	0	0	1
Metastatic melanoma	27	12	7	6	0	2

[a] Assayed by a mixed hemadsorption assay: ++++, > 80% of cells positive; +++, 40-80% positive; ++, 20-40% positive; and +, 5-20% positive.
[b] For a description of melanocytic cells at different stages of melanocytic progression, see Reference 17.

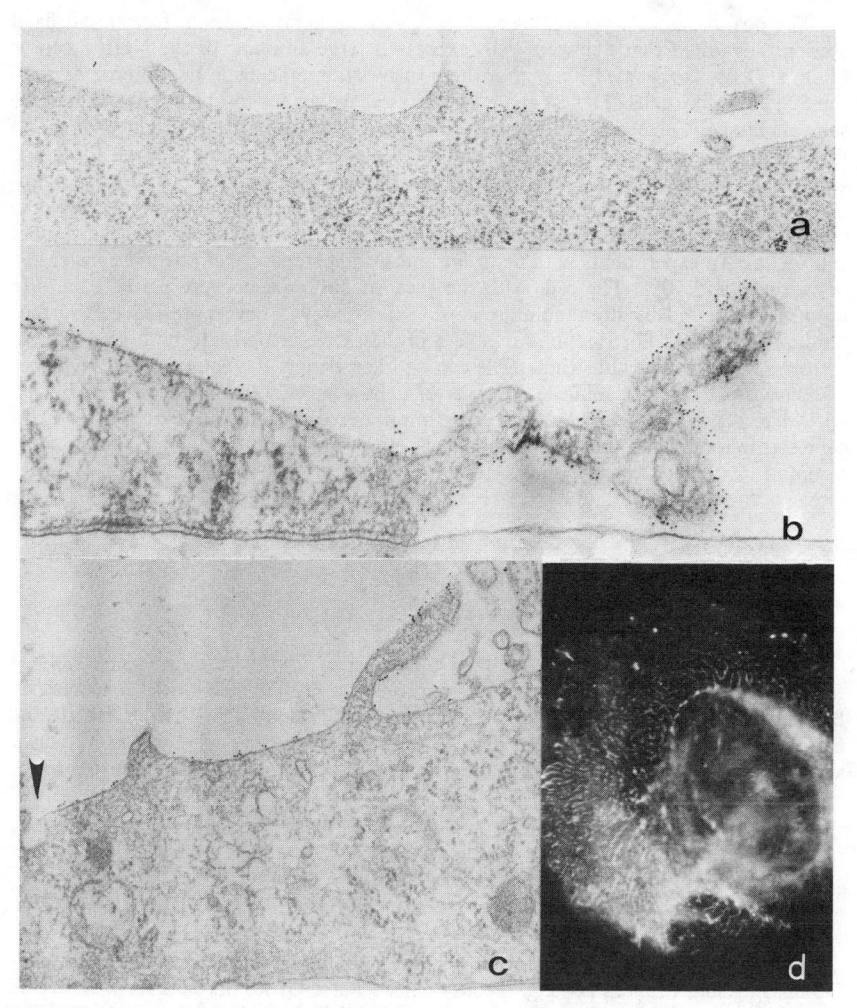

FIGURE 3. Immunolocalization of the NGF receptor on human melanoma A875 cells. (a) Gold particles are distributed in small groups or larger patches over the entire cell surface except where excluded on the growth substrate. × 37,000. (b) Label is concentrated in microvilli. × 53,000. (c) Coated pits remain unlabeled with our growth and fixation conditions (arrow). × 37,000. (d) Immunofluorescent micrograph focused on the cell surface demonstrates the increased localization on microvilli. × 1200.

NGF RECEPTOR IN NORMAL SCHWANN CELLS
AND NEUROFIBROMAS

The positive immunoperoxidase staining of peripheral nerves in frozen and fixed sections suggested that Schwann cells expressed large amounts of the NGF receptor (TABLE 3). It also seemed likely that the positive staining cells in neurofibromas were the Schwann-like cells. To test these hypotheses, we extended our studies to include schwannian cells placed into short-term culture. Cells from a traumatic neuroma and from neurofibromas were grown in culture for several days and assayed for NGF receptor by immunofluorescence microscopy. In both cases, the cells with a Schwann-like morphology were strongly positive for NGF receptor. This property was used to preparatively select for the neurofibroma Schwann-like cells by fluorescence-activated cell sorting. In experiments with neurofibromas, the percentage of positive cells varied between 10 and 70%. The cells with the greatest fluorescence were placed back into culture and tested by immunofluorescence microscopy. They expressed cell surface laminin but lacked fibronectin and gave a proliferative response to both glial growth factor and axolemma; thus these cells can be identified as the Schwann-like cells (see Pleasure et al., in this volume). One set of cells was radioiodinated and solubilized with detergent. The NGF receptor was immunoprecipitated and analyzed by SDS-gel electrophoresis and found to be similar in molecular weight to the melanoma NGF receptor. A detailed comparison is now in progress.

FUTURE DIRECTIONS

Our efforts are now directed toward three goals. First, we have recently isolated the NGF receptor by immunoaffinity chromatography and are now sequencing it. Second, the NGF receptor-bearing transfectant cell lines are being used to isolate and clone the gene for the NGF receptor. Third, we are testing whether an autocrine stimulation of cell growth occurs in diseased cells such as melanoma or neurofibroma.

ACKNOWLEDGMENTS

We thank Allan Rubenstein for his help in obtaining freshly excised neurofibromas; Donna Jackson, Frances Hwang, Geoffry Faust, Peter Grob, Barbara Kreider, David Elder, Carolyn Ernst, Nadia Marano, Joseph Weibel, and Barbara Atkinson for contributing their data for this review; and Marina Hoffman for editorial assistance.

REFERENCES

1. LEVI-MONTALCINI, R. & R. U. ANGELETTI. 1968. Physiol. Rev. 48: 534–569.
2. LEVI-MONTALCINI, R. & B. BOOKER. 1960. Proc. Nat. Acad. Sci. USA 46: 384–391.
3. GORIN, P. D. & E. M. JOHNSON. 1980. Dev. Biol. 80: 313–323.

4. BURGESS, A. & N. NICOLA. 1983. Growth Factors and Stem Cells. Academic Press. New York, N.Y.
5. ALOE, L. & R. LEVI-MONTALCINI. 1979. Proc. Nat. Acad. Sci. USA **76:** 1246-1250.
6. BURSTEIN, D. E. & L. A. GREENE. 1982. Dev. Biol. **94:** 473-482.
7. GROB, P. M., C. H. BERLOT & M. A. BOTHWELL. 1983. Proc. Nat. Acad. Sci. USA **80:** 6819-6823.
8. PUMA, P., S. E. BUXSER, L. WATSON, D. J. KELLEHER & G. L. JOHNSON. 1983. J. Biol. Chem. **258:** 3370-3375.
9. HOSANG, M. & E. M. SHOOTER. 1985. J. Biol. Chem. **260:** 655-662.
10. ROSS, A. H., P. GROB, M. BOTHWELL, D. E. ELDER, C. S. ERNST, N. MARANO, B. F. D. GHRIST, C. C. SLEMP, M. HERLYN, B. ATKINSON & H. KOPROWSKI. 1984. Proc. Nat. Acad. Sci. USA **81:** 6681-6685.
11. GROB, P. M., A. H. ROSS, H. KOPROWSKI & M. BOTHWELL. 1985. J. Biol. Chem. **260:** 8044-8049.
12. FABRICANT, R. N., J. E. DELARCO & G. J. TODARO. 1977. Proc. Nat. Acad. Sci. USA **74:** 565-569.
13. HERLYN, M., Z. STEPLEWSKI, D. HERLYN, W. H. CLARK, A. H. ROSS, M. BLASZCZYK, K. Y. PAK & H. KOPROWSKI. 1983. Cancer Invest. **1:** 215-224.
14. BUXSER, S., P. PUMA & G. L. JOHNSON. 1985. J. Biol. Chem. **260:** 1917-1926.
15. CHAO, M. V., M. A. BOTHWELL, A. H. ROSS, H. KOPROWSKI, A. A. LANAHAN, C. R. BUCK & A. SEHGAL. 1986. Science **232:** 518-521.
16. SMITH, R. M., M. H. COBB, O. M. ROSEN & L. JARRETT. 1985. J. Cell. Physiol. **123:** 167-179.
17. GREENE, M. H., W. H. CLARK, M. A. TUCKER, D. E. ELDER, K. H. KRAMER, D. GUERRY, W. K. WITMER, J. THOMPSON, I. MATOZZO & M. C. FRASER. 1985. N. Engl. J. Med. **312:** 91-94.

Nerve Growth Factor Modification of the Ethylnitrosourea Model for Multiple Schwannomas

STANLEY A. VINORES[a]

Division of Neuropathology
Department of Pathology
University of Virginia School of Medicine
Charlottesville, Virginia 22908

The role of host factors involved in the development of Schwann cell tumors, such as those associated with neurofibromatosis (NF), is not understood. Research in this area has been hampered by the lack of an appropriate animal model. A large number of Schwann cell tumors, particularly in the trigeminal nerves, can be induced in rats by ethylnitrosourea administered during late gestation or shortly after birth.[8,14,36] This report describes the effect that manipulation of the endogenous levels of nerve growth factor has on the incidence of Schwann cell tumors and on early neoplastic proliferation in the Schwann cells of trigeminal nerves.

ETHYLNITROSOUREA CARCINOGENESIS

Ethylnitrosourea (ENU) is a potent transplacental carcinogen which induces neurogenic tumors in a high percentage of rats exposed to a single dose during late gestation or shortly after birth.[8,14,36] The period during which the developing rat nervous system is sensitive to ENU-induced carcinogenesis extends from the 12th day of gestation, prior to which ENU exerts teratogenic rather than carcinogenic consequences, until about two weeks postnatally, following which ENU is still carcinogenic (although a higher dosage is necessary) but without a predilection for the nervous system. The rat central nervous system (CNS) has a maximum sensitivity to ENU carcinogenesis on the 15th day of gestation. Rat CNS tumors resulting from ENU exposure are most often oligodendrogliomas or mixed gliomas (astrocytomas and oligodendrogliomas). Rats treated after this time develop a higher percentage of peripheral nervous system (PNS) schwannomas (neurinomas). The most frequent sites of ENU-induced Schwannomas are the trigeminal nerves, spinal root nerves, lumbar and brachial plexuses, and the sciatic nerves. They rarely occur at other locations. Each structure has its own characteristic peak of sensitivity and latent period before phenotypic changes associated with neoplasia occur. Trigeminal nerve tumors are

[a] Present affiliation: Department of Ophthalmology, University of Virginia School of Medicine, Charlottesville, Va. 22908.

generally the first to appear, followed by other PNS tumors, spinal cord tumors, and lastly, brain tumors.[8,14,34,36]

ENU induces a much broader spectrum of tumors in mice than it does in rats.[6,18,26] Neurogenic tumors do occur in ENU-exposed mice, and although their incidence is strain and age related, it never approaches that found in rats.

NERVE GROWTH FACTOR EFFECT ON ENU CARCINOGENESIS

Nerve growth factor (NGF) is a naturally occurring protein that functions in the development, maintenance, and regeneration of various components of the sensory, sympathetic, and central nervous systems. It can also elicit responses characteristic of neuronal differentiation in a variety of normal and neoplastic neurogenic cell types *in vitro.*[12,13,28] NGF administered to pregnant female rats on day 15 of gestation delays tumor development and increases the life span of the offspring concurrently exposed to 80 mg/kg body weight ENU.[33,34] Neonatal NGF administration (10 days of age) had similar tumor inhibitory effects on rats concurrently treated with ENU. NGF

TABLE 1. Effect of NGF on Neurogenic Tumor Induction in Rats

Treatment	Number	Rats Developing Neurogenic Tumors
Transplacental ENU	11	10 (91%)
Transplacental ENU + NGF	8	2 (25%)
Neonatal ENU	24	21 (88%)
Neonatal ENU + NGF (0.4 mg 7S)	17	9 (53%)
Neonatal ENU + NGF (0.8 mg 7S)	6	2 (33%)

did not prevent tumor formation in transplacentally or neonatally treated rats, but it resulted in the development of more extraneural tumors at the expense of neurogenic tumors (TABLE 1).[22,33,34] Extraneural tumors generally had a fairly long latent period, therefore an increased survival time occurred in NGF-treated rats.

Treatment with antibodies to NGF on postnatal days 1-5, which causes an irreversible degeneration of the sympathetic nervous system,[12,28] prior to ENU exposure on day 10 resulted in earlier tumor appearance.[33,34] This was largely due to an increase in the number of animals with schwannomas in the trigeminal nerves (TABLE 2), which have the shortest latent period of the ENU-induced tumors. Transplacental administration of anti-NGF to rats (days 15-17 of gestation), prior to neonatal ENU treatment, did not significantly alter their survival times, but again resulted in an increased incidence of trigeminal nerve schwannomas. Transplacental anti-NGF promoted longer survival in rats receiving ENU on day 15 of gestation. This appeared to be largely due to the development of more CNS gliomas, which have the longest latent period of ENU-induced tumors.[33,34]

Only a limited number of mice develop neurogenic tumors resulting from ENU treatment.[6,18,26] Twelve percent of Swiss Webster mice, one of the most sensitive strains to ENU-induced neural tumor induction, developed neural tumors following neonatal ENU treatment.[32] Concurrent anti-NGF administration increased this percentage to

TABLE 2. The Effect of NGF Levels on the Induction of Trigeminal Nerve Schwannomas in Rats Receiving 80 mg/kg Neonatal ENU

Treatment	Number	Rats Developing Trigeminal Nerve Schwannomas
ENU only	22	6 (27%)
ENU + neonatal anti-NGF	31	24 (77%)
ENU + transplacental anti-NGF	22	10 (45%)
ENU + NGF	11	2 (18%)

41%, primarily due to an increased incidence of trigeminal nerve schwannomas. Anti-NGF had no effect if administered following ENU exposure. No neurogenic tumors were observed in 12 mice receiving concurrent ENU and NGF, but there was a threefold increase in the number of mice developing extraneural tumors,[32] again suggesting that the NGF-induced resistance of neural cells to ENU carcinogenesis is accompanied by an increased incidence of extraneural tumors.

EARLY NEOPLASTIC PROLIFERATION IN SCHWANN CELLS OF RAT TRIGEMINAL NERVES

The trigeminal nerve is one of the earliest and most consistently involved sites for tumor development in rats presented with a single dose of ENU during late gestation.[24] Sequential studies of the development of trigeminal nerve schwannomas revealed that as early as 20 days after ENU exposure, 50% of the nerves had hypercellularity, hyperchromatism, and increased numbers of mitotic figures in the preganglionic segment at or near the junction between the CNS and PNS. These morphological changes were accompanied by progressive increases in N-acetyl-β-glucosaminidase and β-glucuronidase activities to levels similar to those found in trigeminal nerve schwannomas. Transplantation of affected nerves into syngeneic rats resulted in tumor formation at the implantation site; no tumors resulted from implantation of control nerves. The above results led to the conclusion that the observed hypercellularity represented early neoplastic proliferation (ENP) of the Schwann cells in trigeminal nerves.[23,25]

By 63 days of age, over 70% of the trigeminal nerves of rats exposed to ENU during late gestation contained ENP, and by 90 days, nearly 100% of the trigeminal nerves had ENP or schwannomas. Unexpectedly, at six to seven months, when the peak development of trigeminal nerve schwannomas is anticipated, only 30% of the animals had tumors, suggesting that regression due to unknown factors occurred in the remaining animals.[23-25] Previous studies have failed to show an association between immune mechanisms and neural tumors;[7,15] therefore, it is likely that other host factors, possibly NGF, may play a role in the development of schwannomas.

Ninety percent of the rats exposed to 50 mg/kg ENU on the 21st day of gestation developed ENP or schwannomas (40%) in at least one trigeminal nerve (TABLE 3), and in 70% of these animals, both nerves were involved. NGF administered by multiple inoculations on days 18-20 of gestation or days 7-9 after birth or by a single inoculation on day 7 or day 10 after birth all resulted in a substantial reduction in neoplastic proliferation in trigeminal nerves. The maximal response occurred following daily inoculations of 0.01 mg 7S-NGF on postnatal days 7-9, in which no schwannomas and 44% ENP, only 11% involving both trigeminal nerves, were observed at 90 days.[31] A related study (TABLE 3) in which NGF was administered by osmotic microinfusion pumps (Alza) either transplacentally, prior to ENU treatment, or neonatally, following ENU treatment (20 mg/kg on day 20 of gestation), confirms these findings.[4] Microinfusion of saline beginning on day 14 of gestation or anti-NGF immunoglobulin G (IgG) beginning on day 15 postpartum had no effect on ENU-induced neoplastic proliferation (TABLE 3).

NGF AND NEUROFIBROMATOSIS

Neurofibromatosis (NF) is a hereditary disorder that may occur as a disseminated (peripheral) form or as a central form (characterized by autosomal dominant bilateral acoustic neuromas).[2,17,37] One manifestation of NF is the occurrence of multiple Schwann cell tumors. Research on the pathogenesis of the disease has been hampered by the lack of a good animal model. The association of NGF with NF is not clear, but several interesting observations have been reported. Using a bioassay, nerve growth activity was elevated in the sera of patients with both forms of NF.[20,35] By radioimmunoassay, the sera from disseminated NF patients do not contain elevated NGF, but the sera from patients with the central form of NF had increased levels of NGF.[11,21]

TABLE 3. Effect of NGF on ENU-Induced Neoplastic Proliferation of Schwann Cells in Rat Trigeminal Nerves

Treatment	Number	Tumors	ENP	Affected
ENU[a]	10	4 (40%)	5 (50%)	9 (90%)
ENU[a] + NGF[b] (0.2 mg 7S, days 18–20 of gestation)	13	2 (15%)	7 (54%)	9 (69%)
ENU[a] + NGF[b] (0.03 mg 7S, days 7–9)	9	0 (0%)	4 (44%)	4 (44%)
ENU[a] + NGF[b] (0.08 mg 7S, day 7)	12	3 (25%)	4 (33%)	7 (58%)
ENU[a] + NGF[b] (0.13 mg 7S, day 10)	12	0 (0%)	7 (58%)	7 (58%)
ENU[c]	19	1 (5%)	10 (53%)	11 (58%)
ENU[c] + NGF[d] (total dose = 0.2 mg 2.5S, days 14–21 of gestation)	19	0 (0%)	5 (26%)	5 (26%)
ENU[c] + saline[d] (sham, days 14–21 of gestation)	16	0 (0%)	10 (63%)	10 (63%)
ENU[c] + NGF[d] (total dose = 0.04 mg 2.5S, days 15–22)	18	0 (0%)	5 (28%)	5 (28%)
ENU[c] + anti-NGF IgG[d] (20× serum concentration, total dose = 0.02 ml, days 15–22)	18	1 (6%)	8 (44%)	9 (50%)

[a] 50 mg/kg, day 21 of gestation.
[b] By subcutaneous inoculation.
[c] 20 mg/kg, day 20 of gestation.
[d] By osmotic microinfusin pump.

Of particular prognostic interest was the finding that in three persons at risk for NF, but beyond the usual age of onset, serum NGF levels were normal, but in two of three persons at risk and below the usual age of onset for the disease, NGF levels were elevated.[21] Using a radioreceptor assay, elevated NGF was found in patients with disseminated NF, but normal or low levels were found associated with the central form of the disease.[11] A more recent and more thorough study demonstrated variable serum levels of NGF in both NF patients and controls,[19] but no correlation between serum NGF levels and NF could be established despite the observation that neurofibromas appear to be a rich source of neurite-promoting factors. The somewhat confusing and conflicting reports do not establish whether NGF or related factors play a role in the pathogenesis of NF. A major weakness of these studies is that they all were conducted using mouse NGF for comparison or antibodies to mouse NGF, which has very limited cross reactivity with human NGF.[3,16,35]

DISCUSSION

The reduction in neurogenic tumors following perinatal NGF administration indicates that NGF renders the target cells in the central and peripheral nervous systems more resistant to ENU carcinogenesis, possibly by promoting their maturation. The earlier appearance of tumors that is observed when anti-NGF treatments precede ENU exposure suggests that a reduction in the endogenous levels of NGF may prevent the normal NGF-induced maturation of the target cells, thus increasing the number of ENU-sensitive cells available to the carcinogen.[33,34] In support of this hypothesis is the finding that anti-NGF treatments increase the incidence of ENU-induced neurogenic tumors in mice. Mice have higher endogenous levels of NGF than rats do and their nervous system is not nearly as sensitive to carcinogenesis by ENU; however, the mouse nervous system can be made considerably more sensitive to ENU by the antibody-mediated reduction of the NGF levels.[32]

The reduction in the incidence of gliomas and schwannomas or Schwann cell ENP caused by NGF demonstrates that NGF, directly or indirectly, influences glial and Schwann cells with regard to their sensitivity to ENU carcinogenesis and their rate of proliferation. NGF is capable of acting directly on primitive CNS glia or glial precursor cells as exemplified by the F98 rat anaplastic glioma clone. These cells contain receptors for NGF,[27] and they respond to NGF in vitro by demonstrating increased adhesiveness[27,30] and a decreased growth rate.[29] NGF can also reduce the tumor growth rate of intracranially implanted F98 cells,[29] but with in vivo studies, an indirect mechanism mediated by other NGF-responsive cells cannot be overruled.

It is not clear whether NGF acts directly or indirectly on normal and neoplastic Schwann cells. NGF receptors have been found on normal Schwann cells and on RN6 schwannoma cells,[38] but there is no known response of a pure population of normal or neoplastic Schwann cells to NGF. It is possible that NGF elicits a response from the neurons in the trigeminal nerve, which, in turn, influence the Schwann cells. Schwann cell proliferation is influenced by axonal populations,[1] and NGF has been shown to promote nerve fiber outgrowth from trigeminal nerves of chicks and mice[5,10] and to enhance the survival of neuroblasts in explants of chick trigeminal nerves.[9] The reduction of ENP when NGF treatment follows, as well as precedes, ENU exposure,[4,31] and the increase in metastases of intracerebral implants of an anaplastic schwannoma following anti-NGF treatments[29] demonstrate that NGF can influence the growth of Schwann cells after the initiation phase of ENU-carcinogenesis has occurred as well as before.

Anti-NGF administered prior to perinatal ENU treatment serves as a model for the induction of Schwann cell tumors in rats and to a lesser degree in mice.[32-34] It is not clear whether this is an adequate model for the Schwann cell tumors in NF. Histologically, ENU-induced schwannomas are more anaplastic and invasive than those associated with NF. If this is an appropriate model, the levels or activity of NGF or other neurite-promoting factors should be diminished in NF patients. NGF may possibly be associated with the disease,[11,19-21,35] but the findings are somewhat contradictory and inconclusive and NGF's role has not been established. To resolve this issue will probably require a thorough study using human rather than mouse NGF, which was used in the above studies.

SUMMARY

The administration of ethylnitrosourea (ENU) to pregnant rats late in gestation or to neonatal rats results in the induction of Schwann cell tumors in a high percentage of perinatally exposed animals. Exogenous administration of nerve growth factor (NGF) significantly reduces the number of Schwann cell tumors and other neurogenic tumors developing in ENU-treated rats. Administration of antibodies directed against NGF prior to neonatal ENU exposure results in a substantial increase in the incidence of Schwann cell tumors, particularly in the trigeminal nerves of both rats and mice. Transplacental ENU treatment causes early neoplastic proliferation (ENP) at 90 days of age in the Schwann cell population of trigeminal nerves in nearly all exposed rats. A variety of NGF treatment protocols (single or multiple inoculations or microinfusion prior to or following ENU exposure) resulted in a significant reduction in ENU-induced ENP in trigeminal nerves. These results indicate that NGF may convey protection either directly or indirectly, by an unknown mechanism, to Schwann cells and other supportive neural cells by reducing their sensitivity to ENU-induced neoplastic transformation.

REFERENCES

1. AGUAYO, A. J., J. M. PEYRONNARD, L. C. TERRY, J. S. ROMINE & G. M. BRAY. 1976. Neonatal neuronal loss in rat superior cervical ganglia: retrograde effects on developing preganglionic axons and Schwann cells. J. Neurocytol. 5: 137-155.

2. ALLEN, J. C., R. ELDRIDGE & D. F. YOUNG. 1974. Early-onset acoustic neuroma: genetic, clinical, and nosologic aspects. Birth Defects 10: 171-184.

3. BECK, C. E. & J. R. PEREZ-POLO. 1982. Human β-nerve growth factor does not crossreact with antibodies to mouse β-nerve growth factor in a two-site radioimmunoassay. J. Neurosci. Res. 8: 137-152.

4. CAMP, R. C., A. KOESTNER, S. A. VINORES & C. C. CAPEN. 1984. The effect of nerve growth factor and antibodies to nerve growth factor on ethylnitrosourea-induced neoplastic proliferation in rat trigeminal nerves. Vet. Pathol. 21: 67-73.

5. DAVIES, A. M., A. G. S. LUMSDEN, H. C. SLAVKIN & G. BURNSTOCK. 1981. Influence of nerve growth factor on the embryonic mouse trigeminal ganglion in culture. Dev. Neurosci. 4: 150-156.

6. DENLINGER, R. H, A. KOESTNER & W. WECHSLER. 1974. Induction of neurogenic tumors in C3HeB/FeJ mice by nitrosourea derivatives: observations by light microscopy, tissue culture, and electron microscopy. Int. J. Cancer **13:** 559-571.
7. DENLINGER, R. H., J. A. SWENBERG, A. KOESTNER & W. WECHSLER. 1973. Differential effect of immunosuppression on the induction of nervous system and bladder tumors by *n*-methyl-*n*-nitrosourea. J. Nat. Cancer Inst. **50:** 87-93.
8. DRUCKREY, H., S. IVANKOVIC, R. PREUSSMANN, K. J. ZÜLCH & H. D. MENNEL. 1972. Selective induction of malignant tumors of the nervous system by resorptive carcinogens. *In* Experimental Biology of Brain Tumors. W. M. Kirsch, E. G. Paoletti & P. Paoletti, Eds.: 85-147. Thomas. Springfield, Ill.
9. EBENDAL, T. 1975. Effects of nerve growth factor on the synthesis of nucleic acids and proteins in cultured chick embryo trigeminal ganglia. Zoon **3:** 159-167.
10. EBENDAL, T. & K.-O. HEDLUND. 1975. Effects of nerve growth factor on the chick embryo trigeminal ganglion in cluture. Zoon **3:** 33-47.
11. FABRICANT, R. N. & G. J. TODARO. 1979. Increased levels of a nerve-growth-factor cross-reacting protein in "central" neurofibromatosis. Lancet **2:** 4-7.
12. GREENE, L. A. & E. M. SHOOTER. 1980. The nerve growth factor: biochemistry, synthesis, and mechanism of action. Annu. Rev. Neurosci. **3:** 353-402.
13. HARPER, G. P. & H. THOENEN. 1981. Target cells, biological effects, and mechanism of action of nerve growth factor and its antibodies. Annu. Rev. Pharmacol. Toxicol. **21:** 205-229.
14. KOESTNER, A. 1973. Transplacental carcinogenesis. Proc. 10th Can. Cancer Conf. **10:** 65-75.
15. MORANTZ, R. A., W. SHAIN & H. CRAVIOTO. 1978. Immune surveillance and tumors of the nervous system. J. Neurosurg. **49:** 84-92.
16. PEREZ-POLO, J. R., C. BECK, C. P. REYNOLDS & M. BLUM. 1983. Human nerve growth factor: comparative aspects. *In* Growth and Maturation Factors. G. Guroff, Ed.: 31-54. John Wiley & Sons. New York, N.Y.
17. RICCARDI, V. M. 1981. Von Recklinghausen neurofibromatosis. N. Engl. J. Med. **305:** 1617-1626.
18. RICE, J. M. 1973. The biological behavior of transplacentally induced tumors in mice. IARC Sci. Publ. **4:** 71-83.
19. RIOPELLE, R. J., V. M. RICCARDI, S. FAULKNER & M. C. MARTIN. 1984. Serum neuronal growth factor levels in von Recklinghausen's neurofibromatosis. Ann. Neurol. **16:** 54-59.
20. SHENKEIN, I., E. D. BULKER, L. HELSON, F. AXELROD & J. DANCIS. 1974. Increased nerve-growth-stimulating activity in disseminated neurofibromatosis. N. Engl. J. Med. **290:** 613-614.
21. SIGGERS, D. C., S. H. BOYER & R. ELDRIDGE. 1975. Nerve-growth factor in disseminated neurofibromatosis. N. Engl. J. Med. **292:** 1134.
22. STAHN, R., S. ROSE, S. SANBORN, G. WEST & H. HERSCHMAN. 1975. Effects of nerve growth factor administration on *N*-ethyl-*N*-nitrosourea carcinogenesis. Brain Res. **96:** 287-298.
23. SWENBERG, J. A., N. CLENDENON, R. DENLINGER & W. A. GORDON. 1975. Sequential development of ethylnitrosourea-induced neurinomas: morphology, biochemistry, and transplantability. J. Nat. Cancer Inst. **55:** 147-152.
24. SWENBERG, J. A., A. KOESTNER, W. WECHSLER & R. H. DENLINGER. 1972. Quantitative aspects of transplacental tumor induction with ethylnitrosourea in rats. Cancer Res. **32:** 2656-2660.
25. SWENBERG, J. A., W. WECHSLER & A. KOESTNER. 1972. the sequential development of transplacentally induced neuro-ectodermal tumors. J. Neuropathol. Exp. Neurol. **31:** 202-203.
26. VESSELINOVITCH, S. D., K. V. N. RAO, N. MIHAILOVICH, J. M. RICE & L. S. LOMBARD. 1974. Development of a broad spectrum of tumors by ethylnitrosourea in mice and the modifying role of age, sex, and strain. Cancer Res. **34:** 2530-2538.
27. VINORES, S. A. 1983. Increased adhesion response of anaplastic glioma cells to nerve growth factor and the presence of specific receptors. J. Neurosci. Res. **10:** 381-395.
28. VINORES, S. A. & G. GUROFF. 1980. Nerve growth factor: mechanism of action. Annu. Rev. Biophys. Bioeng. **9:** 223-257.

29. VINORES, S. A. & A. KOESTNER. 1980. The effect of nerve growth factor on undifferentiated glioma cells. Cancer Lett. **10**: 309-318.
30. VINORES, S. A. & A. KOESTNER. 1981. Effect of nerve growth factor producing cells on anaplastic glioma and pheochromocytoma clones: involvement of other factors. J. Neurosci. Res. **6**: 389-401.
31. VINORES, S. A. & A. KOESTNER. 1982. Reduction of ethylnitrosourea-induced neoplastic proliferation in rat trigeminal nerves by nerve growth factor. Cancer Res. **42**: 1038-1040.
32. VINORES, S. A. & J. R. PEREZ-POLO. 1980. The effect of nerve growth factor and antibodies to nerve growth factor on ethylnitrosourea carcinogenesis in mice. J. Cancer Res. Clin. Oncol. **98**: 59-63.
33. VINORES, S. A. & J. R. PEREZ-POLO. 1980. Role of nerve growth factor in ethylnitrosourea-induced neural carcinogenesis. J. Neurosci. Res. **5**: 351-361.
34. VINORES, S. A. & J. R. PEREZ-POLO. 1983. Nerve growth factor and neural oncology. J. Neurosci. Res. **9**: 81-100.
35. WALKER, P., M. E. WEICHSEL, JR. & D. A. FISHER. 1980. Human nerve growth factor: lack of immunocrossreactivity with mouse nerve growth factor. Life Sci. **26**: 195-200.
36. WECHSLER, W., P. KLEIHUES, S. MATSUMOTO, K. J. ZÜLCH, S. IVANKOVIC, R. PREUSS-MANN & H. DRUCKREY. 1969. Pathology of experimental neurogenic tumors chemically induced during prenatal and postnatal life. Ann. N.Y. Acad. Sci. **159**: 360-408.
37. YOUNG, D. F., R. ELDRIDGE & W. S. GARDNER. 1970. Bilateral acoustic neuroma in a large kindred. J. Am. Med. Assoc. **214**: 347-353.
38. ZIMMERMAN, A. & A. SUTTER. 1983. β-Nerve growth factor (βNGF) receptors on glial cells. Cell-cell interaction between neurones and Schwann cells in cultures of chick sensory ganglia. EMBO J. **2**: 879-885.

The Biology of Non-Myelin-Forming Schwann Cells[a]

RHONA MIRSKY AND KRISTJÁN R. JESSEN

Department of Anatomy and Embryology
University College London
Gower Street
London WC1E 6BT, England

INTRODUCTION

Schwann cells ensheathing axons in unmyelinated fibers outnumber those that ensheath and myelinate axons, and therefore constitute an important category of peripheral glia. In comparison with myelin-forming cells, relatively little is known about the specific molecular characteristics of these cells. It is clearly important to establish to what extent these Schwann cells possess a distinctive molecular phenotype and the extent to which this phenotype is controlled by axons or other environmental influences.

In this paper we will focus on three different aspects of the biology of non-myelin-forming Schwann cells. In the first part we will show that non-myelin-forming Schwann cells express several proteins that are also expressed by astrocytes and enteric glial cells. These molecules are not expressed *in situ* by myelin-forming cells, although two of them are expressed by myelin-forming cells when they are removed from axonal contact and placed into dissociated cell culture. Our results suggest that the phenotype of non-myelin-forming Schwann cells, astrocytes, and enteric glia *in situ* is similar, possibly reflecting common functions shared by non-myelin-forming cells of the central and peripheral nervous system.

In the second part we will discuss the expression of the glycosphingolipid galactocerebroside (GC), the major glycolipid of the myelin sheath, by non-myelin-forming Schwann cells *in situ*, and neuronal influences on its expression. In the third part we will consider the ways in which specific Schwann cell-associated molecules respond to changes in the environment that occur when Schwann cells are removed from axonal contact and put into tissue culture.

MATERIALS AND METHODS

Teased-Nerve Preparations

Cervical sympathetic trunk, sciatic nerve, brachial plexus, and dorsal and ventral roots from Sprague-Dawley rats of various ages were excised and partially teased into nerve bundles and individual fibers with fine syringe needles in a small amount of

[a]This work was supported by grants from the Medical Research Council of Great Britain, the Wellcome Trust, and Action Research for the Crippled Child.

phosphate-buffered saline (PBS) on microscope slides. Samples were allowed to dry before immunofluorescent staining.

Frozen Sections

Dorsal root ganglia (DRG), superior cervical ganglia (SCG), dorsal and ventral roots, cervical sympathetic trunk, cerebellum, and proximal colon were removed from Wistar-Furth (W/Fu), or Sprague-Dawley rats of various ages. Frozen sections of 3-7 μm were cut and thawed onto dry polylysine-coated microscope slides. In some experiments sections were briefly rinsed with 0.15% Triton in PBS prior to application of antibodies.

Cell Cultures

Cervical sympathetic trunk and sciatic nerves were removed from Sprague-Dawley rats of various ages, ranging from embryo day 15 to 35 days postnatal. The tissues were dissociated in trypsin alone or trypsin and collagenase and cultured on poly-L-lysine-coated glass coverslips essentially as described previously for sciatic nerve.[1] The nerves from 15-day and 16-day embryos were digested in 0.05% trypsin in minimal Eagle's medium (MEM) plus 0.02 M HEPES, pH 7.4, for 25 minutes at 37°C, before dissociation. Nerves from older embryos and postnatal rats were digested for times ranging from 5 minutes to one hour in 0.15% collagenase (type II, Flow Laboratories Ltd., Irvine, United Kingdom) in minimal Eagle's medium plus 0.02 M HEPES followed by addition of 0.05% trypsin in the same medium for a further 15 minutes before dissociation.

Antibodies

Ascites fluid containing mouse monoclonal antibody A5E3[2] was used at a dilution of 1:500. Hybridoma supernatant of mouse monoclonal anti-Ran-2 characterized by Bartlett et al.[3] was used at a dilution of 1:1. Rabbit antiserum to human glial fibrillary acidic protein (GFAP) was produced by Dr. R. Pruss. Its specificity has been described elsewhere,[4] and it was used at a dilution of 1:1000. Mouse monoclonal antibody, anti-GFAP3, was produced and characterized by Dr. E. Bock.[5] Ascites fluid containing mouse monoclonal antibody to GC was produced and characterized by Dr. B. Ranscht and used at dilutions 1:100 to 1:1000.[6] In some experiments other monoclonal antibodies to GC, produced and characterized by Dr. I. Sommer and Prof. M. Schachner, were used,[7] and a rabbit antiserum to GC produced and characterized by Dr. S. Liebowitz was also used.[6,8] Rabbit antiserum to cow S-100 protein (DAKO Immunoglobulin, a/s, Copenhagen, Denmark) and rabbit antiserum to P_o, produced and characterized by Dr. J. P. Brockes,[9] were also used.

Polyclonal rabbit antibodies to the neural cell adhesion molecules LI and N-CAM (BSP2) were produced and characterized by Professor M. Schachner[10] and Dr. C. Goridis,[11] respectively.

Fluorescein conjugated to goat anti-mouse immunoglobulin (G anti-MIg-F1) (Nordic Laboratories Ltd.), adsorbed with mouse Ig to remove cross-reacting antibodies, was used at a dilution of 1:50. Tetramethyl rhodamine conjugated to goat anti-mouse Ig (G anti-MIg-Rd) (Cappel Labs., Inc.), adsorbed with mouse Ig to remove cross-reacting antibodies, was used at a dilution of 1:50. Control antibodies, either irrelevant monoclonal antibodies of the appropriate IgG subclass or normal rabbit serum suitably diluted, were included in all experiments.

Immunofluorescence

Both single- and double-label immunofluorescence experiments were carried out as described previously on teased nerves,[12] frozen sections,[13] and dissociated cell cultures. S-100 was used as a marker for Schwann cells in culture.[1,2]

Immunoblotting

Brain, sciatic nerve, DRG, SCG, and cervical sympathetic trunk were removed from adult W/Fu or Sprague-Dawley rats. Myenteric plexus from proximal colon of 14-day-old rats was dissected free from smooth muscle as described previously.[14] Tissue extracts were prepared by homogenization for 5 minutes in 2% sodium dodecyl sulfate (SDS), and 2% mercaptoethanol (ME). The homogenate was then boiled for 5 minutes, spun, and the supernatant retained. An aliquot was removed for protein estimation. Samples were subjected to SDS-polyacrylamide gel electrophoresis using 7.5 or 8% total acrylamide slab gels. The separated proteins were then electrophoretically transferred to 0.12 μm pore size nitrocellulose sheets. A transfer time of 2.5 hours was used. After transfer, excess protein binding sites on the sheets were blocked by overnight incubation in PBS containing 5% bovine hemoglobin. The blots were then incubated for 2 hours in 1 μl of rabbit anti-GFAP diluted in 30 ml of PBS containing 3% hemoglobin (PBS-3Hb) or overnight in a 1:3 dilution of mouse anti-GFAP3 supernatant in PBS-3Hb. After incubation blots were washed for 1 hour with five changes of PBS-3Hb and incubated for 1 hour 15 minutes with ^{125}I-labeled sheep anti-rabbit Ig (5 $\times$ 10^6 cpm/blot diluted in 30 ml of PBS-3Hb) in the case of rabbit anti-GFAP, or ^{125}I-labeled rabbit anti-mouse F(ab')$_2$ (15 $\times$ 10^6 cpm/blot diluted in 30 ml of PBS-3Hb) in the case of mouse monoclonal anti-GFAP3. After washing with five changes of PBS, blots were dried and exposed to preflashed x-ray film for 2-21 days in a cassette equipped with an intensifying screen.

GC Synthesis

Synthesis of labeled GC from ^{3}H-galactose was measured in two thin-layer chromatography systems designed to separate, firstly, cerebrosides from all other lipids and, secondly, galactocerebroside from glucocerebroside.[15] Cervical sympathetic trunks or sciatic nerves were dissected from 8- to 10-day-old Sprague-Dawley rats, desheathed, chopped into small fragments, and incubated with 50 μCi of ^{3}H-galactose (Amersham International plc, Amersham, United Kingdom) for 5 hours at 37°C in 95% air/5% CO_2 in a humidified incubator. After removal of excess ^{3}H-galactose, the lipids were extracted and subjected to thin-layer chromatography. After chromatography, carrier lipids were visualized with iodine vapor and the appropriate regions of the plate scraped off and counted in a liquid scintillation counter.

RESULTS

The Molecular Phenotype of Non-Myelin-Forming Schwann Cells

We have identified four molecules that, judging by immunohistochemical experiments, appear to be expressed by non-myelin-forming Schwann cells but not by myelin-forming ones *in situ*. The first of these, glial fibrillary acidic protein, originally considered to be a molecule specific to astrocyte intermediate filaments, we first identified outside the central nervous system in the enteric glia of the gut.[4] It was later found in a minority population of Schwann cells in the sciatic nerve,[16] in the Schwann cells of the olfactory nerve,[17] and in the nerves of the iris.[18] In a survey of a wide variety of rat peripheral nerves, including the cervical sympathetic trunk, the dorsal and ventral roots, brachial plexus, as well as the sciatic nerve, in both teased-nerve preparations and 2-3 μ frozen sections, we have found that in all the nerves surveyed the immunoreactivity is associated with the Schwann cells surrounding the unmyelinated fibers. In older rats it is also present in a minority of satellite cells, in particular those surrounding the cell bodies of the larger neurons in sensory ganglia at the lumbar and cervical levels, and in the satellite cells surrounding about 40-60% of neurons in the superior cervical ganglion. These results suggest that in adult rats this intermediate filament protein is expressed by all the non-myelin-forming Schwann cells of the peripheral nerve trunks, by all enteric glia, and by a minority of satellite cells (FIGURE 1). The GFAP-like immunoreactivity can also be detected immunochemically. Using SDS-polyacrylamide gel electrophoresis and immunoblotting, an immunoreactive band could be detected in extracts from brain, sciatic nerve, dorsal root ganglia, superior cervical ganglia, and cervical sympathetic trunk, as well as in freshly dissected myenteric plexus extracts. In all cases the position of the band, at 49 kd, was indistinguishable from that of rat brain GFAP (FIGURE 1). Interestingly, when a monoclonal antibody to GFAP (anti-GFAP3), was used on frozen sections, immunohistochemically detectable reactivity was seen in astrocytes and a minority of enteric glia, but not in Schwann cells. Immunoblots of brain revealed the expected band at 49 kd, but no band was seen in extracts of sciatic nerve.[13]

Antibodies to the surface proteins Ran-2, A5E3 antigen, and the neural cell adhesion molecule N-CAM show a similar cell-type distribution to GFAP. In double-label immunofluorescence experiments using antibodies to GFAP together with monoclonal antibodies to either Ran-2 or A5E3 antigen on teased-nerve preparations, we have shown that these proteins are present on the surface of non-myelin-forming cells and are absent from myelin-forming ones.[12] Similarly, double-label immunofluorescence experiments using antibodies to Ran-2 and polyclonal antibodies to N-CAM show that this molecule is also present on the surface of non-myelin-forming cells *in situ*, and not detectable on myelin-forming ones.

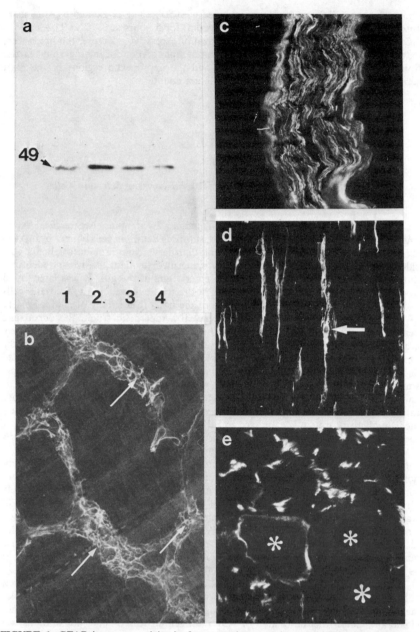

FIGURE 1. GFAP immunoreactivity in frozen sections and immunoblots. (a) Immunoblot using rabbit polyclonal antiserum to GFAP. Track 1, sciatic nerve extract; track 2, extract of superior cervical ganglia; track 3, extract of dorsal root ganglia; track 4, brain extract. Note the presence of an immunoreactive band in all four tracks at 49 kd. (b) Low-power view of GFAP immunoreactivity in the myenteric plexus in a whole-mount preparation of rat colon. The arrows point to cell bodies of enteric glia within ganglia of the plexus. Among the glial cells are unlabeled

In contrast, both the cell surface protein Ran-1,[1] and the neural cell adhesion molecule L1 are detectable on both myelin-forming and non-myelin-forming Schwann cells in teased-nerve preparations, although in both cases the level on the myelin-forming cells appears to be considerably lower than that on the non-myelin-forming cells. In the case of L1 the molecule appears to be present in higher concentrations around the nodes of Ranvier.

Galactocerebroside Expression

In the nervous system, galactocerebroside is normally considered to be associated only with myelin-forming Schwann cells or oligodendrocytes, where it is the major lipid of the myelin sheath. Much interest has therefore focused on the possibility that it has a specific role in the elaboration of myelin sheaths. It is detectable earlier in development than the myelin-associated proteins in both Schwann cells and oligodendrocytes and can be used as a cell type specific marker for oligodendrocytes in dissociated cell cultures from the central nervous system.[8,19] GC can also be demonstrated immunohistochemically in myelin-forming Schwann cells after they have been removed from axonal contact and plated out into tissue culture. Under these conditions, however, Schwann cells, unlike oligodendrocytes, gradually stop expressing immunohistochemically detectable quantities of GC or the myelin-associated proteins P_o, P_1, and P_2 during the first few days *in vitro*, suggesting that axonal contact is required for continuing synthesis of high levels of myelin components in Schwann cells.[19]

The possibility that GC is a universal component of the Schwann cell plasma membrane does not appear to have been seriously investigated before. We have studied GC expression in the rat peripheral nervous system using several different monoclonal antibodies to GC and one polyclonal antibody. In teased-nerve preparations from the sciatic nerve, which contains a mixture of myelinated and unmyelinated fibers, and the cervical sympathetic trunk, in which more than 99% of the axons are unmyelinated, we find that in adult rats both myelin-forming and non-myelin-forming Schwann cells express immunohistochemically detectable amounts of GC (FIGURE 2). In dissociated cell cultures from the cervical sympathetic trunk immunostained after 3 hours in culture, more than 95% express GC (FIGURE 3), although less than 0.5% of the Schwann cells derive from myelin-forming cells (as judged by P_o expression) (FIGURE 4). Like the GC associated with myelin-forming Schwann cells, the molecule disappears rapidly from the surface of non-myelin-forming Schwann cells in culture

---

neuronal cell bodies which are most easily seen in the ganglion at the upper right of the picture. Smooth muscle cells beneath the plexus are unstained. × 60. (c) GFAP immunofluorescence in a 3-4 μm frozen section of cervical sympathetic trunk stained with rabbit anti-GFAP followed by G anti-RIg-Fl. Note staining throughout the width of the nerve. × 84. (d) GFAP immunofluorescence in a 3-4 μm frozen section of dorsal root treated as described in (c). Notice staining of some Schwann cells, one of which is arrowed, lying among many unmyelinated myelinated fibers. × 84. (e) GFAP immunofluorescence in a 3-4 μm frozen section of dorsal root ganglion treated as described in (c). Within the ganglion, three neuronal cell bodies are labeled with asterisks. Notice that the satellite cells around one of them are labeled, while the satellite cells around the other cell bodies are unlabeled. Schwann cells within the ganglion are also stained. (a, d, and e are reproduced from Reference 13 with permission.)

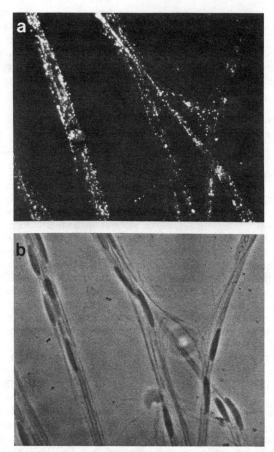

FIGURE 2. Immunofluorescence using antibodies to GC in a teased preparation of cervical sympathetic trunk from 10-day-old rat. (a) Rhodamine optics to visualize GC. (b) Phase contrast. Note the fluorescence in the unmyelinated fiber bundles in which the Schwann cell nuclei can be seen prominently in the phase contrast micrograph (b). × 600.

which suggests that, as in the myelin-forming Schwann cells, an ongoing axonal signal is required to induce and maintain GC synthesis.

To follow the appearance of GC expression during development, dissociated cell cultures were obtained from rats ranging in age from embryonic day 15 to postnatal day 35, and immunostained with GC antibodies after 3 hours in culture. Developmentally, GC is first seen in Schwann cells of the cervical sympathetic trunk at day 19 *in utero*, the proportion of GC-positive cells rising to about 95% at day 10 postnatally. In contrast, GC development in the Schwann cells of the sciatic nerve showed two separate phases of increase. The first occurred between day 18 *in utero* and postnatal day 1, at which time about 60% of the Schwann cells were GC positive, and the second between postnatal days 20 and 35, at which time about 95% of all Schwann cells in the nerve expressed GC (FIGURE 5).

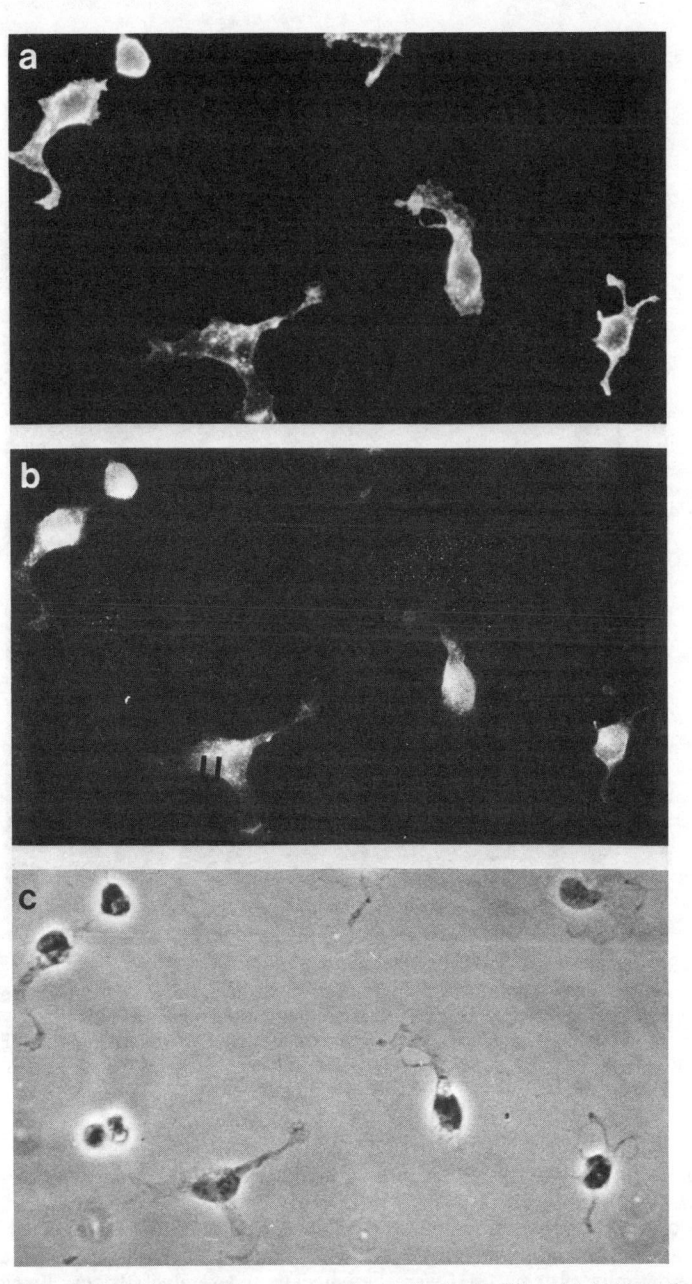

FIGURE 3. Double-label immunofluorescence using antibodies to GC and S-100 in a dissociated cell culture from cervical sympathetic trunk from 10-day-old rats, three hours after plating. (a) Rhodamine optics to visualize GC. (b) Fluorescein optics to visualize S-100. (c) Phase contrast. Note the four GC-positive, S-100-positive Schwann cells, and two GC-negative, S-100-negative cells, presumably fibroblasts. × 600.

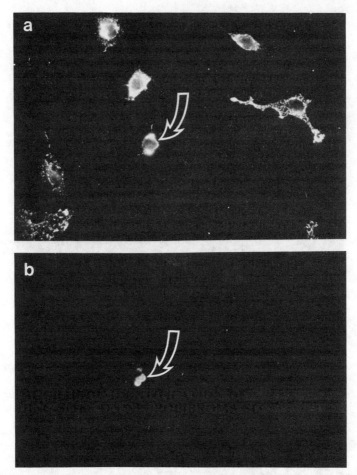

FIGURE 4. Double-label immunofluorescence using antibodies to GC and P_o in a dissociated cell culture from cervical sympathetic trunk from 10-day-old rats, three hours after plating. (a) Rhodamine optics to visualize GC. (b) Fluorescein optics to visualize P_o. Note the single GC-positive, P_o-positive Schwann cell (arrowed), surrounded by several GC-positive, P_o-negative Schwann cells. $\times$ 600.

When the biosynthesis of GC was assayed, by measuring incorporation of ^{3}H-galactose into freshly dissected preparations of sciatic nerves or cervical sympathetic trunks over a 3-hour period, significant quantities of GC were synthesized not only in the sciatic nerves but also in the cervical sympathetic trunks. The two thin-layer chromatography systems used were designed to separate, firstly, cerebrosides from other lipids and, secondly, galactocerebroside from glucocerebroside. In both sciatic nerves and cervical sympathetic trunks, the majority of the ^{3}H-galactose comigrated with the added GC standard, indicating that both nerves could synthesize this molecule.[20]

Regulation of Schwann Cell Phenotype

The phenotype of Schwann cells, both myelin forming and non-myelin forming, appears to be considerably more plastic than that of glia from the central nervous system. This is well illustrated in the case of myelin-forming Schwann cells, which lose all their myelin-related components when they are removed from axonal contact and placed in dissociated cell culture.[19] Similarly, all Schwann cells lose their basal lamina when removed from axonal contact and only reform it when grown together with axons under conditions where complete ensheathment of axons can occur.[21] In the specific case of non-myelin-forming Schwann cells, GC, as mentioned above, is lost when the Schwann cells are removed from axonal contact and placed into culture, with a similar time course to that seen for Schwann cells that *in situ* formed myelin.[20] When the protein molecules restricted to non-myelin-forming Schwann cells *in situ* are considered from this point of view, a somewhat complex picture emerges, which nevertheless reflects the fact that Schwann cells are in general highly sensitive to their environment. Ran-2 disappears from adult Schwann cells in dissociated cell culture over a period of 5-6 days, whereas the perineurial cells which also express Ran-2 continue to express the molecule in culture.

A5E3 is retained by the non-myelin-forming Schwann cells in dissociated cell culture. After 3 days in culture, all Schwann cells in the culture including those derived from myelinated nerves (as judged by P_o expression) express detectable quan-

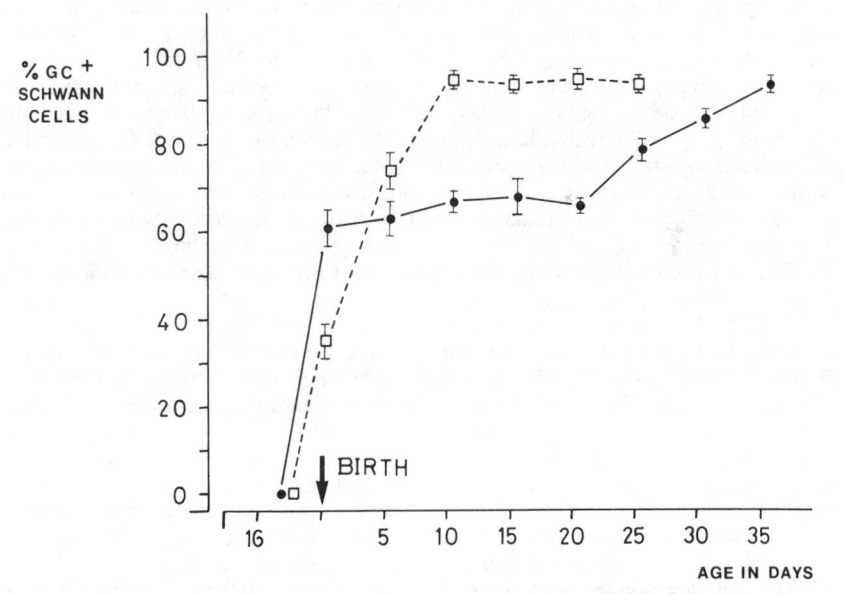

FIGURE 5. Development of GC-positive Schwann cells in sciatic nerve and cervical sympathetic trunk. Sciatic nerves (●) and cervical sympathetic trunks (□) from rats of different ages were dissociated and double labeled with antibodies to GC and S-100 after three hours in culture. The percentage of GC-positive Schwann cells at each time point is shown on the graph. Results at each time point were obtained from a minimum of three experiments, with a total of at least 1000 Schwann cells counted. (Reproduced from Reference 20 with permission.)

.s of A5E3 antigen. It appears that as the myelin-forming Schwann cells stop expressing myelin components, they start expressing A5E3 antigen. The neural cell adhesion molecule N-CAM shows similar behavior. Although it is not detectable on myelin-forming Schwann cells *in situ*, after 4 days in culture all the cells in the culture that derive from myelinated nerves are expressing N-CAM and there is no obvious difference in the levels of immunofluorescence between cells that were making myelin *in situ* and those that were not.

In the case of GFAP, non-myelin-forming Schwann cells retain GFAP expression *in vitro*. Cells that were making myelin *in situ* and therefore not expressing GFAP also appear to develop some GFAP reactivity in culture after 2 days *in vitro*, but much of the fluorescence is not in a filamentous form and it is therefore difficult to be certain that a true switch in phenotypic expression has occurred in this case.

DISCUSSION

It is clear that non-myelin-forming Schwann cells possess a distinctive phenotype of their own. While they express several molecules in common with myelin-forming Schwann cells, including the intracellular molecules vimentin[16] and S100,[1,12] the extracellular molecules Ran-1, L1, and galactocerebroside, and the basal lamina associated components laminin, collagen type IV, entactin, and heparan sulfate proteoglycan,[22,23] they also express molecules not found on myelin-forming Schwann cells. These molecules, which include GFAP, Ran-2, A5E3 antigen,[12] and N-CAM, are all, however, expressed by enteric glia[24] and astrocytes.[2,3,25] Although these molecules, in common with many others, are present on more than one cell type, both inside and outside the nervous system, their distribution is relatively restricted and the phenotype GFAP positive, Ran-2 positive, A5E3 antigen positive, N-CAM positive, is restricted to astrocytes in the central nervous system and to non-myelin-forming Schwann cells and enteric glia in the peripheral nervous system of the adult rat. By analogy with the molecular similarities that exist between oligodendrocytes and myelin-forming Schwann cells, which are related to formation of the myelin sheath, it is possible that the similarities in phenotype between astrocytes and some non-myelin-forming peripheral glia may also reflect common functions shared by these cell types.

The GFAP expressed by non-myelin-forming Schwann cells has a molecular weight in SDS gels indistinguishable from that of astrocytes and appears to be filamentous in form. Differences in GFAP expression are however seen between astrocytes and non-myelin-forming Schwann cells when a monoclonal antibody (anti-GFAP3) is used, suggesting that this antibody recognizes a determinant that is expressed in high quantities in astrocytes, in smaller amounts in enteric glia, and in insignificant amounts in non-myelin-forming Schwann cells. It is possible that this is a phosphorylated determinant, which in the case of monoclonal antibodies to neurofilaments appears to be a favorite site for antibody recognition, but it could also be related to some other difference between the filaments in Schwann cells and astrocytes.

The fact that non-myelin-forming Schwann cells in adult rats express GC is at first sight somewhat surprising. It contradicts the previous consensus of opinion regarding the role and distribution of GC in the nervous system, which holds that this molecule is specifically involved in some event connected with myelin formation.

In our latest studies,[20] the pattern of development of GC expression varied considerably depending on the nerve studied. This variation does, however, seem to be related to differences in patterns of maturation of the two nerves. Our developmental studies show that GC expression is a relatively late maturational event. In the cervical sympathetic trunk, GC is first detectable on day 19 *in utero*. The number of Schwann cells expressing the molecule then rises fairly evenly to level off at day 10 postnatally, when about 95% of the Schwann cells are also GC positive. This time course is similar to that of several other maturational events in the same nerve. Thus axonal diameter, total number of Schwann cells, and the ratio of axons to Schwann cells all show a postnatal phase of rapid development toward mature levels which ends at about day 14. The segregation and enclosure of axons by Schwann cell processes into individual troughs do not coincide with the appearance of GC, since they occur significantly earlier and are to a large extent completed by day 7.[26]

In the sciatic nerve the time course of GC development is quite different from that in the cervical sympathetic trunk. It shows two separate phases of rapid increase: the first between embryonic day 19 and day 1 postnatally, and the second approximately between days 20 and 35, at which stage about 94% of the S-100 positive Schwann cells also express GC. This time course is not similar to that of the appearance of myelin sheaths in this nerve. Myelin sheaths are first seen at day 1 postnatally, and their number increases rapidly during the first week of life and more slowly thereafter.[27–29] As far as can be judged from the literature, however, the first very rapid phase of increase in cells expressing GC coincides with another important development, viz., the period during which most of the axons that will later become myelinated are segregating to achieve a 1:1 relationship with the Schwann cell. The attainment of the 1:1 ratio between axons and Schwann cells is presumed to be accompanied by cessation of division of this Schwann cell population.[29] From several qualitative ultrastructural studies,[26,27,29] it can be inferred that Remak fibers develop significantly later in the sciatic nerve than in the sympathetic trunk. As discussed above, their development in the sympathetic trunk appears to have reached a mature stage at day 15, while at that date only the very first mature Remak fibers are appearing in the sciatic nerve.[27] Similarly, Schwann cell proliferation, which in the trunk is largely over at day 15,[26] is still significant at that date in the sciatic nerve, reaching very low levels by day 28.[27] Comparing our results to those data we suggest that the second rise in the number of GC-positive cells in the sciatic nerve is related to the late emergence of mature Remak fibers in this nerve.

Previous failure to detect GC on non-myelin-forming Schwann cells is probably related to several factors. Several earlier studies concentrated on studying Schwann cells derived from rats ranging in age from embryonic day 18 to postnatal day 5.[6,19,30] During this developmental period, GC expression in Schwann cells in dissociated cell cultures derived from sciatic nerve is largely restricted to Schwann cells that *in situ* are committed to myelin formation. GC expression on non-myelin-forming Schwann cells develops in this nerve after this period, and in Schwann cells from sciatic nerves of 5-day-old rats, GC and P_o are largely coexpressed. Furthermore, in some studies,[19] Schwann cells derived from the superior cervical ganglion were used as a control for non-myelin-forming cells, and as in the sciatic nerve, GC expression in these cells occurs relatively later in development than in the cervical sympathetic trunk. Under the conditions used in our present study, about 10% of the non-myelin-forming Schwann cells from the superior cervical ganglion are GC positive at day 5, attaining maximal levels of GC expression by day 35. In other experiments, when teased-nerve preparations were used to study expression of GC,[30] nerves that were largely unmyelinated were not used; and without markers for the non-myelin-forming Schwann cells, such as GFAP, it is difficult to unequivocally recognize unmyelinated fibers among partially teased bundles of myelinated fibers in mixed nerves like the sciatic nerve.

A clue to how GC expression may be related to other aspects of cellular differentiation comes from studies on oligodendrocytes. In these cells there is good evidence that GC first appears at about the same time as cell division stops in the precursor cell.[31-33] A similar relationship may exist in Schwann cells, irrespective of their differentiation into myelin- or non-myelin-forming cells.

Our results suggest the possibility that an axonal signal is needed to trigger and maintain GC expression in non-myelin-forming Schwann cells, as in myelin-forming cells. Our own more recent denervation experiments *in situ* support this contention. It is therefore likely that, contrary to current thought, the signal that induces GC expression, which may act via elevation of intracellular cyclic AMP levels,[34] can be separated from other events involved in myelin formation, such as induction of the myelin-specific proteins.

Apart from being one of the building blocks of the myelin sheath, the functional role of GC is still unclear. Developmentally, it appears on the surface of non-myelin-forming Schwann cells as they reach maturity, and is expressed by oligodendrocytes and myelin-forming Schwann cells as cell division stops but before the onset of myelination. This points to an involvement in those membrane-membrane interactions that establish the mature relationship between axons and their glial cells, in addition to a specific role in the membrane-wrapping events involved in myelination.

When Schwann cells are compared with astrocytes on one hand, or oligodendrocytes on the other, it is immediately apparent that the Schwann cell phenotype expressed is relatively more dependent on the environment in which the cell finds itself. The loss of basal lamina and of molecules such as GC and Ran-2 by non-myelin-forming Schwann cells, and of GC and myelin proteins by myelin-forming Schwann cells, reflects one aspect of this lability. The increased levels of expression of molecules such as A5E3 antigen and N-CAM when myelin-forming Schwann cells are put into dissociated cell culture suggests that the Schwann cell in culture has a specific phenotype that is closer to that of the non-myelin-forming Schwann cell *in situ* than that of the myelin-forming one. Understanding the control of molecular expression in normal Schwann cells and in particular the mechanisms through which neuronal signals control the Schwann cell phenotype may help us to understand the way in which this control is altered in disease.

ACKNOWLEDGMENTS

We would like to thank Dr. M. J. Brammer and Ms. L. Morgan for invaluable assistance with the experiments on GC; and Drs. J. P. Brockes, C. Goridis, S. Liebowitz, R. Pruss, I. Sommer, and Professor M. Schachner for gifts of antisera.

REFERENCES

1. BROCKES, J. P., K. L. FIELDS & M. C. RAFF. 1979. Studies on cultured rat Schwann cells. I. Establishment of purified populations from cultures of peripheral nerve. Brain Res. **165:** 105-118.
2. MIRSKY, R., J. GAVRILOVIC, P. BANNERMAN, J. WINTER & K. R. JESSEN. 1985. Characterization of a plasma membrane protein in non-myelin forming PNS and CNS glia,

a subpopulation of PNS neurons, perineurial cells and smooth muscle in adult rats. Cell Tissue Res. **240:** 723-733.

3. BARTLETT, P. F., M. D. NOBLE, R. M. PRUSS, M. C. RAFF, S. RATTRAY, & C. A. WILLIAMS. 1981. Rat neural antigen-2 (Ran-2), a cell surface antigen on astrocytes, ependymal cells, Muller cells and leptomeninges defined by a monoclonal antibody. Brain Res. **204:** 339-352.

4. JESSEN, K. R. & R. MIRSKY. 1980. Glial cells in the enteric nervous system contain glial fibrillary acidic protein. Nature. **286:** 736-737.

5. ALBRECHTSEN, M., A. C. VON GERSTENBERG & E. BOCK. 1984. Mouse monoclonal antibodies reacting with human brain glial fibrillary acidic protein. J. Neurochem. **42:** 86-93.

6. RANSCHT, B., P. A. CLAPSHAW, J. PRICE, M. NOBLE & W. SEIFERT. 1982. Development of oligodendrocytes and Schwann cells studied with a monoclonal antibody against galactocerebroside. Proc. Nat. Acad. Sci. USA **79:** 2709-2713.

7. SCHACHNER, M. 1982. Cell type-specific surface antigens in the mammalian nervous system. J. Neurochem. **39:** 1-8.

8. RAFF, M. C., R. MIRSKY, K. L. FIELDS, R. P. LISAK, S. H. DORFMAN, D. H. SILBERBERG, N. A. GREGSON, S. LIEBOWITZ & M. C. KENNEDY. 1978. Galactocerebroside is a specific cell-surface antigenic marker for oligodendrocytes in culture. Nature **274:** 813-816.

9. BROCKES, J. P., M. C. RAFF, D. J. NISHIGUCHI & J. WINTER. 1980. Studies on cultured rat Schwann cells. III. Assays for peripheral myelin proteins. J. Neurocytol. **9:** 67-77.

10. RATHJEN, F. & M. SCHACHNER. 1984. Immunocytological and biochemical characterization of a new neuronal cell surface component (L1 antigen) which is involved in cell adhesion. EMBO J. **3:** 1-10.

11. SADOUL, R., M. HIRN, H. DEAGOSTINI-BAZIN, G. ROUGON & C. GORIDIS. 1983. Adult and embryonic mouse neural cell adhesion molecules have different binding properties. Nature **304:** 347-349.

12. JESSEN, K. R. & R. MIRSKY. 1984. Non myelin forming Schwann cells coexpress surface proteins and intermediate filaments not found in myelin forming cells: a study of Ran-2, A5E3 antigen and glial fibrillary acidic protein. J. Neurocytol. **13:** 923-934.

13. JESSEN, K. R., R. THORPE & R. MIRSKY. 1984. Molecular identity, distribution and heterogeneity of glial fibrillary acidic protein: an immunoblotting and immunohistochemical study of Schwann cells, satellite cells, enteric glia and astrocytes. J. Neurocytol. **13:** 187-200.

14. JESSEN, K. R., M. J. SAFFREY & G. BURNSTOCK. 1983. The enteric nervous system in tissue culture. I. Cell types and their interactions in explants of the myenteric and submucous plexuses from guinea-pig, rabbit and rat. Brain Res. **262:** 17-35.

15. BRAMMER, M. J. 1984. Synthesis of gluco- and galactocerebrosides in bovine neurones and oligodendroglia. J. Neurochem. **42:** 135-141.

16. YEN, S. & K. L. FIELDS. 1981. Antibodies to neurofilament, glial filament and fibroblast intermediate filament proteins bind to different cell types of the nervous system. J. Cell Biol. **88:** 115-126.

17. BARBER, P. C. & R. M. LINDSAY. 1982. Schwann cells of the olfactory nerves contain glial fibrillary acidic protein and resemble astrocytes. Neuroscience 7: 3077-3099.

18. BJÖRKLUND, H., D. DAHL, L. OLSON & A. SEIGER. 1984. Glial fibrillary acidic protein-like immunoreactivity in the iris: development, distribution and reactive changes following transplantation. J. Neurosci. **4:** 978-988.

19. MIRSKY, R., J. WINTER, E. R. ABNEY, R. M. PRUSS, J. GAVRILOVIC & M. C. RAFF. 1980. Myelin-specific proteins and glycolipids in rat Schwann cells and oligodendrocytes in culture. J. Cell Biol. **84:** 483-494.

20. JESSEN, K. R., L. MORGAN, M. BRAMMER & R. MIRSKY. 1985. Galactocerebroside is expressed by non-myelin forming Schwann cells *in situ.* J. Cell Biol. **101:** 1135-1143.

21. BUNGE, M., A. WILLIAMS, P. WOOD, J. UITTO & J. JEFFREY. 1980. Comparison of nerve cell and nerve cell plus Schwann cell cultures, with particular emphasis on basal lamina and collagen formation. J. Cell Biol. **84:** 184-202.

22. CORNBROOKS, C. J., D. J. CAREY, J. A. MCDONALD, R. TIMPL & R. P. BUNGE. 1983.

In vivo and *in vitro* observations on laminin production by Schwann cells. Proc. Nat. Acad. Sci. USA **80:** 3850-3854.

23. BUNGE, R. P. & M. B. BUNGE. 1983. Interrelationship between Schwann cell function and extracellular matrix production. Trends Neurosci. **7:** 499-505.

24. JESSEN, K. R. & R. MIRSKY. 1983. Astrocyte-like glia in the peripheral nervous system: an immunohistochemical study of enteric glia. J. Neurosci. **3:** 2206-2218.

25. HIRN, M., M. S. GHANDOUR, H. DEAGOSTINI-BAZIN & C. GORIDIS. 1983. Molecular heterogeneity and structure evolution during cerebellar ontogeny detected by monoclonal antibody of the mouse cell surface antigen BSP-2. Brain Res. **265:** 87-100.

26. AGUAYO, A. J., L. C. TERRY & G. M. BRAY. 1973. Spontaneous loss of axons in sympathetic unmyelinated nerve fibers of the rat during development. Brain Res. **54:** 360-364.

27. FRIEDE, R. L. & T. SAMORAJSKI. 1968. Myelin formation in the sciatic nerve of the rat. J. Neuropathol. Exp. Neurol. **27:** 546-570.

28. WEBSTER, H. DE F., J. R. MARTIN & M. F. O'CONNELL. 1973. The relationships between interphase Schwann cells and axons before myelination: a quantitative electron microscopic study. Dev. Biol. **32:** 401-416.

29. WEBSTER, H. DE F. & J. T. FAVILLA. 1984. Development of peripheral nerve fibers. *In* Peripheral Neuropathy. P. J. Dyck, P. K. Thomas, E. H. Lambert & R. Bunge, Eds.: 329-359. Saunders. Philadelphia, Pa.

30. WINTER, J., R. MIRSKY & M. KADLUBOWSKI. 1982. Immunocytochemical study of the appearance of P_2 in developing rat peripheral nerve: comparison with other myelin components. J. Neurocytol. **11:** 351-362.

31. ECCLESTON, P. A. & D. H. SILBERBERG. 1984. The differentiation of oligodendrocytes in a serum-free hormone-supplemented medium. Dev. Brain Res. **16:** 1-9.

32. NOBLE, M. & K. MURRAY. 1984. Purified astrocytes promote the *in vitro* division of a bipotential glial progenitor cell. EMBO J. **13:** 2243-2247.

33. WOOD, P. M. & A. K. WILLIAMS. 1984. Oligodendrocyte proliferation and CNS myelination in cultures containing dissociated embryonic neuroglia and dorsal root ganglion neurons. Dev. Brain Res. **12:** 225-241.

34. SOBUE, G. & D. PLEASURE. 1984. Schwann cell galactocerebroside induced by derivatives of adenosine 3′,5′-monophosphate. Science **224:** 72-74.

Pathology of Nerve Sheath Tumors

JAMES C. HARKIN

Department of Pathology
Tulane University School of Medicine
1430 Tulane Avenue
New Orleans, Louisiana 70112

Primary neoplasms of peripheral nerves are usually benign. The tumors have been found in patients in all parts of the world. Generally the patient has a single tumor. A striking difference in the character of peripheral nerve tumors can be found in some of the patients with the genetically determined disorder neurofibromatosis; such patients can have numerous peripheral nerve tumors, bizarre disfiguring tumors, and a greatly increased risk for malignant peripheral nerve tumors when compared to patients without the genetic disorder. Peripheral nerve neoplasms are almost always tumors derived from the nerve sheath cells, not from neoplastic neurons.[1,2] The exception is the neuroblastoma-ganglioneuroma-pheochromocytoma group of tumors generally found on autonomic nerves in the trunk, not in the extremities.

At the end of the description of each tumor a comment indicates how the presence of neurofibromatosis modifies the behavior of the tumor. The nerve sheath tumors can be classified in four general groups: (1) schwannoma, (2) neurofibroma, (3) plexiform neurofibroma, and (4) malignant schwannoma.

SCHWANNOMA

Schwannoma, also known as neurilemoma, is a circumscribed neoplasm composed of Schwann cells. The tumor arises in a nerve and grows to one side of the nerve, allowing the nerve to be saved when the tumor is excised. When the schwannoma involves cranial and spinal nerve roots, it is on *sensory* roots and the lesion expands the entire nerve making it impossible to excise the tumor without destroying the nerve. The schwannoma of the 8th cranial nerve, often called acoustic neuroma, is a good example of such a lesion. Another is the dumbbell tumor found on spinal nerve roots with half adjacent to the spinal cord and half outside. Microscopically a schwannoma is a cellular tumor. Where the elongated nuclei are arranged with their long axis parallel, palisades are created (FIGURE 1). Structures resembling nerve end organs may be found (termed Verocay bodies). Cellular parts of the schwannoma are called Antoni type A pattern; and loose less cellular zones, Antoni type B. Cysts may be found in the tumor. By electron microscopy, the tumor cells have convoluted plasma membranes similar to hyperplastic Schwann cells seen in regenerating nerves (FIGURE 2). A basement membrane encircles each Schwann cell. The extracellular part of a schwannoma contains collagen; in some schwannomas the collagen is aggregated into long spacing collagen or Luse bodies.

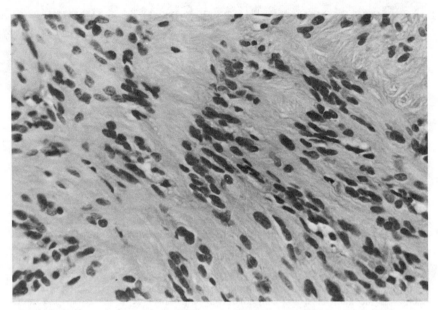

FIGURE 1. Schwannoma, a photomicrograph illustrating elongated nuclei arranged with their long axis parallel. × 300.

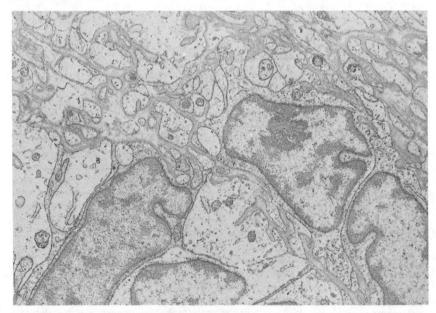

FIGURE 2. Schwannoma, an electron micrograph showing tumor cells with invaginations of the plasma membrane. Tumor cells are each surrounded by a basement membrane. × 8000.

Immunoperoxidase techniques for S-100 protein (named S-100 because the protein is soluble in 100% ammonium sulfate) have been used to identify the neural protein S-100 in Schwann cells and in the tumor cells of schwannoma, adding proof to the identification of the tumor cells as Schwann cells.[3] Parenthetically it should be noted that S-100 protein is found in glial cells, nevus cells, and melanoma cells and can be found in a variety of tissues such as breast carcinoma making the marker limited in its specificity.[4]

Variants include the *ancient schwannoma* with increased cellularity and marked variation in nuclear size. The nuclear atypia should not lead to the erroneous diagnosis of malignant schwannoma. A rare variant is the *plexiform schwannoma* (multinodular schwannoma), a lesion that grossly resembles a plexiform neurofibroma, but microscopically is a typical schwannoma with the same good prognosis as other benign schwannomas.[5]

Relationship to neurofibromatosis: Multiple schwannomas may be found with neurofibromatosis. Bilateral acoustic neuromas (schwannomas) are found only with neurofibromatosis.

NEUROFIBROMA

Neurofibroma is a benign slowly growing localized nonencapsulated neoplasm that contains Schwann cells (or the closely related perineurial cells) and a massive extracellular collagenous matrix (FIGURE 3). Scattered fibrocytes may be found within the

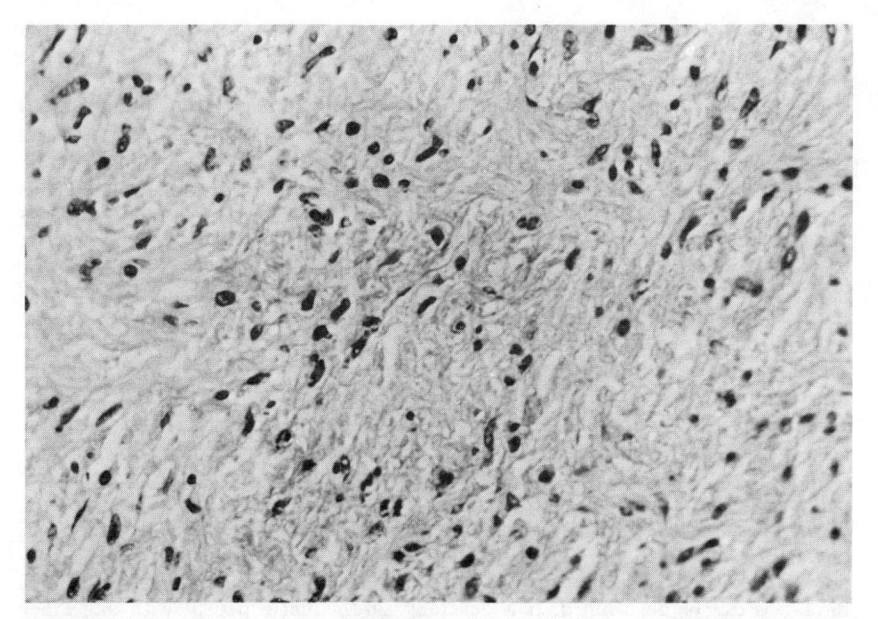

FIGURE 3. Neurofibroma; the photomicrograph is of a tumor with considerable space between nuclei principally extracellular collagen. × 300.

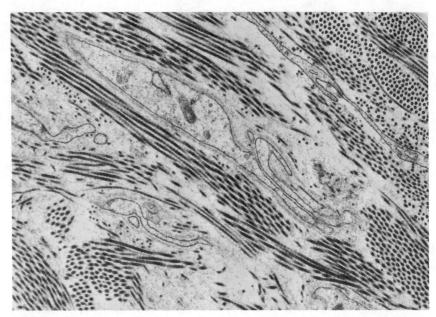

FIGURE 4. Neurofibroma; an electron micrograph illustrates the elongated tumor cells each surrounded by a basement membrane. The collagen in the extracellular region is prominent. × 17,000.

lesion. In the cutaneous neurofibromas the nerve of origin is not seen although a few nerve twigs may be found within the lesion; in neurofibromas arising on large nerves, the nerve can be identified. A neurofibroma is rubbery and may be quite soft. By electron microscopy, the tumor cells are often elongated; most tumor cells are surrounded by a basement membrane (FIGURE 4). The tumor cells react poorly for S-100 protein. Normal perineurial cells are very elongated; they are surrounded by a basement membrane.

Normal perineurial cells react poorly for S-100 protein. The elongated shape of the cells in neurofibroma and the poor reactivity for S-100 protein have been used as evidence that the cells are of perineurial origin rather than of Schwann cell origin.[6] The problem of the origin of the cells in neurofibroma has not been solved, although it is quite clear that the tumor cells are not fibrocytes.

Variants of neurofibroma include two unusual and uncommon lesions: (a) *diffuse neurofibroma* in which broad areas of the dermis are involved; and (b) *symmetrical neurofibroma* in which concentric layers of cells and collagen are formed around each nerve in a fascicle, maintaining the overall structure.[7]

Relationship to neurofibromatosis: The neurofibroma, particularly the cutaneous one, is the characteristic lesion of neurofibromatosis. The majority of dermal neurofibromas removed surgically come from patients who do not have neurofibromatosis, insofar as can be determined. It is generally agreed that a patient with more than three neurofibromas has neurofibromatosis. The very large neurofibromas are found only with neurofibromatosis.

PLEXIFORM NEUROFIBROMA

Plexiform neurofibroma is a specific lesion that should be separated from other neurofibromas. The plexiform neurofibroma grows within a nerve enlarging the nerve fascicles and elongating each fascicle; this growth causes the fascicles to twist on themselves, eventually creating a lesion resembling a tangle of worms. In the early stage of the lesion, hypercellular fascicles are found (FIGURE 5). As the lesion develops there is an increase in number of Schwann cells and/or perineurial cells. A few residual axons that have not been destroyed by the tumor can be found. As the lesion grows the fascicles can become hypocellular and myxomatous in character or become even more cellular; the two patterns can be found side by side in a single lesion. The plexiform neurofibroma can be a small cutaneous lesion that can be completely excised or it can be a large lesion that grows toward the spinal cord, compressing and destroying tissues as it expands. The most serious change in a plexiform neurofibroma is that it may undergo malignant transformation into a malignant schwannoma.

What is the cell of origin of the plexiform neurofibroma? It is uncertain. By electron microscopy, the cells resemble those in cutaneous neurofibromas (FIGURE 6), thus they are Schwann cells or perineurial cells, but not fibrocytes. Most plexiform neurofibromas react poorly to immunoperoxidase preparations for S-100 protein. In one plexiform neurofibroma we studied, the center of the lesion was cellular and resembled a schwannoma by light microscopy and had a positive reaction for S-100 protein. At the periphery of the nodules of the plexiform neurofibroma, the lesion was much less cellular and reacted less intensely with S-100 protein. We have concluded that at least some plexiform neurofibromas may contain Schwann cells that react with

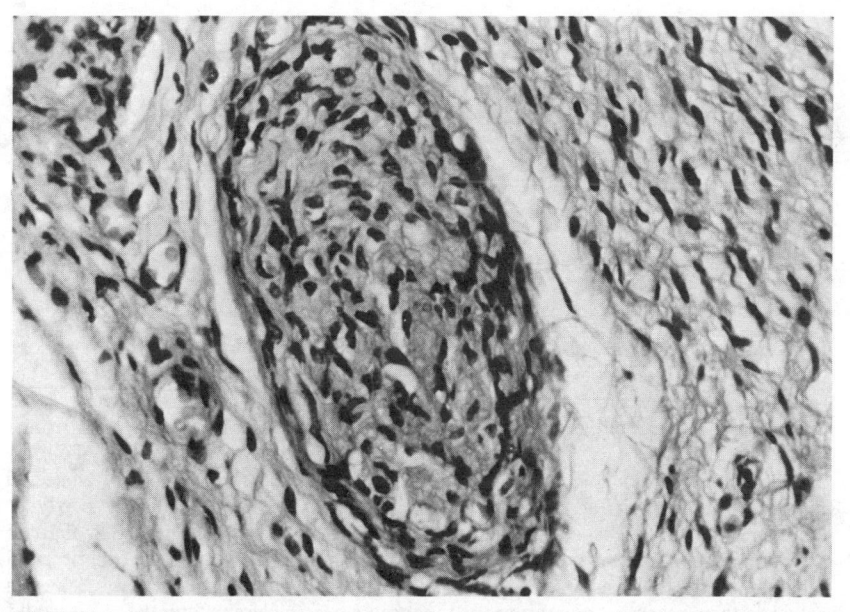

FIGURE 5. Plexiform neurofibroma; in this photomicrograph, the neoplasm is shown with numerous cells within the nerve fascicle. × 300.

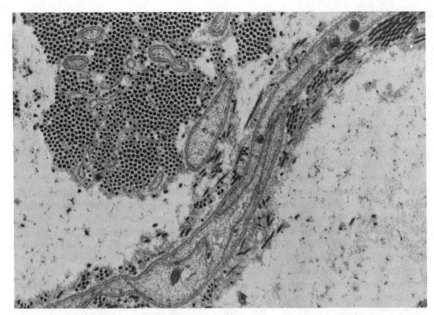

FIGURE 6. Plexiform neurofibroma illustrated in an electron micrograph showing the elongated tumor cells each surrounded by a basement membrane. Many collagen fibrils are present. × 14,000.

S-100. The term composite nerve sheath tumor has been used for those neoplasms that combine features of neurofibroma with those of schwannoma.

Relationship to neurofibromatosis: Plexiform neurofibroma is considered to be found only in patients with neurofibromatosis. Enzinger has questioned if this is invariably true for some of the small cutaneous plexiform neurofibromas.[8]

MALIGNANT SCHWANNOMA

Malignant schwannoma is used as the name for all malignant nerve sheath tumors, neoplasms that arise from Schwann cells or the closely related perinurial cells. The term neurogenic sarcoma has been avoided because malignant nerve sheath neoplasms are not of mesodermal or fibroblastic origin. A malignant schwannoma arises from a nerve or from a plexiform neurofibroma. The tumor is cellular with streams of closely packed cells with elongated nuclei (FIGURE 7). Cell borders are indistinct. Scattered mitotic figures are found. By electron microscopy, the tumor cells are partly or completely encircled by a basement membrane. In poorly differentiated malignant schwannomas, basement membrane may be missing from many cells. In experimental malignant schwannomas produced in rats by ethylnitrosourea, the neoplastic Schwann cells lost their basement membranes as the tumors became less differentiated.[9] It would seem plausible to think the same phenomenon occurs in man. The majority of malignant schwannomas have the pattern described above.[10] The prognosis for patients with malignant schwannoma is poor, although some are cured if the lesion is in an extremity and the limb is amputated. Although it has been alleged that surgical interference with a neurofibroma can precipitate malignant change, the evidence is inconclusive; more likely, the usual condition is that partial resection of a tumor failed to include the tumor that had become malignant.[11]

Variants: Several variants are found: (a) the most common (about 5% of malignant schwannomas) is the malignant epithelioid schwannoma where distinct cell borders are seen around each cell; (b) the malignant triton tumor in which skeletal muscle develops; and (c) the malignant schwannoma with features of malignant mesenchymoma where there are zones of immature tissue, cartilage, and bone; some authors question whether this last tumor is of Schwann cell origin.[12] Some of the malignant nerve sheath tumors would be difficult to recognize histologically as being of nerve origin if it were not known that the lesion had developed from a nerve. Pigmented melanin-containing tumor cells are found in occasional benign and malignant schwannomas and neurofibromas. Malignant melanomas that grow into nerves have been described by Reed and Leonard.[13] We examined one case by light and electron microscopy and immunoperoxidase technique for S-100 protein in which part of the lesion resembled malignant melanoma and part of it a low-grade malignant schwannoma. Although many cells were identified as Schwann cells, it was not possible to exclude the possibility that part of the lesion was a malignant melanoma.

Relationship to neurofibromatosis: Malignant schwannomas are rare tumors, and collected cases fail to provide an adequate estimate of the incidence. Malignant schwannomas are rare in patients with neurofibromatosis but much more common than in patients without the phakomatosis.[14] The incidence of malignant schwannomas has

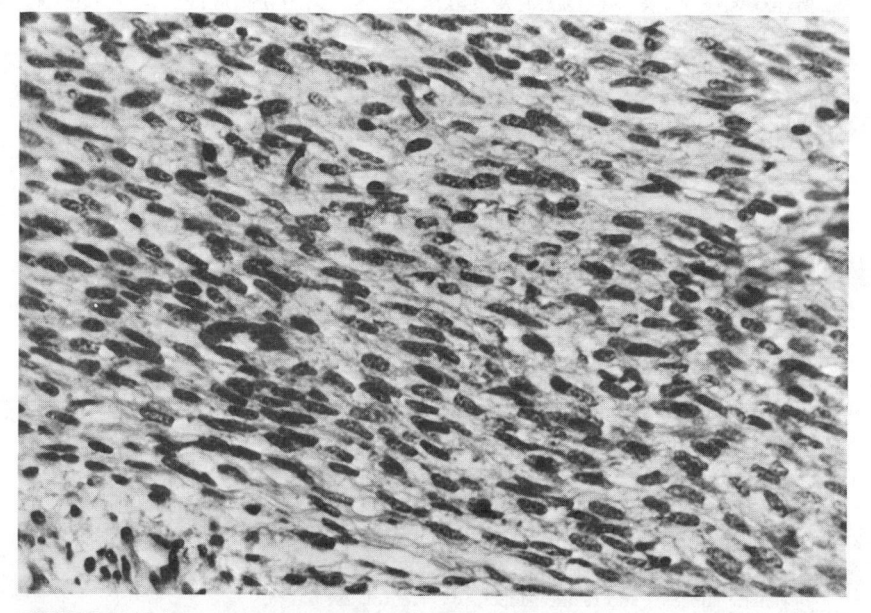

FIGURE 7. Malignant schwannoma seen in this photomicrograph is of the typical histological pattern, cellular with streams of cells. × 300.

been estimated to occur in 2% to 29% of the patients with neurofibromatosis. It probably lies somewhere between 2% and 13%. In children with neurofibromatosis who died from malignant nerve sheath tumors, the average survival time was 1.8 years.[15] In adults fewer than 20% survive 5 years.

COMMENT

The behavior and histopathology of most nerve sheath cell tumors are well documented. The cell of origin of some tumors remains open to question, and because of this a complex and confusing system of nomenclature has arisen. It is unfortunate because almost all pathologists agree on the nature of the tumors, disagreeing only on the name. In the present report we have tried to use a simple terminology, one that has widespread usage, and one that does not require a definitive proof of the origin of each tumor cell.

REFERENCES

1. RUSSELL, D. S. & L. J. RUBENSTEIN. 1977. Pathology of Tumors of the Nervous System. 4th edit. Williams & Wilkins. Baltimore, Md.
2. HARKIN, J. C. & R. J. REED. 1969. Tumors of the peripheral nervous system. In Atlas of Tumor Pathology (second series, fascicle three). Armed Forces Institute of Pathology. Washington, D.C.
3. STEFANSSON, K., R. WOLLMANN & JERKOVIC. 1982. S-100 protein in soft-tissue tumors derived from Schwann cells and melanocytes. Am. J. Pathol. 106: 261-268.
4. KAHN, H. J., A. MARKS, T. HEATHER & R. BAUMAE. 1983. Role of antibody to S-100 protein in diagnostic pathology. Am. J. Clin. Pathol. 79: 341-347.
5. REED, R. J. & J. C. HARKIN. 1983. Tumors of the peripheral nervous system (supplement). In Atlas of Tumor Pathology (second series, fascicle three). Armed Forces Institute of Pathology. Washington, D.C.
6. ERLANDSON, R. A. & J. M. WOODRUFF. 1982. Peripheral nerve sheath tumors. Cancer 49: 273-287.
7. WELLER, R. O. & J. CERVOS-NAVARRO. 1977. In Pathology of Peripheral Nerves: 150-152. Butterworth. London, England.
8. ENZINGER, F. M. & S. W. WEISS. 1983. Benign tumors of peripheral nerves. In Soft Tissue Tumors: 580-624. C. V. Mosby. St. Louis, Mo.
9. CRAVIATO, H., J. F. WEISS, E. DE C. WEISS, H. H. GOEBEL & J. RANSOHOFF. 1973. Biological characteristics of peripheral nerve tumors induced with ethylnitrosourea. Acta Neuropathol. 23: 265-280.
10. GUCCION, J. G. & F. M. ENZINGER. 1979. Malignant schwannoma associated with von Recklinghausen's neurofibromatosis. Virchows Arch. Anat. Pathol. 383: 43-57.
11. SEDDON, H. 1972. Surgical Disorders of the Peripheral Nerves. Williams & Wilkins. Baltimore, Md.
12. ENZINGER, F. M. & S. W. WEISS. 1983. Malignant tumors of peripheral nerves. In Soft Tissue Tumors: 625-656. C. V. Mosby. St. Louis, Mo.
13. REED, R. J. & D. D. LEONARD. 1979. Neurotropic melanoma; a variation of desmoplastic melanoma. Am. J. Surg. Pathol. 3: 301-311.
14. BOLANDE, R. P. 1981. Neurofibromatosis—the quintessential neurocristopathy: pathogenetic concepts and relationships. Adv. Neurol. 29: 67-75.
15. DUCATMAN, B. S., B. W. SCHEITHAUER, D. G. PIEPGRAS, & H. M. REIMAN. 1984. Malignant peripheral nerve sheath tumors in childhood. J. Neuro-Oncol. 2: 241-248.

Sulfated Proteoglycans Produced by Rat Dorsal Root Ganglion Cells

DAVID J. CAREY,[a] HEMLATA MEHTA,[b]
AND MARK S. TODD[a]

[a]Department of Physiology
Milton S. Hershey Medical Center
Pennsylvania State University
Post Office Box 850
Hershey, Pennsylvania 17033

[b]Department of Biochemistry and Molecular Biology
Louisiana State University Medical Center in Shreveport
Post Office Box 33932
Shreveport, Louisiana 71130

Proteoglycans and glycosaminoglycans are constituents of the extracellular matrix (ECM) of many tissues, where they fulfill a variety of functions, ranging from maintenance of a permeability barrier to plasma proteins in the glymerular basement membrane[1] to regulation of branching morphogenesis during the development of tissues such as the salivary gland.[2,3] Of considerable interest recently are heparan sulfate-containing proteoglycans which are found in basal laminae[4-6] and plasma membranes[7,8] of several cell types.

The ECM deposited by primary cultures of embryonic rat Schwann cells and nerve cells obtained from the dorsal root ganglion provides a convenient system for studying the biosynthesis, regulation, and function of ECM components. This matrix consists of a basal lamina with associated small-diameter fibrils which covers the outer surface of the Schwann cells.[9] In cultures that contain fibroblasts (organotypic cultures), the number and diameter of the fibrils are greater; with extended time in culture a perineurium is formed, with associated basal laminae.[10] The deposition of the Schwann cell basal lamina in culture is regulated by nerve cells and certain soluble media components.[11-14] Moreover, this ECM appears to be important for normal development, in that perturbation of ECM deposition in Schwann cell-nerve cell cultures blocks the subsequent ensheathment and myelination of axons by Schwann cells.[11,15]

Until now, biochemical studies on this ECM have focused on the protein components. Schwann cells have been shown to synthesize collagen types I, III, IV, and V as well as laminin.[9,14,16] Fibroblasts, in contrast, produce collagen types I and III and fibronectin.[16] The suspected importance of proteoglycans in other tissues has led us to investigate the biosynthesis and potential functions of proteoglycans in primary organotypic cultures of embryonic rat dorsal root ganglia. In this paper we provide evidence that these cultures synthesize several species of sulfated proteoglycans, and that inhibition of proteoglycan biosynthesis alters the development of the ganglionic nonneuronal cells.

MATERIALS AND METHODS

Cell Culture

Primary organotypic cultures were established from dorsal root ganglia of late embryonic rats. The roots and capsules were removed, and 2–4 ganglia were placed onto a substratum of pepsinized calf-skin collagen in dishes identical to the Aclar minidishes previously described.[17] The cultures were fed a medium consisting of 85% Eagles minimum essential medium, 10% human placental serum, 5% chick embryo extract, 6 mg/ml glucose, and 10 units/ml nerve growth factor.

To examine the effects of 4-methylumbelliferyl-β-D-xyloside the compound (obtained from Sigma Chemical Co., St. Louis, Mo.) was dissolved in dimethylsulfoxide at a concentration of 100 mM and diluted into culture medium to a final concentration of 1.0 mM. On day 7 and thereafter the cultures were fed medium containing 1 mM xyloside. Cultures established from the same litter of embryos and fed identical medium but lacking the xyloside derivative served as controls.

Radiolabeling

Cultures were labeled in Ham's F-12 medium supplemented with 10% dialyzed human placental serum containing 200 μCi/ml $^{35}SO_4$ (carrier free, from New England Nuclear, Boston, Mass.) for 48 hours. The medium was removed, and the cells were rinsed with 0.05 M Na-phosphate, 0.15 M NaCl, 2.5 mM phenylmethylsulfonyluoride, 10 mM EDTA, pH 7.4. The cell layers were extracted with 4 M guanidine-hydrochloride (GuHCl), 0.1% Triton X-100, 0.05 M Na-acetate, 4 mM benzamidine, 10 mM EDTA, pH 5.0.

Proteoglycan Analysis

Culture media and GuHCl extracts were applied to a 1 × 50 cm column of Sephadex G-50 and eluted with GuHCl buffer. The void volume fractions were pooled and then subjected to CsCl density gradient centrifugation in GuHCl buffer and an initial density of 1.45 g/ml. Centrifugation was in a Beckmen SW50.1 rotor at 10°C and 37,000 rpm for 65 hours. The gradients were pooled in three fractions designated low density (< 1.35 g/ml), medium density (1.35–1.45 g/ml), and high density (> 1.45 g/ml). Recoveries from gradients were greater than 90%.

These fractions were subjected to preparative gel filtration chromatography on a 1 × 100 cm column of Sepharose CL-4B eluted with GuHCl buffer. The pooled $^{35}SO_4$ peaks recovered from this column were further purified by DEAE-cellulose chromatography. Samples were dialyzed into 0.05 M tris-Cl, 4 M urea, 2 mM EDTA, 4 mM benzamidine, 0.05% Triton X-100, pH 7.4 and applied to a 1 × 16 cm column of DEAE-cellulose equilibrated in the same buffer. The column was eluted with a linear gradient of 0 to 1 M NaCl in column buffer.

Glycosaminoglycans were released from proteoglycan core proteins by hydrolysis in 0.05 M NaOH-1 M NaBH$_4$ at 45°C for 24 hours. Glycosaminoglycan fractions were subjected to specific chemical and enzymatic degradation procedures. For nitrous acid hydrolysis samples were mixed with 0.75 M sodium nitrite and 5.7 acetic acid, and incubated at room temperature for 80 minutes.[18] Chondroitinase ABC (Sigma Chemical Co., St. Louis, Mo.) digestions were performed in 0.1 M tris-Cl, 0.1 M sodium acetate, pH 7.3 at an enzyme-to-substrate ratio of 0.1 unit/mg for 2 hours at room temperature.[19] Testicular hyaluronidase (Miles Laboratories, Elkhart, Ind.) digestion was done in 0.1 M sodium phosphate, 0.15 M NaCl, pH 5.3 at a ratio of enzyme to substrate of 100 μg/mg for 18 hours at 37°C.[19] The degree of hydrolysis by these enzymes was determined by Sephadex G-50 chromatography.

Analytical gel filtration chromatography before and after alkaline hydrolysis was performed on a Sepharose CL-4B column eluted with GuHCl buffer. The column was calibrated with chondroitin sulfate chains as described by Wasteson.[20] Chondroitin sulfate was determined spectrophotometrically.[21]

Light Microscopy

Cultures were examined and photographed using a Nikon diaphot inverted microscope. In some cases cultures were fixed and stained with Sudan Black B (Fisher Scientific, Pittsburgh, Pa.) as described by Wood.[22]

RESULTS

$^{35}SO_4$ Labeling of Cultures

Primary dorsal root ganglion cultures contain sensory neurons, Schwann cells, and fibroblasts. Metabolic labeling of these cultures resulted in the incorporation of significant amounts of $^{35}SO_4$ into molecules eluting in the void volume of a Sephadex G-50 column. When cultures labeled for 48 hours were fractionated into medium, 4 M GuHCl extract of cells, and nonextractable residue, the distribution of macromolecular $^{35}SO_4$ shown in TABLE 1 was obtained. Approximately 30% of the total incorporated radioactivity was found in the medium. Of the 70% associated with the cells, approximately 75% (53% of the total $^{35}SO_4$ incorporated) was extracted by 4 M GuHCl.

The glycosaminoglycan compositions of the culture medium and 4 M GuHCl extracted $^{35}SO_4$-labeled material were determined following mild alkaline hydrolysis and selective enzymatic or chemical degradation. As shown in TABLE 2, the culture medium and 4 M GuHCl extracts of cells had similar glycosaminoglycan compositions, containing approximately 30% heparan sulfate, 65% chondroitin sulfate, and 5% dermatan sulfate. The sum of the percentages represented by each glycosaminoglycan species approximated 100% of the total incorporated $^{35}SO_4$, indicating that sulfated glycosaminoglycans (or proteoglycans) comprised nearly all of the incorporated $^{35}SO_4$. This conclusion was confirmed by sodium dodecyl sulfate (SDS)-gel electrophoresis and autoradiography (data not shown).

TABLE 1. Distribution of Macromolecular $^{35}SO_4{}^a$

Compartment	Counts per Minute per Explant	Percent of Total $^{35}SO_4{}^b$
Culture medium	1.3×10^5	30 ± 12
4 M GuHCl extract of cells	3.1×10^5	53 ± 8
Residue	0.9×10^5	17 ± 0.4

^{a} Cultures were labeled for 48 hours; average of three experiments.
^{b} Percent distribution $\pm$ standard deviation (SD).

CsCl Density Gradient Centrifugation

The $^{35}SO_4$-labeled macromolecules present in 4 M GuHCl extracts were subjected to CsCl density gradient centrifugation in the presence of 4 M GuHCl. The density distribution of $^{35}SO_4$-labeled molecules is shown in TABLE 3. The highest concentration of $^{35}SO_4$-labeled material appeared at the top of the gradient, at densities $< 1.35 g/$ ml. Only approximately 10% of the $^{35}SO_4$ material appeared in the high-density fraction (> 1.45 g/ml). That the majority of the $^{35}SO_4$-labeled material of all densities was glycosaminoglycan (presumably bound to proteoglycan) was demonstrated by the fact that the amounts of each fraction degraded by nitrous acid and chondroitinase ABC totaled approximately 100% (TABLE 3).

The density distributions of heparan sulfate and chondroitin sulfate are also shown in TABLE 3. The low-density fraction contained 84% of the total GuHCl-extractable $^{35}SO_4$-labeled heparan sulfate, whereas the high-density fraction contained only 7%. Similar to the heparan sulfate only 13% of the $^{35}SO_4$-labeled chondroitin sulfate was found in the high-density fraction, the remainder being distributed in the low- and medium-density fractions.

TABLE 2. Glycosaminoglycan Compositions of Medium and 4 M GuHCl Extracted Sulfated Proteoglycans

Compartment	Percent of Total $^{35}SO_4$ in Compartment^a		
	HS^b	CS^c	DS^d
Culture medium	29	67	5
4 M GuHCl extract of cells	28	63	6

^{a} Results are averages of three experiments.
^{b} Heparan sulfate, calculated from percent of counts per minute (cpm) susceptible to nitrous acid hydrolysis.
^{c} Chondroitin sulfate, calculated from percent of cpm susceptible to testicular hyaluronidase digestion.
^{d} Dermatan sulfate, calculated as difference between cpm digested by chondroitinase ABC and testicular hyaluronidase.

Proteoglycan Purification

The low-, medium-, and high-density fractions obtained by CsCl density gradient centrifugation were subjected to gel filtration chromatography on Sepharose Cl-4B in 4 M GuHCl buffer. FIGURE 1 shows the ^{35}S elution profiles obtained. Each fraction displayed a unique pattern of two or more peaks of radioactivity, with K_{av} ranging from 0 to 0.63.

Some of the ^{35}SO$_4$-labeled peaks obtained by Sepharose Cl-4B chromatography were further purified by DEAE-cellulose chromatography. With one exception each sample bound to DEAE-cellulose and produced a single peak of radioactivity eluting between 0.4 and 0.6 M NaCl. The low-density peak (K_{av} = 0.35) was resolved by DEAE-cellulose chromatography into two peaks of radioactivity.

TABLE 3. Density Distribution of ^{35}SO$_4$-Labeled Guanidine-HCl Extracted Macromolecules

Density (g/ml)	Percent Total^a ^{35}SO$_4$	Percent Digested by		Percent of Total Extractable Glycosaminoglycan^b	
		Nitrous Acid	Chondroitinase ABC	HS	CS
< 1.35	48	39	62	84	38
1.35–1.45	40	5	94	9	49
> 1.45	12	12	86	7	13

^{a} Of total radioactivity recovered from CsCl gradient, overall recovery was > 90%.
^{b} HS: heparan sulfate; CS: chondroitin sulfate.

Analysis of Glycosaminoglycan Chains

The ^{35}SO$_4$-labeled materials purified by DEAE-cellulose chromatography were further analyzed to determine the size and identity of the component glycosamino-glycan chains. A portion of each sample was applied directly to a 1.0 × 100 cm column of Sepharose Cl-4B equilibrated with 4 M GuHCl buffer. The remainder of each sample was subjected to mild alkaline/ borohydride hydrolysis, and a portion of each hydrolyzed sample was chromatographed on the same Sepharose Cl-4B column. The results obtained are shown in FIGURE 2. In each case, the alkaline hydrolyzed products obtained from the column eluted as single peaks which eluted later than the original unhydrolyzed samples. These results indicate the parent molecules are proteoglycans each possessing glycosaminoglycan side chains of a single size class. The K_{av} of these glycosaminoglycans ranged from 0.51 to 0.64. Calibration of the Sepharose Cl-4B column with chondroitin sulfate indicated that these represented M_r ranging from 10,000 to 40,000.

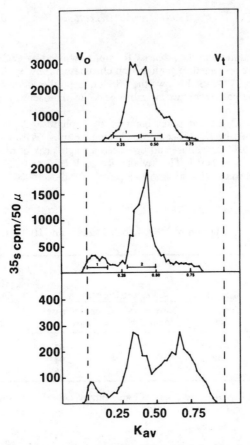

FIGURE 1. Sepharose Cl-4B chromatography of $^{35}SO_4$-labeled molecules of various densities obtained from GuHCl extracts of cells. Radiolabeled molecules of low, medium, or high density obtained by CsCl density gradient centrifugation were subjected to preparative gel filtration chromatography on Sepharose Cl-4B as described in Materials and Methods. Fraction sizes were 1 ml. Fractions were pooled as indicated in the figure. The dashed vertical lines to the left and right of each figure indicate the positions of the void volume (V_o) and total volume (V_t), respectively. Top panel, low density; middle panel, medium density; lower panel, high density.

The identities of the glycosaminoglycans released by alkaline hydrolysis from the purified proteoglycans were determined by subjecting separate aliquots to nitrous acid hydrolysis and chondroitinase ABC digestion. Representative data for one of the major species, a low-density proteoglycan which eluted from Sepharose Cl-4B at a $K_{av} = 0.35$, are shown in FIGURE 3. The data for the remaining glycosaminoglycans are summarized in TABLE 4. Of the five proteoglycans that were examined, one contained predominantly heparan sulfate; the other four contained predominantly chondroitin sulfate. All of these chondroitin sulfate-containing proteoglycans contained, in addition, some heparan sulfate, ranging from 20% to 30% of the total ^{35}S in each proteoglycan. These five species accounted for approximately 75% of the total GuHCl extractable ^{35}S.

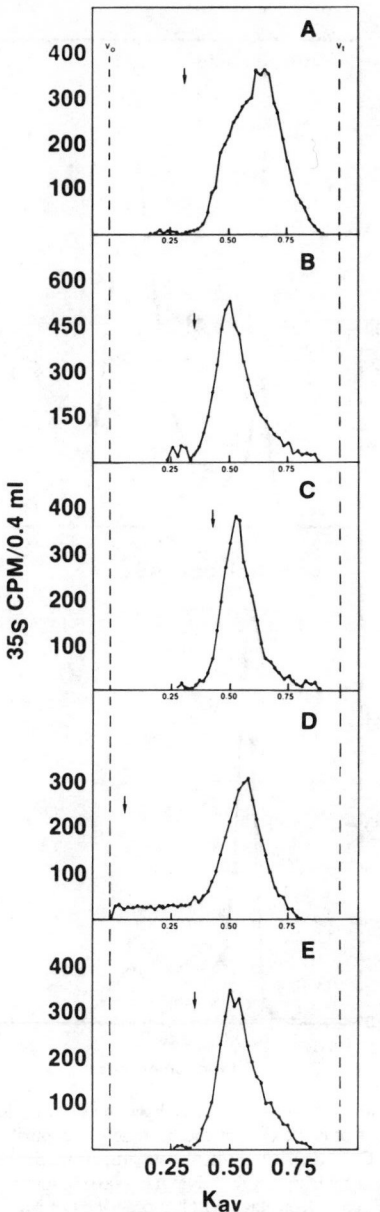

FIGURE 2. Sepharose Cl-4B chromatography of $^{35}SO_4$-labeled glycosaminoglycans. The $^{35}SO_4$-labeled proteoglycans obtained after DEAE-cellulose chromatography were hydrolyzed in NaOH/NaBH$_4$ as described in Materials and Methods, and a portion applied to a Sepharose Cl-4B column equilibrated and eluted with GuHCl buffer. Fraction sizes were 1 ml. The dashed vertical lines to the left and right of each figure indicate the void volume (V_o) and the total volume (V_t) of the column, respectively. Vertical arrows indicate the positions of elution of the purified samples before alkaline hydrolysis. Panels a, b, and c were obtained from low-density proteoglycans, panels d and e from medium-density proteoglycans.

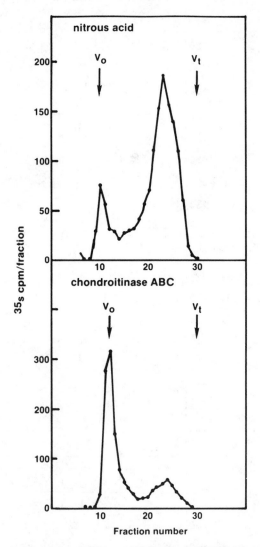

FIGURE 3. Nitrous acid and chondroitinase ABC digestion of $^{35}SO_4$-labeled glycosaminoglycan obtained from GuHCl extract of cells. One of the proteoglycans purified from a GuHCl extract of $^{35}SO_4$-labeled cultures by CsCl density gradient centrifugation, Sepharose Cl-4B, and DEAE-cellulose chromatography was hydrolyzed with $NaOH/NaBH_4$, and separate aliquots incubated either in nitrous acid or with chondroitinase ABC as described in Materials and Methods. After these incubations the material was applied to a Sephadex G-50 column. The sample illustrated is obtained from the low-density fraction of the GuHCl extract, which eluted in the first peaks after Sepharose Cl-4B and DEAE-cellulose chromatography. The vertical arrows to the left and right indicate the void volume (V_0) and the total volume (V_t) of the column. Fraction sizes were 1 ml.

TABLE 4. Properties of Sulfated Proteoglycans Extracted with Guanidine HCl from Dorsal Root Ganglion Cultures

	Proteoglycan	Glycosaminoglycan		
Density[a]	K_{av} on Sepharose Cl-4B	K_{av} on Sepharose Cl-4B	Composition[b]	Percent of Total $^{35}SO_4$[c]
Medium	0.36	0.53	CS:HS(4:1)	30
Low	0.44	0.54	CS:HS(4:1)	20
Low	0.35	0.64	HS:CS(4:1)	10
Low	0.35	0.51	CS:HS(4:1)	10
Medium	0.06	0.57	CS:HS(4:1)	5

[a] From CsCl density gradient centrifugation; see Materials and Methods for definitions.
[b] CS, chondroitin sulfate; HS, heparan sulfate; ratio in parentheses.
[c] Percent of total in GuHCl extract.

Effect of 4-Methylumbelliferyl-β-D-xyloside

To determine whether the production of these proteoglycans is important for the development of dorsal root ganglion cells, we tested the effects of adding to the medium of these cultures an inhibitor of proteoglycan bisynthesis, 4-methylumbelliferyl-β-D-xyloside. The drug was added on day 7, and the cells were grown for an additional three weeks. The effect of the xyloside derivative on the accumulation of $^{35}SO_4$-labeled macromolecules in the cultures is shown in TABLE 5. Xyloside caused a nearly twofold increase in the amount of macromolecular ^{35}S in the culture medium and an approximately 80% reduction in macromolecular ^{35}S in GuHCl extracts of cells. A similar effect of β-D-xyloside derivatives has been noted for other cells.[3,23]

In xyloside-treated cultures all of the ^{35}S radioactivity in the medium eluted on Sepharose Cl-4B as a single peak ($K_{av} = 0.7$) representing free glycosaminoglycans. No material eluting as proteoglycans was observed. In the GuHCl-extracted material, approximately half of the ^{35}S radioactivity eluted as free glycosaminoglycans ($K_{av} = 0.7$) with the remainder eluting at earlier positions (FIGURE 4). These earlier eluting molecules in xyloside-treated cultures could be either proteoglycans or sulfated glycoprotein (e.g., laminin). Assuming these are proteoglycans, this result and the data in TABLE 5 indicate that $^{35}SO_4$-labeled proteoglycan accumulation in the ECM of these cultures was inhibited by 90%.

TABLE 5. Effect of 4-Methylumbelliferyl-β-D-xyloside on the Accumulation of $^{35}SO_4$-Labeled Macromolecules

	Macromolecular $^{35}SO_4$[a] (cpm/culture)		
Compartment	Control	Xyloside[b]	Xyloside/Control
Culture medium	9.23×10^5	1.66×10^6	1.8
Guanidine extract of cells	1.24×10^6	2.18×10^5	0.18

[a] Cultures labeled for 48 hours with $^{35}SO_4$ beginning on day 21 in culture.
[b] Treated with 1 mM 4-methylumbelliferyl-β-D-xyloside from day 7 to day 23 in culture.

We next examined cultures to determine what, if any, developmental abnormalities were produced. Treatment with xyloside had no observable effect on the nerve cells. For example, neither nerve cell survival nor the extent or rate of neurite growth in the presence of the drug was significantly altered compared to controls (data not shown).

During the growth of these ganglia in culture, fibroblast-like cells migrate out of the ganglia and proliferate, forming a carpet of cells that eventually covers the entire

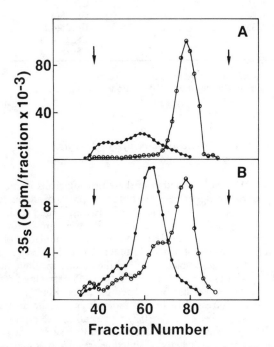

FIGURE 4: Effect of 4-methylumbelliferyl-β-D-xyloside on proteoglycan biosynthesis. Beginning on day 7 cultures were fed medium containing 1 mM 4-methylumbelliferyl-β-D-xyloside. After an additional two weeks, the cultures were labeled with $^{35}SO_4$ in the presence of the drug, and the radiolabeled macromolecules in the culture medium (panel a) and 4 M guanidine-HCl extracts (panel b) were subjected to Sepharose Cl-4B chromatography as described in Materials and Methods. Sibling cultures treated identically but not given the drug served as controls. Equal amounts of $^{35}SO_4$-labeled macromolecules from drug-treated ($\bigcirc$) and control cultures ($\bullet$) were chromatographed on the same column. The arrows indicate excluded and included volumes of the column.

surface of the culture dish. Some of these cells eventually form a perineurium around the nerve fiber–Schwann cell bundles.[10] In two-week-old control cultures, the extent of radial migration of this carpet of cells was reduced slightly by the drug.

In addition, these cells exhibited altered morphology. In control cultures these cells tended to be elongated, aligning themselves parallel to the nerve fiber bundles (FIGURE 5c). In cultures treated with xyloside these cells were less elongated and more cuboidal and were oriented in a more random manner in relation to the nerve fiber bundles (FIGURE 5d). In xyloside-treated cultures the fiber bundles themselves

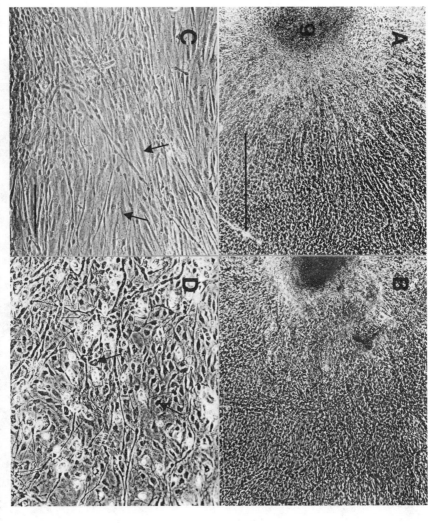

FIGURE 5: Effect of β-D-xyloside on organotypic dorsal root ganglion cultures. Control cultures (a and c) and cultures treated with 1 mM β-D-xyloside (b and d) were photographed with phase contrast optics in the living state at two weeks in culture. Note the more random pattern of fiber growth and altered morphology of fibroblastic cells in xyloside-treated cultures. G = ganglion; arrows, fibroblastic cells. Bar in (a) equals 1 mm; Bar in (c) equals 100 μm.

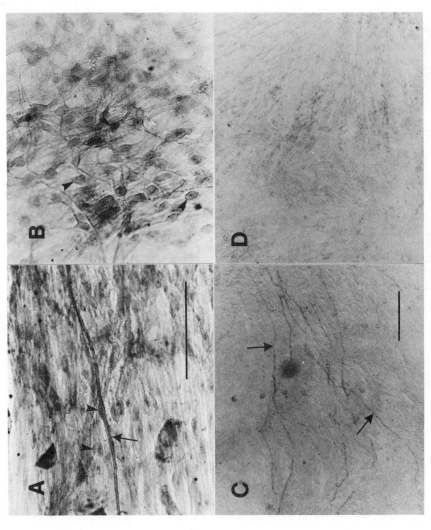

FIGURE 6. Effect of β-D-xyloside on myelin formation. Control cultures (a, c) and cultures treated with 1 mM β-D-xyloside beginning on day 7 (b, d) were analyzed for myelin formation at three weeks (a, b) and four weeks (c, d). The three-week cultures were fixed and stained with Sudan Black B. Four-week-old cultures were photographed with bright field optics in the living state. Arrows, myelin segments; arrowheads, Schwann cell nuclei. Note the absence of myelin in xyloside-treated cultures. Bar in (a) equals 100 μm; Bar in (c) equals 200 μm.

exhibited a less ordered pattern of growth compared to control cultures (FIGURE 5a-d, FIGURE 6a and b).

In control organotypic cultures, myelination of axons by Schwann cells was visible with the light microscope at approximately three weeks in culture (FIGURE 6a), and by four weeks in culture the amount of myelin formed was significant (FIGURE 6c). In cultures treated with 1 mM β-D-xyloside, however, we observed no myelin formation up to four weeks in culture (FIGURE 6b and d), the longest period examined.

DISCUSSION

The results presented in this paper demonstrate that cultured cells obtained from the embryonic peripheral nervous system synthesize and incorporate into the ECM a variety of sulfated proteoglycans. Evidence obtained from $^{35}SO_4$ labeling, CsCl density gradient centrifugation, and Sepharose C1-4B chromatography suggests the presence of as many as eight distinct proteoglycan species in 4 M GuHCl extracts of cells. Approximately 30% of the total $^{35}SO_4$ was incorporated into heparan sulfate, with the remainder present mostly in chondroitin sulfate. Five of the major ^{35}S-labeled proteoglycans, together comprising three-fourths of the total $^{35}SO_4$ incorporated, were further analyzed. One of these contained predominantly heparan sulfate; the others contained predominantly chondroitin sulfate. It should be pointed out that while the cell extractions were performed in the presence of protease inhibitors and in denaturing solvents, it is possible that several of the chondroitin sulfate proteoglycans observed were derived by proteolysis from a single larger species. The similarities of glycosaminoglycans of several of the purified proteoglycans are consistent with this possibility. Further structural and biosynthetic studies will be required to clarify this point.

The data presented here extend previous studies which have shown that the ECM produced in culture is essential for normal Schwann cell development.[11,12,15] The experiments in which proteoglycan biosynthesis was inhibited by 4-methylumbelliferyl-β-D-xyloside suggest a possible role for proteoglycans in the development of endoneurial and/or perineurial fibroblasts as well as in myelin formation by Schwann cells. A precise description of the roles played by proteoglycans in these processes, however, must await further experimentation. Functions ascribed to proteoglycans in other tissues include maintenance of a permeability barrier in the glomerular basement membrane,[4] regulation of morphogenesis in branched epithelial tissue,[2,3] and activity as a neurite-outgrowth-promoting factor for a variety of neurons.[23]

Experiments in which the individual cell types present in dorsal root ganglia have been cultured either alone or in combination have shown that Schwann cells synthesize collagen types I, III, IV, and V[9,14] and laminin[16] and that fibroblasts synthesize collagen types I and III (Carey, Eldridge, and Bunge, unpublished observations) and fibronectin.[16] Sensory neurons in culture do not synthesize significant amounts of any of these ECM components although their presence is required for formation of this endoneurial-like ECM in culture.[13] Experiments to determine which cells in the cultures are responsible for synthesizing the individual proteoglycans are under way. For example, in cultures of Schwann cells and neurons (devoid of fibroblasts), the low-density heparan sulfate proteoglycan extracted by GuHCl is present whereas the two medium-density chondroitin sulfate proteoglycans are absent.[24]

The structural heterogeneity of proteoglycans raises several interesting questions concerning their biosynthesis, e.g., do different cells use the same or different core proteins to produce structurally similar but not identical proteoglycans? Also, what regulates such factors as the length and number of glycosaminoglycan side chains? The availability of this culture system should allow us to begin to address some of these important questions concerning regulation of proteoglycan metabolism and the functions of proteoglycans.

SUMMARY

Primary organotypic cultures of embryonic rat dorsal root ganglia, which contain sensory neurons, Schwann cells, and fibroblasts, produce an extensive extracellular matrix. These cultures actively incorporated $^{35}SO_4$ into glycosaminoglycans, of which 30% were heparan sulfate, 65% chondroitin sulfate, and 5% dermatan sulfate. Sulfate-labeled proteoglycans made by these cells were extracted with 4 M guanidine-hydrochloride and purified by CsCl density gradient centrifugation, gel filtration chromatography, and DEAE-cellulose chromatography. Eight individual species were resolved, of which five were subjected to further analysis. One low-density (< 1.35 g/ml) proteoglycan, with a K_{av} on Sepharose Cl-4B $= 0.34$ contained heparan sulfate chains of $M_r = 20,000$. The other four proteoglycans, with K_{av} on Sepharose Cl-4B of 0.04, 0.35 (two), and 0.44, contained predominantly chondroitin sulfate chains with M_r ranging from 30,000 to 40,000. To determine possible functions of these proteoglycans, cultures were grown in medium containing 1 mM 4-methyl-umbelliferyl-β-D-xyloside. The drug inhibited $^{35}SO_4$ proteoglycan accumulation in the cell layer by approximately 90%. Drug-treated cultures exhibited several developmental abnormalities, including decreased migration of fibroblast-like cells, abnormal morphology of these cells, and decreased myelination of axons by Schwann cells.

REFERENCES

1. KANWAR, Y., A. LINKER & M. FARQUHAR. 1980. J. Cell. Biol. **86:** 688-693.
2. BERNFIELD, M. & S. BANNERJEE. 1982. Dev. Biol. **90:** 291-305.
3. THOMPSON, H. & B. SPOONER. 1982. Dev. Biol. **89:** 417-424.
4. KANWAR, Y. & M. FARQUHAR. 1979. Proc. Nat. Acad. Sci. USA **76:** 1303-1307.
5. HASSELL, J., P. ROBEY, H. BARRACH, J. WILCZEK, S. RENNARD & G. MARTIN. 1980. Proc. Nat. Acad. Sci. USA **77:** 4494-4498.
6. LAURIE, G. W., C. P. LeBLOND & G. MARTIN. 1980. J. Cell. Biol. **95:** 340-344.
7. OLDBERG, A., L. KJELLEN & M. HOOK. 1979. J. Biol. Chem. **254:** 8505-8510.
8. RAPRAEGER, A. & M. BERNFIELD. 1983. J. Biol. Chem. **258:** 3632-3636.
9. BUNGE, M., A. WILLIAMS, P. WOOD, J. UITTO & J. JEFFREY. 1980. J. Cell Biol. **84:** 184-202.
10. BUNGE, M., R. BUNGE, E. PETERSON & M. MURRAY. 1967. J. Cell biol. **32:** 439-466.
11. MOYA, F., M. BUNGE & R. BUNGE. 1980. Proc. Nat. Acad. Sci. USA **77:** 6902-6906.
12. CAREY, D. & R. BUNGE. 1981. J. Cell Biol. **91:** 666-672.
13. BUNGE, M., A. WILLIAMS & P. WOOD. 1982. Dev. Biol. **92:** 449-460.
14. CAREY, D., C. ELDRIDGE, C. CORNBROOKS, R. TIMPL & R. BUNGE. 1983. J. Cell Biol. **97:** 493-479.
15. COPIO, D. & M. BUNGE. 1980. J. Cell Biol. **87:** 114 (abstr).

16. CORNBROOKS, C., D. CAREY, J. MCDONALD, R. TIMPL & R. BUNGE. 1983. Proc. Nat. Acad. Sci. USA **80:** 3850-3854.
17. BUNGE, R. & P. WOOD. 1973. Brain Res. **57:** 261-276.
18. GLIMELIUS, B., B. NORLING, B. WESTERMARK & A. WASTESON. 1978. Biochem. J. **172:** 443-456.
19. YANAGISHITA, M. & V. HASCALL. 1979. J. Biol. Chem. **254:** 12354-12355.
20. WASTESON, A. 1971. J. Chromatogr. **59:** 87-97.
21. GOLD, E. 1979. Anal. Biochem. **99:** 183-188.
22. WOOD, P. 1976. Brain Res. **115:** 361-375.
23. LANDER, A., D. FUJII, D. GOSPODAROWICZ & L. REICHARDT. 1982. J. Cell Biol. **94:** 574-585.
24. MEHTA, H, C. ORPHE, M. S. TODD, C. J. CORNBROOKS & D. J. CAREY. 1985. J. Cell Biol. **101:** 660-666.

Schwann Cell Proliferation *In Vitro*

An Overview

NANCY RATNER,[a,b] RICHARD P. BUNGE,[a]
AND LUIS GLASER[b]

[a]Department of Anatomy and Neurobiology
[b]Department of Biological Chemistry
Division of Biology and Biomedical Sciences
Washington University School of Medicine
St. Louis, Missouri 63110

Neurofibromas are characterized by an abnormal proliferation of Schwann cells and accumulation of extracellular matrix material in peripheral nerves. Schwann cells ordinarily undergo proliferation during two stages of functional expression: (1) in development during population of peripheral nerves with Schwann cells prior to myelination;[1,2] and (2) following damage to the peripheral nerve, in the process of Wallerian degeneration.[3] During the developmental phase, Schwann cells are also active in producing extracellular matrix material.[4]

The use of an *in vitro* system in which pure populations of primary Schwann cells proliferate at a very low level until stimulated by mitogen has enabled characterization of several Schwann cell mitogens. We have been studying factors that regulate normal Schwann cell proliferation, and have characterized mitogenic molecules for Schwann cells present on the surface of neurons. One of these molecules is a heparan sulfate proteoglycan, presumably related in structure to materials present in the extracellular matrix. We are hopeful the mitogen we are studying in tissue culture may correspond to mitogen(s) that stimulate Schwann cell division during embryogenesis. In this brief paper we will review methods used to study Schwann cell mitogens, discuss both soluble and insoluble mitogens, and review known responses of Schwann cells to these agents. The unexpected finding of proteoglycan involvement in mitogenesis raises the question of a possible linkage between abnormal Schwann cell proliferation and extracellular matrix deposition in neurofibromatosis, as we will discuss below.

METHODS OF SCHWANN CELL PREPARATION

All of the *in vitro* work on Schwann cell division that we will discuss has been carried out using embryonic or neonatal Schwann cells obtained from rodents. The Schwann cell populations usually are 95-99% pure, with fibroblasts as the major contaminant. The latter can be recognized on the basis of their large size (relative to Schwann cells) and their ability to be stained by antibodies to thy1.1[5] and fibronectin.[6]

Three procedures have been designed to obtain purified Schwann cell populations. In the first,[7,8] embryonic rat dorsal root ganglia (from embryonal day 15 to 20) are removed from the animal and allowed to form a neuritic outgrowth in the presence of the antimitotic agent fluorodeoxyuridine, which kills rapidly dividing fibroblasts (and some Schwann cells) but not postmitotic neurons. After 1-2 weeks, such ganglia are transplanted onto fresh substrate and allowed to regenerate neurites. Schwann cells resident within the explant which have escaped the antimitotic treatment emerge from the ganglia and populate the outgrowing neurites. After about one month, removal of the explant (and thus all neuronal cell bodies) from this type of culture provides, after harvest of the outgrowth zone, a Schwann cell population of approximately 10^5 cells. Schwann cells can be identified by their alignment with neurite bundles (when present), staining with antilaminin antibodies,[6] and their ensheathment and myelination of neurons.[8] In the other two types of preparations, Schwann cells are isolated from neonatal rat or mouse sciatic nerves. Brockes and his colleagues enzymatically dissociate rat sciatic nerves,[5] which are approximately 85% Schwann cells at this age,[1] plate the derived cells, and kill many of the fibroblasts present by treatment for three days in 10^{-5} M cytosine arabinoside. Residual fibroblasts are killed by treatment with anti-thy1.1 antibody and rabbit complement.[5] A typical preparation of this type yields a minimum of 10^6 purified Schwann cells (up to 99.5% pure) per 20 sciatic nerves after only 4 days. These Schwann cells can be passaged *in vitro;* after several passages they retain their ability to interact with and myelinate dorsal root ganglion (DRG) neurons.[9] Both these methods have been criticized because the use of antimitotic agents may select a subpopulation of slowly dividing Schwann cells, but it should be noted that Schwann cells, subsequent to this treatment, are able to express all known Schwann cell functions, including myelination.[8,9] Pleasure and his collaborators have utilized the fact that fibroblasts in sciatic nerve preparations adhere more firmly to polylysine-covered glass than do Schwann cells to enrich for nonadherent Schwann cells, which can be replated onto poly-D-lysine and shown by immunofluorescent criteria to be at least 95% pure;[10] manipulation of media components is used to inhibit fibroblast proliferation.[11]

Schwann cells isolated by these three methods all divide very slowly in tissue culture, with a doubling time of 8 days[12] to 2 weeks[11] in the presence of 10% fetal calf serum, indicating that potential mitogens present in serum are insufficient to stimulate Schwann cell proliferation.

SCHWANN CELL PROLIFERATION ASSAY

The response of Schwann cells to mitogens is usually measured by the incorporation of [^{3}H]thymidine into DNA, determined either by autoradiography (fraction of cells with labeled nuclei) or by measurement of acid-insoluble radioactivity. These assays measure the ability of the mitogen to bring the cell into the S phase of growth. A more direct assay of mitogenicity is the more tedious measurement of increase in cell numbers, and most investigators have attempted to demonstrate that cell number increases on addition of mitogen in at least some experiments. Direct counting of Schwann cells using a hemocytometer,[12] or counting of fixed and stained Schwann cells,[13] which allows simultaneous demonstration of cell type using anti-Schwann cell antibody staining, corroborates results of experiments in which [^{3}H]thymidine is used as a marker for newly synthesized DNA. In these experiments, 24-48 hours following the addition of labeled thymidine, cells are either solubilized[14] or trypsinized from the substrate[11] and counted on filters in a scintillation cocktail. This technique generates data that can be misleading if cell number varies from sample to sample for any reason, and are liable to misinterpretation if cultures retain dividing fibroblasts. Therefore, several groups have analyzed the incorporation of [³H]thymidine into Schwann cell DNA by fixation of cultures followed by whole-mount autoradiography.[14–17] The percent of Schwann cells incorporating label is presented as a percentage of the total cells counted; contaminating fibroblasts, if present, can be identified and excluded from the count. Finally, DeVries et al. used the fluorescently activated cell sorter to demonstrate that when Schwann cells are stimulated to incorporate [³H]thymidine, the fraction of cells in the population in the S phase of the cell cycle also increases, with a concomitant decrease in the percent of cells in the G_o/G_1 phase,[17] thereby demonstrating that DNA repair mechanisms cannot account for uptake of [³H]thymidine into Schwann cell nuclei.

AGENTS THAT ARE NOT SCHWANN CELL MITOGENS

In addition to growth factors present in serum such as epidermal growth factor (EGF), platelet-derived growth factor (PDGF), and fibroblast growth factor (FGF),[18] many hormones, growth factors, and compounds known to stimulate cell division in other systems have been tested as potential Schwann cell mitogens. In one study, Concanavalin A, phytohemagglutinin, nerve growth factor (NGF), EGF, FGF, acetylcholine, norepinephrine, insulin, proinsulin, dexamethasone, PGF_{28}, arachidonic acid, ouabain, and trypsin were all found to be inactive.[8] Raff et al. were unable to show any mitogenic activity of luteotropic hormone, follicle-stimulating hormone, thyroid-stimulating hormone, growth hormone, adrenocorticotropic hormone, vasopressin, prolactin, luteinizing hormone, prostaglandin E_1, or isoproterenol at concentrations up to 50 μg/ml.[12] DeVries et al. showed that gangliosides (mixed, from bovine brain), heparin, cGMP, myelin basic protein, and plasma membranes from rat liver were also not mitogenic for isolated Schwann cells.[17] Sobue et al. isolated membrane fractions from rat skeletal muscle, erythrocytes, and mitochondria; none of these membrane fractions was mitogenic for Schwann cells.[13] Particulate fractions from fibroblasts (3T3) cells and from several neuroblastomas, as well as from embryonic central nervous system (CNS), were also nonmitogenic.[19]

Recently, however, we have found that particulate fractions from embryonic CNS are mitogenic, although less mitogenic than DRG-derived membranes.[26] Pure pituitary FGF also appears to be mitogenic for Schwann cells when assayed in the presence of serum.

MEMBRANE-ASSOCIATED SCHWANN CELL MITOGENS

Most mitogenic molecules that have been well characterized are soluble; an example is platelet-derived growth factor.[20] In contrast, the surface of neurons and/or their axons contain one or more molecules mitogenic for Schwann cells.[19] The original observations establishing this extraordinary intercellular signaling were made on rat sensory neurons[21] and on chick autonomic neurons[22] cocultured with Schwann cells. The motivation for testing various membrane fractions for their mitogenicity came from the results of Wood and Bunge, who demonstrated that growing dorsal root ganglia neurities would stimulate the incorporation of [³H]thymidine into quiescent Schwann cells.[21] This observation was followed by the demonstration that a permeable collagen membrane interposed between neuron and Schwann cell prevented transmission of the mitogenic signal, implying that a membrane-associated mitogen on the surface of the neuron was responsible for stimulating Schwann cell division.[19] This hypothesis was strengthened by a series of experiments in which membranes derived from dorsal root ganglia neurites were shown to mimic the effect of the intact neuron in stimulating Schwann cell division.[15] In FIGURE 1 we illustrate the results of an

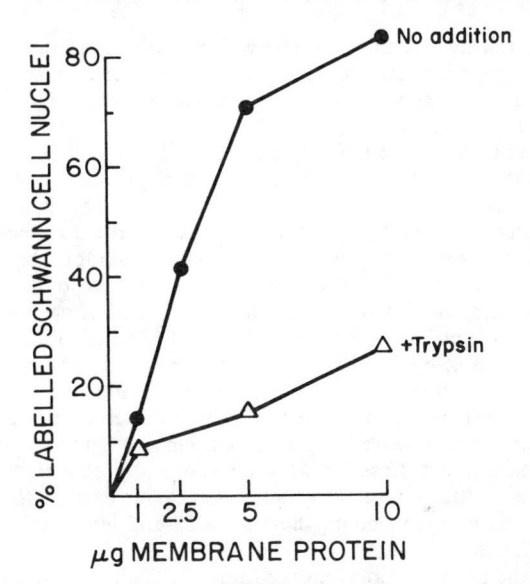

FIGURE 1. Schwann cell response to DRG-derived membranes. Dorsal root ganglion were dissociated and grown in culture for one month as described.[24] Membranes were prepared from these neurons either without (no addition) or following (+ trypsin) digestion of the cell surface with 0.1% trypsin in Ca^{2+}-Mg^{2+} free Hanks salt solution for 30 minutes at 35°C. Enzyme digestion was stopped by addition of a 10-fold excess of soybean trypsin inhibitor prior to isolation of membranes. Freshly prepared membranes were added to replated Schwann cells, isolated by the procedure of Brockes *et al.*,[5] and Schwann cell nuclei incorporating [³H]thymidine from 16-40 hours after initial membrane addition were assayed by autoradiography as described.[16]

experiment to show the effect of neurite membranes on Schwann cell proliferation. This experiment demonstrates that treatment of the neuronal cell surface with trypsin prior to isolation of membranes inhibits the mitogenicity of the membranes, indicating that the mitogen is located on the cell surface and that it is sensitive to trypsin.[14–16] This system is unique in several ways. First, growth of Schwann cells will be constrained to the vicinity of appropriate axons. Second, it is one of the few well-characterized examples where specific cell-cell contact is required to elicit a metabolic response.

We have recently shown that a neuronal cell surface heparan sulfate proteoglycan is a component of the mitogenic signal by using a class of biosynthetic inhibitors (the

β-D-xylosides) that inhibit the addition of glycosaminoglycan chains to proteoglycan core proteins,[23] and appear to inhibit the transport of the core protein to the cell surface.[24] Treatment of cultures of Schwann cells and neurons with 4-me-umbelliferyl-β-D-xyloside abolishes the mitogenic response (FIGURE 2). A series of experiments demonstrates that the effect of the β-D-xyloside is on the neuron rather than the Schwann cell, implying that a proteoglycan on the neuronal surface is required for the mitogenic response.[24] Treatment of neurons with heparitinase decreases their mitogenicity, suggesting that the neuronal mitogen requires a cell surface heparan sulfate for activity. Membranes from β-D-xyloside-treated neurites or heparatinase-treated neurons elicit a diminished mitogenic response. Whether the heparan-containing proteoglycan is the mitogen on the neuronal surface or is part of a macro-molecular complex required to elicit the mitogenic response requires purification of this molecule.

To initiate purification of this molecule we have solubilized the mitogenic activity from dorsal root ganglion neurons, and purified the molecule 100-fold over crude membranes; the molecule appears to remain soluble after removal from the membrane, as expected for a proteoglycan.[25]

Although axons within the CNS do not normally contact Schwann cells, it has been observed that neurites of embryonic retinal ganglion cells in culture can stimulate Schwann cell proliferation.[26] It is possible that some CNS cell types, as yet unidentified, could be stimulated to divide by the presence of the neuronal surface mitogen. Axo-lemmal membranes derived from myelinated axons from adult rat brain also stimulate Schwann cell proliferation.[13,14,17,27-30] The extent of inactivation of the axolemmal fraction by heat treatment is somewhat variable. Sobue *et al.* show a 60% decrease in activity after 1 minute at 70°C,[13] similar to the 60-70% inactivation shown by Cassel *et al.* after 10 minutes of heat treatment,[14] but DeVries *et al.* observed no diminution of activity after 10 minutes at 100°C.[17] The brain axolemmal fraction is unable to stimulate Schwann cell proliferation in the absence of serum, while the dorsal root ganglia-derived mitogen is active[14] in the Bottenstein and Sato[31] serum-free, hormon-ally supplemented medium. Cassel *et al.* show essentially no activity of bovine axo-lemma membranes in the absence of serum,[14] and Sobue *et al.*, although they claim some activity in serum-free medium, show 3- to 20-fold less activity than in any of their other experiments.[13]

The cells of the pheochromocytoma cell line, PC12, in response to nerve growth factor, extend axons.[32] Schwann cells align along these neurites,[33] and are stimulated to divide in the presence or absence of serum in the medium.[16] However, membrane fractions derived from these cells are essentially nonmitogenic in the absence of serum.[16] It therefore seems plausible that, during isolation of membranes from PC12 cells and perhaps also bovine axolemma, a component of the mitogen becomes lost or inacti-vated. An indication of partial inactivation of the axolemmal mitogen during isolation is the lack of enrichment of mitogenic activity in the axolemmal fraction over brain or white matter homogenate.[13,14]

ARE MEMBRANE-ASSOCIATED SCHWANN CELL
MITOGENS IDENTICAL?

Three membrane-associated mitogens have been identified: (1) the mitogen from sensory neurons, which is sensitive to heat and trypsin, is active in the absence of

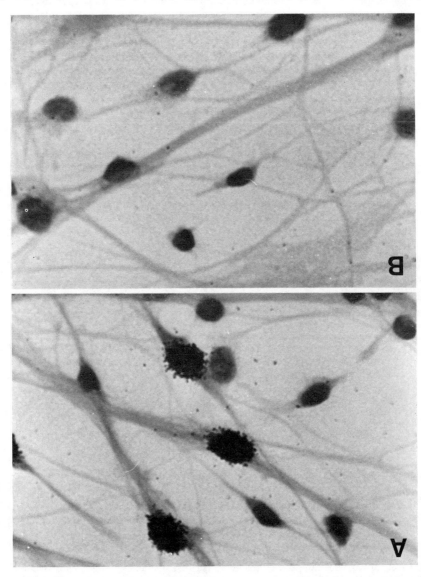

FIGURE 2. Treatment with 1 mM 4-methylumbelliferyl-β-D-xyloside decreases the fraction of proliferating Schwann cells in neuron-Schwann cell cultures. (A) Bright field photomicrograph of toluidine blue-stained autoradiograph of a control neuron-Schwann cell culture. Neurite bundles are shown, with Schwann cell nuclei, both labeled and unlabeled, associated with fascicles. (B) Parallel culture treated for 72 hours with 1 mM 4-methylumbelliferyl-β-D-xyloside prior to fixation and autoradiography. Schwann cells are associated with neurites as in the control, yet few labeled nuclei are observed.

serum, is an intrinsic membrane protein, and has a proteoglycan component; (2) the mitogen from adult CNS myelinated axons, which is partially sensitive to heat and trypsin, is probably an intrinsic membrane protein since it is very resistant to solubilization, and is inactive in the absence of serum; and (3) the PC12 mitogen, which is sensitive to heat and trypsin, is an intrinsic membrane protein, but loses its ability to stimulate Schwann cell division in the absence of serum when it is presented as a membrane fraction rather than as intact cells. The data in TABLE 1 demonstrate that the mitogen on the surface of PC12 cells is at least in part sensitive to the inhibitor 4-methylumbelliferyl-β-D-xyloside, another indication that this molecule is similar to the dorsal root ganglion mitogen.

The mitogen active during the development of the peripheral nervous system is probably that present on sensory neurons in culture; the identity of this molecule with similar molecules derived from PC12 cells and adult axolemma has yet to be rigorously demonstrated.

TABLE 1. Inhibition of PC12 Cell-Stimulated Schwann Cell Proliferation by an Inhibitor of Proteoglycan Biosynthesis[a]

| | Percent Labeled Schwann Cells | | | |
| | Exp. 1 | Exp. 2 | Exp. 3 | |
	3 Days	3 Days	3 Days	7 Days
Control	11.5	17.6	22.1	17.9
+ 1 mM 4-methylumbelliferyl-β-D-xyloside	4.2	9.7	9.6	6.9
Percent control	36.5	55.1	43.4	38.5

[a] PC12 cells were plated onto ammoniated rat tail collagen and allowed to grow neurites in the presence of serum-free media with NGF for 2 weeks. Schwann cells derived from dorsal root ganglia or sciatic nerves were then added to cultures for 5–7 days. Inhibitor was added to duplicate cultures for the indicated number of days. [³H]Thymidine was added for the final 24 hours of coculture prior to fixation and autoradiography as described.[24] For comparison, dorsal root ganglion neurons in coculture with Schwann cells are inhibited over 80% by 3-day exposure to β-D-xyloside.[24] Schwann cells not contacted by PC12 neurites had labeling indices of less than 0.8% in all experiments.

In the developing nerve, Schwann cells remain in close apposition to the outgrowing neurites, adhere to the neurites, and are stimulated to divide. Adhesion between neuron and Schwann cell is a specific interaction separable from mitogenicity and demonstrable by cell-cell interactions in tissue culture for DRG neurons,[8,15,19,21] PC12 cells,[16] spinal cord neurons,[26] and retinal neurons.[26] Specific adhesion between neuronal membranes and Schwann cells can be demonstrated by autoradiography in that [¹²⁵I]-axolemmal fragments bind only to Schwann cells, and not to fibroblasts in the same culture,[30] which may be an *in vitro* model of the *in vivo* cell-cell interaction. The mitogenic and cell adhesion molecules on the neurite surface may be different, based on the fact that in the presence of the drug 4-methylumbelliferyl-β-D-xyloside, the proteoglycan required for the mitogenic response is present in greatly reduced amounts (10–20% of control levels) on the neuronal cell surface, yet adhesion between neuron and Schwann cell is, as judged by morphological observations, normal.[24]

SCHWANN CELL DIVISION DURING WALLERIAN DEGENERATION

The mitogen that stimulates Schwann cell proliferation during Wallerian degeneration appears to be distinct from membrane-associated mitogens. Following crushes of peripheral nerves, Schwann cells proliferate, and more proliferation occurs in more highly myelinated nerves.[34,35] Salzer and Bunge have shown, in an *in vitro* model of Wallerian degeneration, that it is the myelin-associated Schwann cells that incorporate [³H]thymidine following nerve injury.[8] Furthermore, several groups have shown that isolated CNS-derived myelin fractions are mitogenic for isolated Schwann cells.[14,27,29] This myelin fraction stimulates Schwann cell proliferation with a different initial rate than does axolemma and is sensitive to a lysosomal inhibitor, ammonium chloride, whereas axolemmal-stimulated proliferation is not.[29] Furthermore, saturating concentrations of myelin stimulate Schwann cell proliferation to a level only 50% that observed at saturating concentrations of axolemmal fragments. While a mechanistic interpretation of these observations is not yet possible, taken together they indicate that a component that fractionates with CNS myelin provides the stimulus for Schwann cell division during Wallerian degeneration, and is probably unrelated to the developmentally expressed mitogens.

EXTRACELLULAR MATRIX AND SCHWANN CELL PROLIFERATION

A third class of Schwann cell mitogens has been studied in the laboratory of Monique Dubois-Dalcq. Since it has been shown that Schwann cells in culture secrete basal lamina components,[6,36-40] and the Schwann cell-neuron unit is surrounded by a basal lamina *in vivo*, the influence of several basal lamina components on Schwann cell growth was investigated. Both fibronectin[41] and laminin[42] have been reported to generate increases in numbers of isolated rat Schwann cells. Levels of laminin necessary to stimulate cell division were quite high (50-250 μg/ml),[42] much higher levels than are necessary to optimally stimulate neurite outgrowth (10 μg/ml), for example.[43] It is also clear that the laminin found on Schwann cell surfaces in tissue culture[6,42] and the fibronectin on primary rat fibroblasts in the same culture dishes[6] are insufficient to stimulate Schwann cell division. However, the proliferation of many cells is influenced by contact with extracellular matrix.[44] Isolated oligodendrocytes, the myelin-producing cells of the CNS, are stimulated to divide when in contact with extracellular matrix material from bovine corneal epithelial cells.[45] Results from this laboratory have shown that Schwann cells can also be stimulated to divide when plated onto the extracellular matrix provided by embryonic rat Reichert's membrane.[46] Since *in vivo* Schwann cells do not proliferate when in contact with their own basal lamina (except, as discussed above, during Wallerian degeneration), these results do not appear to be related to normal Schwann cell proliferation. In neurofibromatosis, however, abnormal basal lamina is formed close to Schwann cells, which expand in number. It would be of some interest to determine whether this extracellular matrix material contains components mitogenic for Schwann cells, whether these be related to the developmental mitogen, a heparan sulfate proteoglycan (heparan sulfate proteoglycans are components of most basal lamina), or other proteins such as laminin or fibronectin, which apparently can stimulate Schwann cell division under some circumstances.

SOLUBLE SCHWANN CELL MITOGENS

Acid extracts of brain and pituitary were found to contain activity that stimulated the proliferation of primary cultures of "glial" cells.[47] This activity has been purified 100,000-fold to apparent homogeneity by Lemke and Brockes from bovine pituitary glands,[48] and can be eluted from polyacrylamide gels as an active 31,000-dalton protein. This protein, called glial growth factor, is distinct from other characterized polypeptide growth factors such as platelet-derived growth factor (which is unable to stimulate Schwann cell proliferation), although it shares molecular weight, heat stability, sensitivity to disulfide reducing agents, and basic isoelectric point with PDGF.[20,48] Glial growth factor (GGF) stimulates the proliferation not only of Schwann cells but also of astrocytes,[49] but not of oligodendrocytes and microglia; rat muscle fibroblasts can also be stimulated to divide in the presence of GGF.[50] The function of GGF is unknown, but it has been postulated to stimulate astrocyte proliferation during development or after injury[51] or, as a neuronal secretory product, influence blastemal cell proliferation during limb regeneration.[52] In vitro, GGF has proved of considerable utility in the amplification of primary Schwann cell cultures. A crude carboxymethylcellulose fraction of the ammonium sulfate-precipitated acid extract of bovine pituitaries is generally used at a concentration of approximately 10 μg/ml,[53] since the pituitary extract prior to ion exchange chromatography can be toxic for Schwann cells.[54] Amplification of Schwann cell numbers is often accomplished using a combination of crude GGF and cholera toxin.[12]

Another soluble protein isolated from bovine brain is glia maturation factor (GMF).[55] Lim and colleagues have purified a 14,000-dalton protein which stimulates Schwann cell proliferation and in vitro causes a morphological change to spindle shape. GMF has an apparent size of 14,000 daltons and an isoelectric point of 5.2. An antibody has been raised against this protein.

Because cyclic AMP has been suggested as a mediator of developmental changes in the Schwann cell, cholera toxin, which irreversibly ADP-ribosylates the catalytic subunit of adenylate cyclase and thereby raises intracellular cyclic AMP levels, was added to cultured Schwann cells. Cholera toxin alters Schwann cells from a typical bipolar morphology to a more fibroblastic shape and, at concentrations as low as 10 ng/ml, stimulates Schwann cell proliferation.[12,14] Cyclic AMP analogues (and cyclic AMP itself) can also stimulate Schwann cell proliferation.[8,12,14,28]

SCHWANN CELL RESPONSE TO MITOGENS

Since cholera toxin can stimulate Schwann cell division, it was postulated that cyclic AMP might be a second messenger for the effect of Schwann cell mitogens. Cholera toxin itself raises intracellular cyclic AMP levels in Schwann cells 10-fold from 2-20 hours after addition to the culture media, as assayed by radioimmunoassay; the greatest increase was observed at 6 hours (13.9-fold).[12] However, when crude GGF was added to Schwann cells, no increase in intracellular cyclic AMP was observed at any of the three times assayed. Since these growth factors increase Schwann cell number synergistically, these data were interpreted to mean that two separate pathways, one independent of cyclic AMP, can mediate Schwann cell division. The ability of the membrane-associated Schwann cell mitogens to raise intracellular cyclic AMP levels in Schwann cells has also been studied. Sixteen hours following the addition of DRG neuron-derived membranes or PC12 cell membranes, cyclic AMP levels rose 3- to 4-fold.[16] Heat treatment, which inactivates the mitogenic effect of the membranes, also prevented the rise in cyclic AMP levels.[16] In these experiments the cholera toxin-induced rise in cyclic levels was, on the average, 37-fold. Membranes from both bovine axolemma and myelin have also been added to Schwann cells for 3, 6, and 9 hours prior to radioimmunoassay for cyclic AMP.[28] These authors observed a 5-fold increase in response to cholera toxin at 6 hours, and no response at 9 hours; neither myelin nor axolemmal fragments increased cyclic AMP levels in the Schwann cells. A possible explanation of these results may be found in the observation that axolemmal fragments are not saturably bound to Schwann cells until 4 hours after their addition to the culture medium,[30] and induction of mitosis requires contact of membrane fragments with Schwann cells for a minimum of 6-8 hours.[30] Therefore, at later times it might be possible to determine accurately whether increases in cyclic AMP actually occur. In addition, since cyclic AMP levels are known to rise and fall during the cell cycle in other cell types,[56] it is essential to study the time course of cyclic AMP changes in parallel with the onset of DNA synthesis in target cells and other early changes known to occur in mitogen-stimulated cells, such as ion fluxes,[57] in order to determine the optimal time to definitively ask whether or not a cyclic AMP-dependent pathway is activated by a mitogen. In light of these problems, it remains an open question whether an elevation in cyclic AMP levels is required for Schwann cell proliferation. In fact, Sobue *et al.* found no synergy in the response of Schwann cells to axolemmal fractions plus cholera toxin,[13] a possible indication that these mitogens do work through a similar pathway; however, effects of axolemma and GGF were additive, again suggesting that GGF represents a separate class of Schwann cell mitogen.

Meodor-Woodruff *et al.* also examined the effects of altering intracellular Ca^{++} on Schwann cell response to particulate axolemmal and myelin-derived fractions.[28] A decrease in intracellular calcium generated by either 2.5 mM extracellular citrate (a calcium chelator) or 10 μM trifluoperazine (which inactivates the calcium-binding protein calmodulin) caused 80% and 90% decreases of the Schwann cells' response to the membrane fractions. High levels of the tumor-promoting phorbol ester, phorbol 12-myristate-13-acetate (10^{-8} M), in some experiments increased the mitogenicity of membranes 2- to 3-fold. Given the multiplicity of effects of phorbol esters, the interpretation of these data is not obvious.

Another interesting finding which might bear on the transduction of the mitogenic signal is that Schwann cells and neurons in culture can secrete the enzyme plasminogen activator.[58] Secretion of plasminogen activator in chicken spinal cord cultures has been shown to be related to clustering of neuronal cell bodies, fasciculation of neurites, and enhanced migration and proliferation of Schwann cells along neurite fascicles.[59] Schwann cells stimulated to proliferate by GGF secrete 8-fold more plasminogen activator than do cells in serum alone.[60] Controlled proteolysis, regulated by plasminogen activator secretion, could therefore be involved at some stage of neuron-Schwann cell interaction. In tissue culture, neurons and Schwann cells carry out the developmental interactions of Schwann cell proliferation along neurites in the absence of serum;[61] these cultures have, therefore, no source of plasminogen, the substrate of plasminogen activator. It therefore seems unlikely that the mitogenic neuron-Schwann cell interaction is mediated through plasminogen activator directly. GGF stimulation of Schwann cell division occurs only in the presence of serum, however, although a provocative abstract suggests that this serum requirement may be replaced by plasminogen.[62] PC12 membranes[16] and axolemmal membranes[13,14] also show very little mitogenicity in the absence of serum. It is not yet known whether these requirements for serum can also be replaced with plasminogen. The levels of serum required for maximal response are very high (10% or more), perhaps in excess of what one might anticipate from a plasminogen requirement. If this model has any validity, then the dorsal root ganglion neuron can be hypothesized to contain a membrane-associated plasminogen-like molecule, rendering membranes derived from dorsal root ganglion neurons mitogenic in the absence of serum. Secretion of plasminogen activator by tumor cells can be correlated in some instances with their invasiveness;[63] altered proliferation of Schwann cells in neurofibromas could result from altered regulation of the normal use of this secreted enzyme.

REFERENCES

1. ASBURY, A. K. 1967. J. Cell Biol. **34:** 735-743.
2. TERRY, L. C., G. M. BRAY & A. J. AGUAYO. 1974. Brain Res. **69:** 144-148.
3. ABERCROMBIE, M. & M. L. JOHNSON. 1946. J. Anat. **80:** 37-50.
4. BUNGE, M. B. & R. P. BUNGE. Ann. N.Y. Acad. Sci. (This volume.)
5. BROCKES, J. P., K. L. FIELDS & M. C. RAFF. 1979. Brain Res. **165:** 105-118.
6. CORNBROOKS, C. J., D. J. CAREY, J. G. MCDONALD, R. TIMPL & R. P. BUNGE. 1983. Proc. Nat. Acad. Sci. USA **80:** 3850-3854.
7. WOOD, P. 1976. Brain Res. **115:** 361-375.
8. SALZER, J. L. & R. P. BUNGE. 1980. J. Cell Biol. **84:** 739-752.
9. PORTER, S., M. B. CLARK, L. GLASER & R. P. BUNGE. J. Neurosci. (In press.)
10. KREIDER, B. Q., A. MESSING, H. DOAN, S. U. KIM, R. P. LISAK & D. E. PLEASURE. 1981. Brain Res. **207:** 433-444.
11. KREIDER, B. Q., J. COREY-BLOOM, R. P. LISAK, H. DOAN & D. E. PLEASURE. 1982. Brain Res. **237:** 238-243.
12. RAFF, M. C., E. ABNEY, J. P. BROCKES & A. HORNBY-SMITH. 1978. Cell **15:** 813-822.
13. SOBUE, G., B. KREIDER, A. ASBURY & D. PLEASURE. 1983. Brain Res. **280:** 263-275.
14. CASSEL, D., P. M. WOOD, R. P. BUNGE & L. GLASER. 1982. J. Cell. Biochem. **18:** 433-445.
15. SALZER, J. L., A. K. WILLIAMS, L. GLASER & R. P. BUNGE. 1980. J. Cell Biol. **84:** 753-766.
16. RATNER, N., L. GLASER & R. P. BUNGE. 1984. J. Cell Biol. **98:** 1150-1155.
17. DEVRIES, G. H., L. N. MINIER & B. L. LEWIS. 1983. Dev. Brain Res. **9:** 87-92.
18. JAMES, R. & R. B. BRADSHAW. 1984. Annu. Rev. Biochem. **53:** 259-292.
19. SALZER, J. L., R. P. BUNGE & L. GLASER. 1980. J. Cell Biol. **84:** 767-778.
20. STILES, C. D. 1983. Cell **33:** 653-655.
21. WOOD, P. M. & R. P. BUNGE. 1975. Nature **256:** 662-664.
22. MCCARTHY, K. D. & L. M. PARTLOW. 1976. Brain Res. **114:** 415-426.
23. ROBINSON, H. C., M. J. BRETT, P. J. TRALAGGAN, D. A. LOWTHER & M. OKAYAMA. 1975. Biochem. J. **148:** 25-34.
24. RATNER, N., R. P. BUNGE & L. GLASER. 1985. J. Cell Biol. **101:** 744-754.
25. RATNER, N., D. HONG, R. P. BUNGE & L. GLASER. J. Neurosci. Abstr. (In press.)
26. RATNER, N., P. W. WOOD, R. P. BUNGE & L. GLASER. In Neuronal-Glial Interactions. Plenum Press. New York, N.Y. (In press.)
27. DEVRIES, G. H., J. L. SALZER & R. P. BUNGE, 1982. Dev. Brain Res. **3:** 295-299.
28. MEADOR-WOODRUFF, J. H., B. L. LEWIS & G. H. DEVRIES. 1984. Biochem. Biophys. Res. Commun. **122**(1): 373-380.
29. YASHINO, J. E., M. P. DINNEEN, B. L. LEWIS, J. H. MEADOR-WOODRUFF & G. H. DEVRIES. 1984. J. Cell Biol. **99:** 2309-2313.
30. SOBUE, G. & D. PLEASURE. 1985. J. Neurosci. **5**(2): 379-387.
31. BOTTENSTEIN, J. E. & G. H. SATO. 1979. Proc. Nat. Acad. Sci. USA **76:** 514-517.
32. GREENE, L. A. & A. S. TISCHLER. 1982. Adv. Cell. Neurobiol. **3:** 373-414.
33. COCHRAN, M. & M. M. BLACK. 1985. Exp. Brain Res. **17:** 105-116.

34. BRADLEY, W. G. & A. ASBURY. 1970. Exp. Neurol. **26:** 275-282.
35. ROMINE, J. S., G. M. BRAY & A. J. AGUAYO. 1976. Arch. Neurol. **33:** 49-54.
36. BUNGE, M. B., J. JEFFREY & P. WOOD. 1977. J. Cell Biol. **75:** 161a.
37. BUNGE, M. B., A. K. WILLIAMS, P. M. WOOD, J. UITTO & J. J. JEFFREY. 1980. J. Cell Biol. **84:** 184-202.
38. CAREY, D. J. & R. P. BUNGE. 1981. J. Cell Biol. **91:** 666-672.
39. BUNGE, M. B., A. K. WILLIAMS & P. M. WOOD. 1982. Dev. Biol. **92:** 449-460.
40. CAREY, D. J., C. F. ELDRIDGE, C. J. CORNBROOKS, R. TIMPL & R. P. BUNGE. 1983. J. Cell Biol. **97:** 473-479.
41. BARON-VAN EVERCOOREN, A., H. K. KLEINMAN, H. E. J. SEPPA, B. RENTIER & M. DUBOIS-DALCQ. 1982. J. Cell Biol. **93:** 211-216.
42. MCGARVEY, M. L., A. B.-V. EVERCOOREN, H. K. KLEINMAN & M. DUBOIS-DALCQ. 1984. Dev. Biol. **105:** 18-28.
43. EDGAR, D., R. TIMPL & H. THOENEN. 1984. EMBO J. **3:** 1463-1468.
44. GOSPODAROWITZ, D., G. GREENBERG & C. R. BIRDWELL. 1978. Cancer Res. **38:** 4155-4165.
45. OVADIA, H., I. LUBETZKI-KORN, T. BRENNER, O. ABRAMSKY, R. FRIDMAN & I. VLODAVSKY. 1984. Brain Res. **322:** 93-100.
46. ELDRIDGE, C. & R. P. BUNGE. Unpublished observations.
47. GOSPODAROWICZ, D. 1974. Nature **249:** 123-127.
48. LEMKE, G. E. & J. P. BROCKES. 1984. J. Neurosci. **4**(1): 75-83.
49. BROCKES, J. P., G. E. LEMKE & D. R. BALZER. 1980. J. Biol. Chem. **255:** 8374-8377.
50. BROCKES, J. P. & G. E. LEMKE. 1981. *In* Development in the Nervous System. J. D. Feldman & G. R. Garrod, Eds.: 309-327. Cambridge University Press. Cambridge, England.
51. BROCKES, J. P., K. J. FRYXELL & G. E. LEMKE. 1981. J. Exp. Biol. **95:** 215-230.
52. BROCKES, J. P. 1984. Science **225:** 1280-1287.
53. BROCKES, J. P., G. E. LEMKE & D. R. BALZER. 1980. J. Biol. Chem. **255:** 8374-8377.
54. RATNER, R., R. P. BUNGE & L. GLASER. Unpublished observations.
55. LIM, R., J. F. MILLER, D. J. HICKLIN & A. A. ANDRESEN. 1985. Biochemistry **24:** 8070-8074.
56. WHITFIELD, J. F., A. L. BOYNTON, J. P. MACMANNS, R. H. RIXON, M. SIKORSKA, B. TSANG & P. R. WALKER. 1980. Ann. N.Y. Acad. Sci. **339:** 216-240.
57. REUSS, L., D. CASSEL, P. ROTHENBERG, B. WHITELEY, D. MANUCSO & L. GLASER. Curr. Top Membr. Transp. (In press.)
58. KRYSTOSEK, A. & N. A. SEEDS. 1984. J. Cell Biol. **98:** 773-776.
59. KALDERON, N. 1979. Proc. Nat. Acad. Sci. USA **76**(11): 5992-5996.
60. KALDERON, N. 1984. Proc. Nat. Acad. Sci. USA **81:** 7216-7220.
61. MOYA, F., R. P. BUNGE & M. B. BUNGE. 1980. Proc. Nat. Acad. Sci. USA **77:** 6902-6906.
62. KALDERON, N. 1983. Trans. Soc. Neurosci. **9**(2): 841a (abstr.).
63. MULLINS, D. E. & S. T. ROHRLICH. 1983. Biochim. Biophys. Acta **695:** 177-214.

Influences of Peripheral Nerve Components on Axonal Growth[a]

P. M. RICHARDSON

Division of Neurosurgery
McGill University
1650 Cedar Avenue
Montreal, Quebec, Canada H3G 1A4

R. J. RIOPELLE

Division of Neurology
Queen's University
146 Stuart Street
Kingston, Ontario, Canada K7L 3N6

INTRODUCTION

One function of sheath cells (Schwann cells and endoneurial fibroblasts) is to promote the regeneration of injured axons. Sheath cells are associated with several molecules that support neurite extension *in vitro* including one agent very similar to classical nerve growth factor (NGF).[1,2] In this essay, evidence will be summarized that NGF is normally synthesized by sheath cells and acts on receptors along the course of axons in nerve trunks. Two types of action of sheath cells on regenerating neurons will be described with the suggestion that two classes of molecules are involved.

NGF AND SHEATH CELLS

The cellular origin of NGF has remained elusive because of technical difficulties in measuring the very low concentrations of NGF in physiologically appropriate sites. Bioassay[1,2] and two-site immunoassay[3] are now sensitive enough to detect the small amounts of NGF in normal rodent nerves. For example, the culture system illustrated in FIGURE 1 detects neurotrophic agents exuding from nerve segments to neurons in adjacent chick sympathetic ganglia. In such an assay, NGF from a nerve needs to

[a]The authors' laboratories are supported by the National Institutes of Health, the Medical Research Council of Canada, the Multiple Sclerosis Society of Canada, and the Physicians' Services Incorporated Foundation of Ontario.

182

diffuse through only 10-20 μl of gel to reach a ganglion that displays neurite outgrowth in the presence of NGF at 100 pg/ml (4 pM). Because more than one neurotrophic agent is present in nerve[1,2] (FIGURE 1), the concentration of NGF in tissues can be measured only by comparing similar cultures with or without antibodies to NGF. An important disadvantage of bioassays is their semiquantitative nature: an advantage is the small chance of falsely positive results when bioactivity suppressed by antibodies to NGF is measured.

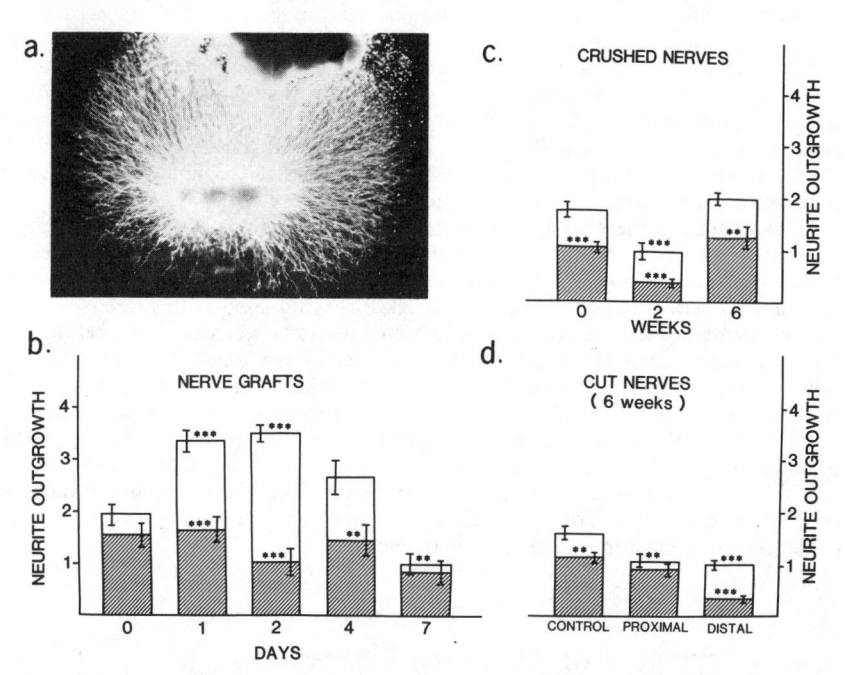

FIGURE 1. Endoneurial fragments of rat sciatic nerve, 1-2 mm long, were usually killed by freezing (to prevent *in vitro* synthesis of NGF) and placed in supplemented collagen gels 1 mm away from viable chick sympathetic ganglia.[2] Two days later, neurite outgrowth from the ganglia was scored blindly from 0 (under basal conditions) to 5 (βNGF at 10 ng/ml). For each group of nerve fragments, mean scores ($\pm$ standard error of the mean) in the absence of anti-NGF (upper bar) and presence of NGF (lower bar) are plotted. The distance between the two bars yields a semiquantitative estimate of NGF concentration. Asterisks indicate significant change in total activity as compared to control nerves (upper bars) or significant suppression by anti-NGF (lower bars): **, $p < 0.01$; ***, $p < 0.001$. (a) Profuse halo of neurite outgrowth from sympathetic ganglia beside a viable nerve fragment. (b) Sciatic nerves were cut at five levels and the four isolated grafts left in the thigh for 0-7 days before bioassay; $n = 12$-20 fragments from 6 nerves. (c) Nerves were crushed and allowed to regenerate for 2 or 6 weeks before sampling distal to the crush site; $n = 19$-21 fragments from 4 nerves. (d) Nerves were cut in midthigh and the two ends clipped and widely separated to minimize regeneration. At 6 weeks, samples were taken proximal or distal to the cut; $n = 53$-58 fragments from 18-30 nerves.

By enzyme immunoassay, normal rat sciatic nerves contain approximately 30 pg NGF per cm length,[4] or 50-100 pM if NGF were distributed uniformly in extracellular and intracellular compartments of the nerve. In fact, much of the NGF in normal nerves is probably in transit within axons because the concentration of NGF is subnormal in the proximal stump of a divided nerve.[4] Therefore, the extracellular concentration of NGF in the endoneurium is difficult to estimate.

Peripheral nerve segments contain not only NGF but also cells that can synthesize NGF. NGF is released by viable nerve explants *in vitro* and accumulates in nerve grafts *in vivo*[2] (FIGURES 1a and b). The elegant demonstration that mRNA for NGF is found in sciatic nerve extracts[5] constitutes virtual proof that NGF is synthesized in normal nerves *in vivo*. An important unanswered question is whether NGF is derived from all Schwann cells, some Schwann cells, or endoneurial fibroblasts. NGF is probably also produced by some cell population in the central nervous system (CNS).[5-7] However, arguments to support the common belief that NGF is produced by target cells contacted by peripheral axons are not entirely convincing. For example, the presence of NGF and the capacity to synthesize NGF in the iris and other richly innervated peripheral tissues[3,5,8-10] could well be the result rather than the cause of the many nerves in these tissues. In peripheral tissues, NGF immunoreactivity is restricted to nerves and has not been seen in any target cells.[6,11]

Fluctuations in the endoneurial concentration of NGF after nerve injury tempt speculation about the regulation of NGF synthesis. In nerve grafts isolated in the thigh, NGF accumulates at a mean rate of 1-2 pg/cm nerve per hour for the first 48 hours[12] (FIGURE 1b). It is possible that NGF is synthesized at this rate by sheath cells in normal nerves and is merely sequestered in grafts because normal retrograde transport is eliminated. It is also possible that the rate of synthesis of NGF by Schwann cells increases transiently during Wallerian degeneration as does the rate of mitosis.[13] Axonal signals control proliferation, myelination, and protein synthesis by Schwann cells[14-20] and could be involved in the regulation of NGF synthesis. The additional possibility of a feedback control is raised by the finding of NGF receptors on Schwann cells.[21] Such a mechanism could account for observations that the concentration of NGF in the distal stumps of chronically injured nerves is relatively normal regardless of the degree of regeneration (FIGURES 1c and d).

NGF RECEPTORS ON AXONS

The biological functions of NGF are mediated through binding to specific receptors in the membrane of responsive neurons. The biochemistry of such receptors has been studied in cultured fetal and neoplastic cells of neural crest origin;[22-24] their regional and cellular distributions have been examined by retrograde axonal tracing and receptor radioautography.[25-28]

Dissociated embryonic sensory neurons possess two receptors for NGF with dissociation equilibrium constants, 20 pM and 2 nM, differing by a factor of 100.[22] The high-affinity site, probably responsible for neurite outgrowth and for the internalization of NGF,[22,29] is reported to be a sialoglycoprotein with a molecular weight of 75,000[30] or 150,000.[24] Unless the retrograde transport of NGF is entirely an epiphenomenon, the NGF-receptor complex can be assumed to have some function after entering the cell. However, knowledge about the intracellular mechanisms by which the internalized NGF-receptor complex modifies gene expression and/or posttranslational events[31,32] is incomplete.

In adult animals, high-affinity NGF receptors on axons in peripheral nerves are difficult to study because of additional binding at lower affinity probably to Schwann cells.[21] Fortuitously, NGF receptors are also present on the spinal projections of primary sensory neurons[27,28] where they are more amenable to biochemical study. Analysis of the binding of radioiodinated NGF to membrane fractions from the dorsal third of the spinal cord indicates some receptor sites with a dissociation equilibrium constant (K_d) of 20-40 pM.[33] On this basis, one can reasonably assume that information regarding NGF receptors on fetal cells pertains to adult sensory neurons as well. Also, the concentration of NGF in the endoneurium and the K_d of its receptor are of the same order of magnitude as expected where a polypeptide ligand reacts physiologically with its receptor.

A decade ago, radioiodinated NGF was shown to be taken up selectively at or near the terminals of sympathetic and sensory axons and transported retrogradely to their cell bodies.[25,26] Recent modifications of such transport experiments for sensory neurons indicate that NGF receptors are also found along nonterminal segments of

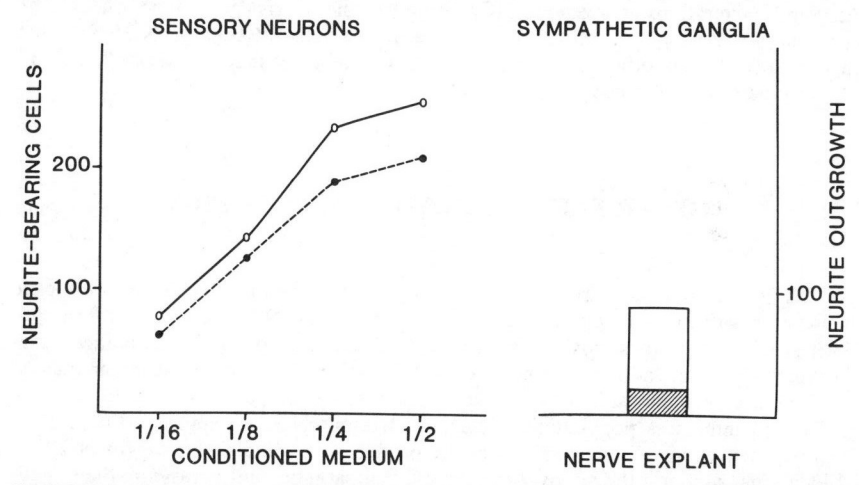

FIGURE 2. Neurotrophic activity released *in vitro* by viable nerve fragments is estimated by two bioassays. **Left:** culture media, conditioned for 20 hours with washed and minced nerves (2 cm/ml), were serially diluted for assay with dissociated sensory neurons. Process-bearing neurons were counted blindly and the results normalized to responses with NGF on the same day. Upper and lower lines show scores without or with anti-NGF; $n = 9$. Most responses to conditioned medium exceed those to NGF and most of the activity is not suppressed by anti-NGF. **Right:** bioassay with sympathetic ganglia (FIGURE 1) beside viable nerve fragments. Responses are less than those to NGF (100%), and most of the activity is suppressed by anti-NGF.

peripheral process and on the intraspinal projections.[27,28] Presumably, NGF receptors are synthesized in the cell bodies of dorsal root ganglion (DRG) neurons, anterogradely transported in central and peripheral axons, and inserted along the axolemma of both processes. However, synthesis and anterograde transport of the NGF receptor have not been directly documented or quantified.

Among peripheral neurons, NGF receptors are present on sympathetic and some sensory neurons but not motor or parasympathetic neurons. Even with optimal concentrations of NGF, survival of cultured sensory neurons is submaximal and can be augmented by additional neurotrophic activity from peripheral nerve or elsewhere[1] (FIGURE 2). During the development of chick DRG, effects of NGF on survival and differentiation are more obvious on small dorsomedial neurons than on large ventrolateral neurons.[34] Small DRG neurons tend to be more responsive to NGF than large neurons in mature rats also. In radioautographs of lumbar DRG containing retrogradely transported radioiodinated NGF, a disproportionately small number of large neurons were labeled (FIGURE 3). When NGF receptors were localized in the spinal cord by receptor radioautography, labeling was densest in superficial layers of the dorsal horn where unmyelinated and small myelinated axons might be expected to terminate.[33] However, some large DRG neurons projecting to the dorsal column nuclei do take up radioiodinated NGF.[27] Not all mature sensory neurons respond to NGF; those with NGF receptors tend to be smaller than those without receptors.

Observations about the synthesis of NGF by sheath cells and distribution of NGF receptors along axons are consistent with the hypothesis that NGF normally acts in a paracrine manner within the endoneurium.[35] In addition to its possible functions during regeneration, endogenous NGF supports the survival and function of sympathetic and sensory neurons in normal, mature animals.[36,37] Because NGF does not act on all neurons, other neurotrophic factors supporting motor neurons and some sensory neurons are presumed to exist.

OTHER FACTORS IN THE ENDONEURIUM

Within the endoneurium are found two broad categories of molecules that influence neurite growth in tissue culture. Diffusible proteins like NGF permit specific populations of neurons to survive, differentiate, and extend processes. Immobilized glycoproteins promote adhesion of neurites to cell surfaces or to an extracellular matrix.

The neurotrophic activity in nerve fragments is only partially blocked by anti-NGF and influences populations of neurons without NGF receptors[1,2] (FIGURE 1). "Ciliary neuronotrophic factor," an acidic protein with a molecular weight of 20-25 kilodaltons, supports the survival of sensory, sympathetic, and parasympathetic neurons in tissue culture and has been extracted from several avian and mammalian tissues including normal nerves and sheath cell tumors.[38-42] This second neurotrophic factor appears to be released by sheath cells[43] (FIGURE 2) and not in nerves merely because it is being transported from peripheral tissues. However, observations regarding bioactivity in nerve fragments after chronic injury with or without regeneration (FIGURES 1c and d) suggest that axons might regulate synthesis of non-NGF neurotrophic factor(s). Physiological studies of "ciliary neuronotrophic factor" await its further purification and availability in larger quantities.

In addition to humoral neurotrophic factors, Schwann cells[44,45] synthesize laminin and other components of the extracellular matrix that can provide a substratum for neurite outgrowth in tissue culture.[46-50] Interactions between axons and sheath cells may be mediated by a family of adhesion molecules found on cell surfaces;[51-53] antibodies to neuronal cell adhesion molecules interfere with the fasciculation and attachment of neurites.[53,54]

In tissue culture, growth cones are guided by adhesive, bound molecules as they move along cell surfaces or other pathways[55-57] and can also be attracted or repelled by diffusible factors.[58-60] Observations about neurite growth *in vitro* suggest possible mechanisms of axon regeneration but must be cautiously extrapolated to a situation where the growth is greatly prolonged in time and space. Molecules present in the endoneurium with known potential to stimulate neuronal growth seem likely to participate in peripheral nerve regeneration.

SHEATH CELLS IN REGENERATION

Sheath cells act by two distinct mechanisms to promote axon regeneration—as a favorable terrain for elongating axons and as a source of retrograde signals that activate the nerve cell body.

For successful regeneration, viable Schwann cells must be present in the region of growth.[61,62] Axon tips extend for only a short distance without ensheathment, usually

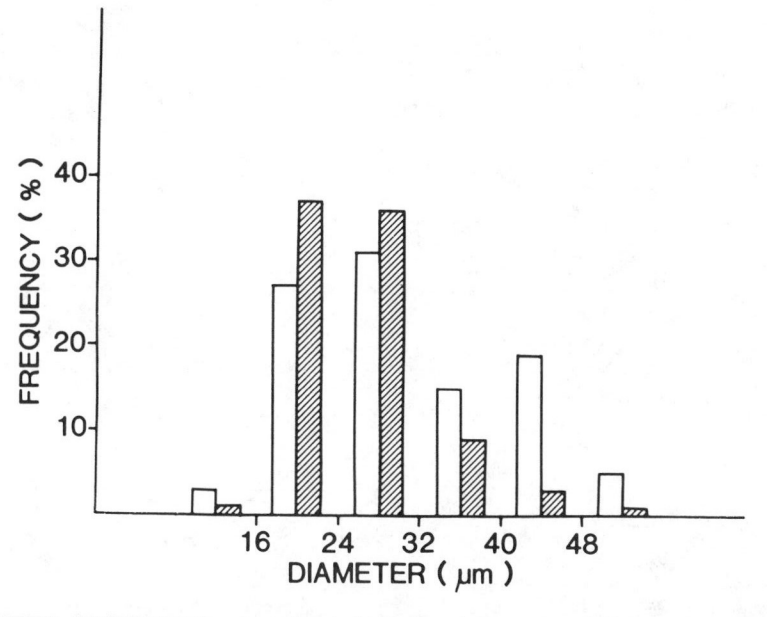

FIGURE 3. ^{125}I-NGF (10 ng) was injected into the sciatic nerve; and 11 hours later, the L5 DRG was removed, fixed, and embedded in plastic for light microscope radioautography.[27] In selected sections, cell diameters were measured for all neurons with visible nucleoli and histograms were prepared for labeled (hatched columns $n = 142$) and unlabeled (white columns, $n = 264$) neurons. Axons from very few large neurons took up ^{125}I-NGF.

less than 1 mm,[63-65] and the success of acellular prostheses probably depends on Schwann cell migration into the field of growth.[66-68] The fact that regenerating axons are closely apposed to Schwann cells suggests that axons adhere to molecules on the cell surface or immediately adjacent extracellular matrix. After nerve injury, axons form topographically accurate reconnections only when guided mechanically by preserved elements of the endoneurium,[62,69] and selective cues like those along the pathways of developing axons[70] are not apparent in regeneration. The attraction of regenerating axons to Schwann cells is specific only to the extent that two defined cell types are involved. Peripheral nerve grafts promote the regeneration of axons from central neurons,[71,72] grafts from purely sensory nerves transmit regenerating motor fibers, and Schwann cells from an unmyelinated nerve accept and myelinate other axons after cross-union.[14,20] Observed local actions of Schwann cells on regenerating axons can still be largely explained by a nonselective "contact guidance,"[73] perhaps mediated by laminin and/or cell surface molecules. An additional role for selective chemotactic effects during regeneration has been neither proved nor disproved.

The regenerative behavior of an interrupted axon depends on events in the nerve cell body as well as the environment at the site of growth.[74,75] Under some circumstances, for example after dorsal root crush,[76] axons regenerate for several centimeters without any apparent morphological or biochemical change in the nerve cell body. However, the central regeneration of primary sensory neurons is strongly enhanced by injury to their peripheral branch.[77] Furthermore, transection of a peripheral nerve is a much greater stimulus to regeneration than is crush (FIGURE 4) despite the fact

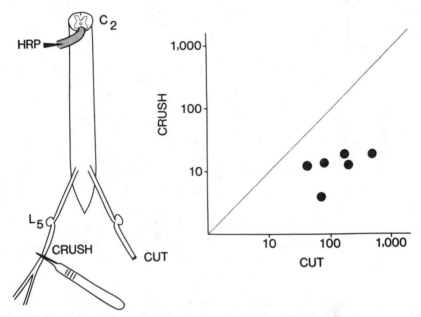

FIGURE 4. In 6 rats, the dorsal columns were cut and a segment of the right sciatic nerve was grafted to the cord. The left sciatic nerve was crushed. Two months later, neurons in the L4+L5 DRG with axons regenerating into the grafts were retrogradely labeled with horseradish peroxidase (HRP). For each animal, the abscissa and ordinate are the number of labeled neurons in the L4+L5 DRG on the right and left sides respectively. Nerve transection is 10 times as effective as nerve crush in evoking central regeneration from primary sensory neurons and 100 times as effective as no sciatic nerve injury.[77]

that either injury interrupts virtually all the axons in a nerve and prevents contact with target tissues for at least two weeks. The discrepancy between the effects of crush and cut strongly suggests that retrograde signals activating the nerve cell body are triggered by events within the endoneurium and not by disconnection from target tissues. Either uptake and retrograde transport of an adventitious injury factor[78] or interruption of normal retrograde transport of neurotrophic molecules from distal sheath cells could be responsible for intraneuronal changes that favor regeneration. Whether the initial endoneurial event is positive or negative, the enhancement phenomenon can be taken as evidence for a second influence of Schwann cells on injured neurons.

A propensity to regenerate is one of many reactions of neurons when their axons are cut. Several degenerative changes in sympathetic and sensory neurons following section of their axons have now been linked to perikaryal deprivation of NGF. Neuronal death,[79] synaptic disconnection,[80] and fall in substance P and acid phosphatase[81,82] after nerve transection can all be mitigated by administration of exogenous NGF. Each of these changes is less severe after nerve crush versus transection, perhaps because perikaryal deprivation of NGF is less prolonged and less severe when regenerating axons quickly reestablish contact with NGF-releasing sheath cells. Is the enhanced regenerative activity of sensory neurons with cut axons also related to their NGF depletion?[83] Although such an inverse correlation between intraneuronal NGF concentration and tendency to regenerate appears paradoxical, anti-NGF administered during development has recently been shown to increase the number of unmyelinated fibers in dorsal roots.[84] However, administration of NGF to the proximal stump of the cut sciatic nerve did not conclusively modify the regeneration of the corresponding central axons into a peripheral nerve graft.[83] Further knowledge of the mechanisms of action of NGF and the regulaton of its receptors is required to clarify possible retrograde and local effects of NGF on injured neurons.

CONCLUSIONS

Two types of interaction between sheath cells and regenerating neurons can be discerned and correlated with two classes of neurite-promoting molecules. As a working hypothesis, we suggest that molecules in or near the Schwann cell membrane provide local nonselective guidance to axon tips while diffusible neurotrophic molecules like NGF are involved in retrograde signals that regulate the regenerative response of the nerve cell body. Because NGF can be purified in sufficient quantities for radioiodination, preparation of antibodies, or infusion, several approaches to studying its physiology are feasible. Such studies indicate that NGF is released by sheath cells and might serve as a marker in peripheral nerve tumors. Purification of other neurotrophic molecules derived from sheath cells is an urgent requirement for more complete understanding of molecular events in normal and abnormal nerves.

ACKNOWLEDGMENTS

Valerie Verge and Monica Altares provided excellent technical assistance.

REFERENCES

1. RIOPELLE, R. J., R. J. BOEGMAN & D. A. CAMERON. 1981. Peripheral nerve contains heterogeneous growth factors that support sensory neurons in vitro. Neurosci. Lett. **25:** 311-316.
2. RICHARDSON, P. M. & T. EBENDAL. 1982. Nerve growth activities in rat peripheral nerve. Brain Res. **246:** 57-64.
3. KORSCHING, S. & H. THOENEN. 1983. Nerve growth factor in sympathetic ganglia and

corresponding target organs of the rat: correlation with density of sympathetic innervation. Proc. Nat. Acad. Sci. USA **80:** 3513-3516.

4. KORSCHING, S. & H. THOENEN. 1983. Quantitative demonstration of the retrograde axonal transport of endogenous nerve growth factor. Neurosci. Lett. **39:** 1-4.

5. SHELTON, D. L. & L. F. REICHARDT. 1984. Expression of the β-nerve growth factor gene correlates with the density of sympathetic innervation in effector organs. Proc. Nat. Acad. Sci. USA **81:** 7951-7955.

6. AYER-LELIEVRE, C. S., T. EBENDAL, L. OLSON & A. SEIGER. 1983. Localization of nerve growth factor-like immunoreactivity in rat nervous tissue. Med. Biol. **61:** 296-304.

7. CRUTCHER, K. A. & F. COLLINS. 1982. In vitro evidence for two distinct hippocampal growth factors: basis of neuronal plasticity? Science **217:** 67-68.

8. EBENDAL, T., L. OLSON, A. SEIGER & K-O. HEDLUNG. 1980. Nerve growth factors in the rat iris. Nature **286:** 25-28.

9. BARTH, E.-M., S. KORSCHING & H. THOENEN. 1984. Regulation of nerve growth factor synthesis and release in organ cultures of rat iris. J. Cell Biol. **99:** 839-843.

10. HEUMANN, R., S. KORSCHING, J. SCOTT & H. THOENEN. 1984. Relationship between levels of nerve growth factor (NGF) and its messenger RNA in sympathetic ganglia and peripheral target tissues. EMBO J. **3**(13): 3183-3189.

11. RUSH, R. A. 1984. Immunohistochemical localization of endogenous nerve growth factor. Nature **312:** 364-367.

12. RICHARDSON, P. M., T. EBENDAL & R. J. RIOPELLE. 1985. Nerve growth and nerve growth factor within peripheral nervous tissue. In Neural Grafting in the Mammalian CNS. A Björklund & U. Stenevi, Eds.: 319-327. Elsevier Science Publishers. Amsterdam, Holland.

13. BRADLEY, W. G. & A. K. ASBURY. 1970. Duration of synthesis phase in neurilemma cells in mouse sciatic nerve during degeneration. Exp. Neurol. **26:** 275-282.

14. AGUAYO, A. J., J. EPPS, L. CHARRON & G. M. BRAY. 1976. Multipotentiality of Schwann cells in cross-anastomosed and grafted myelinated and unmyelinated nerves: quantitative microscopy and radioautography. Brain Res. **104:** 1-20.

15. BROCKES, J. P. 1984. Mitogenic growth factors and nerve dependence of limb regeneration. Science **225:** 1281-1287.

16. CAREY, D. J., C. F. ELDRIDGE, C. J. CORNBROOKS, R. TIMPL & R. P. BUNGE. 1983. Biosynthesis of type IV collagen by cultured rat Schwann cells. J. Cell Biol. **97:** 473-479.

17. MÜLLER, H. W., P. J. GEBICKE-HÄRTER, D. H. HANGER & E. M. SHOOTER. 1985. A specific 37,000-dalton protein that accumulates in regenerating but not in nonregenerating mammalian nerves. Science **228:** 499-501.

18. PODUSLO, J. F., C. T. BERG & P. J. DYCK. 1984. Schwann cell expression of a major myelin glycoprotein in the absence of myelin assembly. Proc. Nat. Acad. Sci. USA **81:** 1864-1866.

19. SOBUE, G., B. KREIDER, A. ASBURY & D. PLEASURE. 1983. Specific and potent mitogenic effect of axolemmal fraction on Schwann cells from rat sciatic nerves in serum-containing and defined media. Brain Res. **280:** 263-275.

20. WEINBERG, H. J. & P. S. SPENCER. 1975. Studies on the control of myelinogenesis. I. Myelination of regenerating axons after entry into a foreign unmyelinated nerve. J. Neurocytol. **4:** 395-418.

21. ZIMMERMANN, A. & A. SUTTER. 1983. β-Nerve growth factor (βNGF) receptors on glial cells. Cell-cell interaction between neurones and Schwann cells in cultures of chick sensory ganglia. EMBO J. **2**(6): 879-885.

22. SUTTER, A., R. J. RIOPELLE, R. M. HARRIS-WARRICK & E. M. SHOOTER. 1979. Nerve growth factor receptors. J. Biol. Chem. **254**(13): 5972-5982.

23. RIOPELLE, R. J., T. HALIOTIS & J. C. RODER. 1983. Nerve growth factor receptors of human tumors of neural crest origin: characterization of binding site heterogeneity and alteration by theophylline. Cancer Res. **43:** 5184-5189.

24. HOSANG, M. & E. M. SHOOTER. 1985. Molecular characteristics of nerve growth factor receptors on PC12 cells. J. Biol. Chem. **260**(1): 655-662.

25. HENDRY, I. A., K. STÖCKEL, H. THOENEN & L. L. IVERSEN. 1974. The retrograde axonal transport of nerve growth factor. Brain Res. **68:** 103-121.

26. SCHWAB, M. & H. THOENEN. 1977. Selective trans-synaptic migration of tetanus toxin

after retrograde axonal transport in peripheral sympathetic nerves: a comparison with nerve growth factor. Brain Res. **122:** 459-474.

27. RICHARDSON, P. M. & R. J. RIOPELLE. 1984. Uptake of nerve growth factor along peripheral and spinal axons of primary sensory neurons. J. Neurosci. **4**(7): 1683-1689.

28. YIP, H. K. & E. M. JOHNSON. 1984. Developing dorsal root ganglion neurons require trophic support from their central processes. Proc. Nat. Acad. Sci. USA **81:** 6245-6249.

29. BERND, P. & L. A. GREENE. 1984. Association of ^{125}I-nerve growth factor with PC12 pheochromocytoma cells. J. Biol. Chem. **259**(24): 15509-15516.

30. CHAO, M. V., M. A. BOTHWELL, A. H. ROSS, H. KOPROWSKI, A. A. LANAHAN, C. R. BUCK & A. SEHGAL. 1986. Gene transfer and molecular cloning of the human NGF receptor. Science **232:** 518-521.

31. YANKNER, B. A. & E. M. SHOOTER. 1982. The biology and mechanism of action of nerve growth factor. Annu. Rev. Biochem. **51:** 845-868.

32. ROHRER, H., T. SCHÄFER, S. KORSCHING & H. THOENEN. 1982. Internalization of nerve growth factor by pheochromocytoma PC12 cells: absence of transfer to the nucleus. J. Neurosci. **2:** 687-697.

33. RICHARDSON, P. M., V. M. K. VERGE ISSA & R. J. RIOPELLE. Distribution of neuronal receptors for nerve growth factor in the rat. J. Neurosci. (In press.)

34. HAMBURGER, V., J. K. BRUNSO-BECHTOLD & J. W. YIP. 1981. Neuronal death in the spinal ganglia of the chick embryo and its reduction by nerve growth factor. J. Neurosci. **1**(1): 60-71.

35. VARON, S. S. & R. P. BUNGE. 1978. Trophic mechanisms in the peripheral nervous system. Annu. Rev. Neurosci. **1:** 327-361.

36. GOEDERT, M., K. STOECKEL & U. OTTEN. 1981. Biological importance of the retrograde axonal transport of nerve growth factor in sensory neurons. Proc. Nat. Acad. Sci. USA **78:** 5895-5898.

37. SCHWARTZ, J. P., J. PEARSON & E. M. JOHNNSON. 1982. Effect of exposure to anti-NGF on sensory neurons of adult rats and guinea pigs. Brain Res. **244:** 378-381.

38. BONYHADY, R. E., I. A. HENDRY & C. E. HILL. 1982. Reversible dissociation of a bovine cardiac factor that supports survival of avian ciliary ganglionic neurones. J. Neurosci. Res. **7:** 11-21.

39. EBENDAL, T., M. BELEW, C.-O. JACOBSON & J. PORATH. 1979. Neurite outgrowth elicited by embryonic chick heart: partial purification of the active factor. Neurosci. Lett. **14:** 91-95.

40. BARBIN, G., M. MANTHORPE & S. VARON. 1984. Purification of the chick eye ciliary neuronotrophic factor. J. Neurochem. **43:** 1468-1478.

41. WILLIAMS, L. R., M. MANTHORPE, G. BARBIN, M. NIETO-SAMPEDRO, C. W. COTMAN & S. VARON. 1984. High ciliary neuronotrophic specific activity in rat peripheral nerve. Int. J. Dev. Neurosci. **2:** 177-180.

42. DOSTALER, S., R. J. RIOPELLE & P. M. RICHARDSON. 1985. Partial characterization of a novel neurotrophic factor from peripheral nerve tumors. Soc. Neurosci. Abstr. **11:** 1082.

43. VARON, S., S. D. SKAPER & M. MANTHORPE. 1981. Trophic activities for dorsal root and sympathetic ganglionic neurons in media conditioned by Schwann and other peripheral cells. Dev. Brain Res. **1:** 73-87.

44. CORNBROOKS, C. J., D. J. CAREY, J. A. McDONALD, R. TIMPL & R. P. BUNGE. 1983. In vivo and in vitro observations on laminin production by Schwann cells. Proc. Nat. Acad. Sci. USA **80:** 3850-3854.

45. PALM, S. L. & L. T. FURCHT. 1983. Production of laminin and fibronectin by schwannoma cells: cell-protein interactions in vitro and protein localization in peripheral nerve in vivo. J. Cell Biol. **96:** 1218-1226.

46. CARBONETTO, S. 1984. The extracellular matrix of the nervous system. Trends Neurosci. **7:** 382-387.

47. MANTHORPE, M., E. ENGVALL, E. RUOSLAHTI, F. M. LONGO, G. E. DAVIS & S. VARON. 1983. Laminin promotes neuritic regeneration from cultured peripheral and central neurons. J. Cell Biol. **97:** 1882-1890.

48. ROGERS, S. L., P. C. LETOURNEAU, S. L. PALM, J. McCARTHY & L. T. FURCHT. 1983.

Neurite extension by peripheral and central nervous system neurons in response to substratum-bound fibronectin and laminin. Dev. Biol. **98:** 212-220.

49. EDGAR, D., R. TIMPL & H. THOENEN. 1984. The heparin-binding domain of laminin is responsible for its effects on neurite outgrowth and neuronal survival. EMBO J. **3:** 1463-1468.

50. LANDER, A. D., D. K. FUJII & L. F. REICHARDT. 1985. Laminin is associated with the "neurite outgrowth-promoting factors" found in conditioned medium. Proc. Nat. Acad. Sci. USA **82:** 2183-2187.

51. GRUMET, M., S. HOFFMAN & G. M. EDELMAN. 1984. Two antigenically related neuronal cell adhesion molecules of different specificities mediate neuron-neuron and neuron-glial adhesion. Proc. Nat. Acad. Sci. USA **81:** 267-271.

52. SCHACHNER, M., A. FAISSNER, J. KRUSE, J. LINDNER, D. H. MEIER, F. G. RATHJEN & H. WERNECKE. 1983. Cell-type specificity and developmental expression of neural cell-surface components involved in cell interactions and of structurally related molecules. Cold Spring Harbor Symp. Quant. Biol. **48:** 557-568.

53. RUTISHAUSER, U. 1983. Molecular and biological properties of a neural cell adhesion molecules. Cold Spring Harbor Symp. Quant. Biol. **48:** 501-514.

54. RIOPELLE, R. J., R.C. MCGARRY, S. MIRSKI & J. C. RODER 1984. Some substrate interactions of neurons in vitro are mediated by a family of surface proteins related to and including myelin associated glycoprotein. Soc. Neurosci. Abstr. **10:** 41.

55. FALLON, J. R. 1985. Preferential outgrowth of central nervous system neurites on astrocytes and Schwann cells as compared with non-glial cells in vitro. J. Cell Biol. **100:** 198-207.

56. LETOURNEAU, P. C. 1975. Cell-to-substratum adhesion and guidance of axonal elongation. Dev. Biol. **44:** 92-101.

57. WESSELLS, N. K., P. C. LETOURNEAU, R. P. NUTTALL, M. LUDUEÑA-ANDERSON & J. M. GEIDUSCHEK. 1980. Responses to cell contacts between growth cones, neurites and ganglionic non-neuronal cells. J. Neurocytol. **9:** 647-664.

58. CAMPENOT, R. B. 1982. Development of sympathetic neurons in compartmentalized chambers. Dev. Biol. **93:** 1-12.

59. GUNDERSEN, R. W. & J. N. BARRETT. 1979. Neuronal chemotaxis: chick dorsal root axons turn towards high concentrations of nerve growth factor. Science **206:** 1079-1080.

60. EBENDAL, T. 1982. Orientational behaviour of extending neurites. *In* Cell Behaviour. R. Bellairs, A. Curtis & G. Dunn, Eds.: 281-295. Cambridge University Press. Cambridge, England.

61. ZALEWSKI, A. A. & A. K. GULATI. 1982. Evaluation of histocompatibility as a factor in the repair of nerve with a frozen nerve allograft. J. Neurosurg. **56:** 550-554.

62. THOMAS, P. K. 1974. Nerve injury. *In* Essays on the Nervous System. R. Bellairs & E. G. Gray, Eds.: 44-70. Clarendon Press. Oxford, England.

63. MORRIS, J. H., A. R. HUDSON & G. WEDDELL. 1972. A study of degeneration and regeneration in the divided rat sciatic nerve based on electron microscopy. Z. Zellforsch. **124:** 103-130.

64. BRAY, G. M., J.-M. PEYRONNARD & A. J. AGUAYO. 1972. Reactions of unmyelinated nerve fibers to injury. An ultrastructural study. Brain Res. **42:** 297-309.

65. IDE, C., K. TOHYAMA, R. YOKOTA, T. NITATORI & S. ONODERA. 1983. Schwann cell basal lamina and nerve regeneration. Brain Res. **288:** 61-75.

66. LUNDBORG, G., L. B. DAHLIN, N. DANIELSEN, R. H. GELBERMAN, F. M. LONGO, H. C. POWELL & S. VARON. 1982. Nerve regeneration in silicone chambers: influence of gap length and of distal stump components. Exp. Neurol. **76:** 361-375.

67. POLITIS, M. J., K. EDERLE & P. S. SPENCER. 1982. Tropism in nerve regeneration in vivo. Attraction of regenerating axons by diffusible factors derived from cells in distal nerve stumps of transected peripheral nerves. Brain Res. **253:** 1-12.

68. WILLIAMS, L. R., H. C. POWELL, G. LUNDBORG & S. VARON 1984. Competence of nerve tissue as distal insert promoting nerve regeneration in a silicone chamber. Brain Res. **293:** 201-211.

69. HORCH, K. 1979. Guidance of regrowing sensory axons after cutaneous nerve lesions in the cat. J. Neurophysiol. **42:** 1437-1449.

70. GOODMAN, C. S., M. J. BASTIANI, C. Q. DOE, S. DU LAC, S. L. HELFAND, J. Y. KUWADA

& J. B. THOMAS. 1984. Cell recognition during neuronal development. Science **225:** 1271-1279.
71. RICHARDSON, P. M., U. M. MCGUINNESS & A. J. AGUAYO. 1980. Axons from CNS neurones regenerate into PNS grafts. Nature **284:** 264-265.
72. RICHARDSON, P. M., V. M. K. ISSA & A. J. AGUAYO. 1984. Regeneration of long spinal axons in the rat. J. Neurocytol. **13:** 165-182.
73. WEISS, P. & A. C. TAYLOR. 1944. Further experimental evidence against "neurotropism" in nerve regeneration. J. Exp. Zool. **95:** 233-257.
74. MCQUARRIE, I. M. & B. GRAFSTEIN. 1973. Axon outgrowth enhanced by a previous nerve injury. Arch. Neurol. **29:** 53-55.
75. GRAFSTEIN, B. & I. M. MCQUARRIE. 1978. Role of the nerve cell body in axonal regeneration. *In* Neuronal Plasticity. C. W. Cotman, Ed.: 155-195. Raven Press. New York, N.Y.
76. PERRY, G.W., S. R. KRAYANEK & D. L. WILSON. 1983. Protein synthesis and rapid axonal transport during regrowth of dorsal root axons. J. Neurochem. **40:** 1590-1598.
77. RICHARDSON, P. M. & V. M. K. ISSA. 1984. Peripheral nerve injury enhances central regeneration of primary sensory neurones. Nature **309:** 791.
78. KRISTENSSON, K. & Y. OLSSON. 1976. Retrograde transport of horseradish peroxidase in transected axons. 3. Brain Res. **115:** 201-213.
79. HENDRY, I. A. & J. CAMPBELL. 1976. Morphometric analysis of rat superior cervical ganglion after axotomy and nerve growth factor treatment. J. Neurocytol. **5:** 351-360.
80. PURVES, D. & A. NJÅ. 1976. Effect of nerve growth factor on synaptic depression following axotomy. Nature **260:** 535-536.
81. CSILLIK, B., M. SCHWAB & H. THOENEN. 1985. Transganglionic regulation of central terminals of dorsal root ganglion cells by nerve growth factor. Brain Res. **331:** 11-15.
82. FITZGERALD, M., P. D. WALL, M. GOEDERT & P. C. EMSON. 1985. Nerve growth factor counteracts the neurophysiological and neurochemical effects of chronic sciatic nerve section. Brain Res. **332:** 131-141.
83. RICHARDSON, P. M. & V. M. K. VERGE. The induction of a regenerative propensity in sensory neurons following peripheral axonal injury. J. Neurocytol. (In press.)
84. HULSEBOSCH, C. E., R. E. COGGESHALL & J. R. PEREZ-POLO. 1984. Increased numbers of thoracic dorsal root axons in rats given antibodies to nerve growth factor. Science **225:** 525-526.

Characterization of a Laminin-Containing Neurite-Promoting Factor and a Neuronotrophic Factor from Peripheral Nerve and Related Sources[a]

GEORGE E. DAVIS, MARSTON MANTHORPE,
LAWRENCE R. WILLIAMS, AND SILVIO VARON

Department of Biology
School of Medicine
University of California, San Diego
La Jolla, California 92093

INTRODUCTION

The proper development of the peripheral nervous system (PNS) requires that embryonic neural crest cells, which are the precursor cells for neurons and glial cells in the PNS, will differentiate at appropriate times and positions in the developing embryo.[1,2] These events are regulated via neural crest cell genetic programs but also by environmental signals supplied from adjacent neural crest or other cells and extracellular matrices. Distinctive cell behaviors appear to be important in these events and include cell migration,[3,4] proliferation, differentiation, and adhesion to other cells[5] and extracellular matrices.[6] It has been suggested that neurofibromatosis is a disorder of this neural crest cell developmental scheme since its characteristic clinical manifestations[7] (i.e., multiple neurofibromas, café-au-lait spots, pigmented iris hamartomas) are thought to arise from cell types with neural crest progenitors. Neurofibromas, by histologic examination, contain cellular elements that resemble those present in peripheral nerve (i.e., Schwann and fibroblast-like cells, and neurites) as well as extracellular matrix elements such as collagen, acid mucopolysaccharides, and basement membranes.[8,9] The mechanism behind the generation of neurofibromas is unknown, but may involve an abnormal communication among these peripheral nerve elements and/or between the corresponding neural crest cells and their extracellular environment.

We have been particularly interested in understanding neuron-glial cell interactions and have focused on what glial cells contribute to neuronal performances.[10-12] Since we have not addressed this problem in the context of neurofibromatosis, it is not clear

[a]This work has been supported by National Institutes of Health Grant NS-16349 and U.S. Public Health Service Grant GM-07198.

to what extent our findings will have relevance to the pathogenesis of the disease. Recent data will be presented concerning the characterization of two protein factors that influence distinct neuronal behaviors *in vitro;* one that is required for neuronal survival and the other that acts in a substratum-bound manner to promote neurite outgrowth.

NEURONOTROPHIC VERSUS NEURITE-PROMOTING FACTORS

Cultured embryonic or newborn PNS neurons can be shown to require specific protein factors for their survival. These survival-promoting agents, often designated as neuronotrophic factors (NTFs), have been observed in various glial cell conditioned media or in the extracts of various tissues. To date, four NTFs for PNS neurons have

TABLE 1. Comparison of Purified Neuronotrophic Factors

	NGF	BDNF[a]	Chick CNTF	Rat CNTF
Physical properties				
Biologically active subunit:				
a. Molecular weight (kD)	13	12.3	24	28
b. Isoelectric point	9.3	10.2	5.0	5.7
Ganglionic neurons supported				
E8 chick dorsal root	+	−	−	−
E10 chick dorsal root	+	+	+	+
Newborn mouse dorsal root	+	NR	+	+
E11 chick sympathetic	+	−	+	+
Newborn rat superior cervical	+	NR	+	+
E8 chick ciliary	−	−	+	+

[a] NR = not reported.

been purified and characterized, namely, nerve growth factor (NGF),[13] brain-derived neurotrophic factor (BDNF),[14] and two ciliary neuronotrophic factors (CNTFs)—one from selected intraocular tissues (i.e., the innervation territory of the ciliary ganglion) of the embryonic chick[15] and the other from adult rat sciatic nerve.[16,47] These NTFs differ with respect to their subunit molecular weights, isoelectric points, and ability to support sensory, sympathetic, and parasympathetic neurons (TABLE 1).

Substratum-binding neurite-promoting factors (NPFs) were first observed in various cell conditioned media.[17-19] These factors were found to bind readily to polycationic substrata and were easily distinguished from survival factors also present in the conditioned media on the basis of such an affinity as well as the fact that the NPFs had no survival influence by themselves.[17,18] Recently, the purified extracellular matrix glycoprotein laminin has been found to be a very potent substratum-binding neurite-promoting factor,[20-23] mimicking at least qualitatively NPF activities from conditioned media. More recently, laminin has been reported to be a component of many of the conditioned medium NPFs,[24-26] although these factors do not appear to consist solely of laminin (see next section). FIGURE 1 illustrates the separate and distinct influences

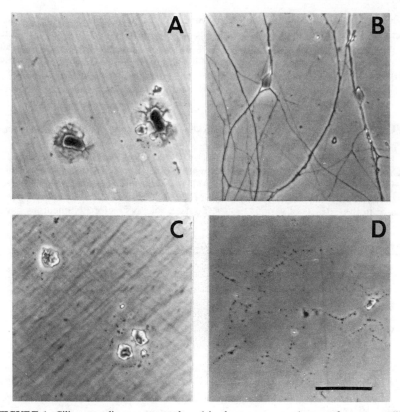

FIGURE 1. Ciliary ganglion neurons cultured in the presence or absence of rat nerve ciliary neuronotrophic factor (CNTF)[16] and rat schwannoma neurite-promoting factor (NPF).[25] Polyornithine tissue culture substrata (6 mm wells) were treated with 50 μl of a 1 μg/ml solution of rat schwannoma NPF in buffered saline or with buffered saline alone for 2 hours at 37°C. Serum-containing culture medium either contained 50 trophic units of purified rat nerve CNTF or was unsupplemented. The culture wells were seeded with ciliary neurons, were fixed after 24 hours of culture, and were stained with 0.1% toluidine blue. Cultures shown contained (A) CNTF alone; (B) CNTF plus an NPF-treated substratum; (C) neither factor; and (D) an NPF-treated substratum alone. Bar equals 50 μm.

of a purified NPF from rat RN22 schwannoma cell conditioned media and a purified NTF from adult rat sciatic nerve extracts on embryonic ciliary ganglion neuronal performances *in vitro*. The following sections will discuss in more detail the characterization of the rat schwannoma NPF and the rat sciatic nerve CNTF.

RAT RN22 SCHWANNOMA NEURITE-PROMOTING FACTOR

As mentioned above, substratum-binding NPF activities are synthesized by many cell types including Schwann, astroglial, endothelial, and muscle cells.[19] In addition, in an *in vivo* silicone chamber model of rat peripheral nerve regeneration, a fluid surrounding the regenerating nerve acquires a substratum-binding NPF activity.[27] In all of these cases, it is likely that the "conditioned medium" reflects what is shed from cell surfaces or what is released by cells for the purpose of binding to cell surfaces and/or extracellular matrices. The rat RN22 schwannoma cell line (derived from a chemically induced peripheral nerve tumor)[28] was found to be an excellent conditioned medium source of NPF activity and hence was chosen as a model system for the characterization of this type of factor.

With the discovery that purified laminin is also a potent NPF it seemed reasonable to suggest that laminin itself might be the active component in the neurite-promoting activities within different conditioned media. Initial experiments discouraged this view since antilaminin antibodies, which totally interfere with the neurite-promoting activity of laminin, had no effect on NPF activities from schwannoma, Schwann, astroglia, and oligodendroglia conditioned media[22] or the *in vivo* chamber fluid activity.[27] This distinction prompted further investigations of the properties of the schwannoma NPF and resulted in a detailed comparison between this factor and purified laminin.

The schwannoma NPF was isolated from conditioned medium using a three-step procedure (DE52 ion-exchange chromatography→cesium chloride equilibrium gradient centrifugation→sucrose density gradient centrifugation).[25] Between 10 and 60 μg of protein is obtained from 1.5 liters of conditioned medium. When the preparation is run on sodium dodecyl sulfate-polyacrylamide gel electrophoresis (SDS-PAGE) with reduction, it exhibits predominant doublet bands at approximately 200 kD (migrating closely to the 200 kD subunit of laminin); and without reduction, a band at approximately 900 kD which runs slightly faster than nonreduced laminin (FIGURE 2). Other minor bands are routinely observed in the preparation at 130-150 kD and 35 kD. If these bands are blotted to nitrocellulose, antilaminin antibodies can be shown to bind to both the 200 and 900 kD bands in the schwannoma preparation (FIGURE 3). The schwannoma NPF can also be shown to copurify with laminin antigens (using enzyme-linked immunoassays) and to be removed from solution by immobilized an-

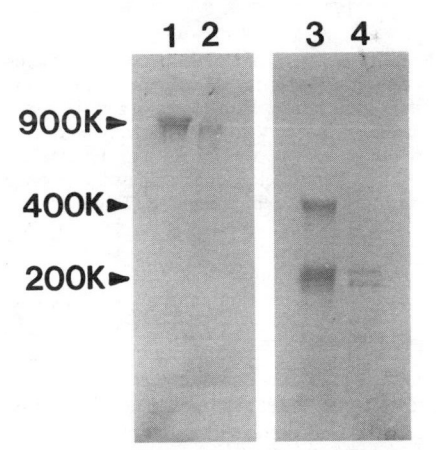

FIGURE 2. SDS-PAGE analysis of rat schwannoma neurite-promoting factor and rat laminin. Ten micrograms of laminin or 5 μg of schwannoma NPF was added per lane in a 2-10% polyacrylamide gel with (lanes 3 and 4) or without (lanes 1 and 2) reduction with 2-mercaptoethanol. Lanes 1 and 3, rat laminin; lanes 2 and 4, rat schwannoma NPF. Gels were stained with Coomassie Blue.

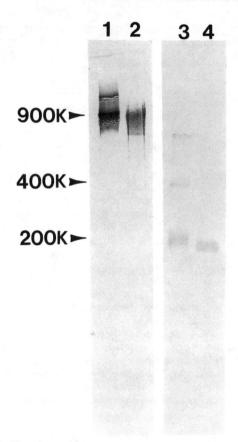

FIGURE 3. Immunoblot of rat schwannoma neurite-promoting factor and laminin with anti-laminin antisera. One microgram of either the schwannoma NPF or laminin was added per lane in a 2-10% polyacrylamide gradient gel with (lanes 3 and 4) and without (lanes 1 and 2) reduction with 2-mercaptoethanol. The proteins were electrophoretically blotted to nitrocellulose, the blots incubated with rabbit antisera to laminin and a peroxidase-conjugated secondary antibody as described,[25] and then were reacted for peroxidase activity with chloronaphthol. Lanes 1 and 3, rat laminin; lanes 2 and 4, rat schwannoma NPF.

tilaminin antibodies. The neurite-promoting activities of the schwannoma NPF and laminin were also compared using various parameters of neuritic growth from ciliary ganglion neurons.[29] The two factors were virtually indistinguishable in their effects, suggesting that they are likely to possess very similar neurite-promoting "active sites." Taken together, these data provide compelling evidence that laminin is the active neurite-promoting component in the schwannoma neurite-promoting factor. However, more studies will be necessary to confirm this point.

   Recently, purified laminin as well as other extracellular matrix proteins has been examined by rotary shadowing electron microscopy.[30] Laminin has a characteristic cross-shaped appearance with one long arm and three short arms, and several studies have attempted to correlate different functional domains with different regions of the rotary-shadowed structure.[31-33] One very recent study suggested that the active neurite-promoting site within the laminin molecule resides in the heparin-binding globular domain at the end of the long arm.[33] This site was found to be distinct from sites previously reported for cell-adhesion domains in the short-arm region of the structure. The schwannoma NPF preparation was also examined by rotary shadowing and found to have cross-shaped images of similar dimensions to purified laminin[25,26] (FIGURE 4). Nearly all of the images appeared to have intact long arms but to have one altered (truncated or missing) short arm. Also seen in the preparation were structures resembling published images of proteoglycans,[34] and occasionally these were found in apparent association with the laminin images[25,26] (not shown).

The biochemical characteristics of the schwannoma NPF (e.g., strong binding to DE52 ion-exchange columns, increased buoyant density)[25] suggest that there are likely to be glycosaminoglycan or proteoglycan materials in the factor. In support of this idea are recent data showing that a highly sulfated material (detected by $^{35}SO_4$ labeling) is associated with the factor.[26] The majority of this sulfated material can be degraded with nitrous acid suggesting that it is heparan sulfate. The schwannoma preparation also cross-reacts with an antibody prepared against a purified basement membrane heparan sulfate proteoglycan even in the presence of excess amounts of laminin. This provides evidence that the highly sulfated material is probably heparan sulfate proteoglycan and that the schwannoma NPF likely to be a laminin-heparan sulfate proteoglycan complex. However, it remains to be determined whether the heparan sulfate is associated solely with a proteoglycan core protein or whether it might be similarly linked to the laminin component. In any case, this laminin-containing NPF is distinct from purified laminin and further experiments are necessary to ascertain whether these differences have significance for the presentation of biologically active laminin *in vitro* and *in vivo*.

Recent data from another study corroborate these findings by demonstrating that an NPF from bovine corneal endothelial conditioned medium contains laminin, heparan sulfate proteoglycan, and a 150 kD protein which might be entactin.[24] In

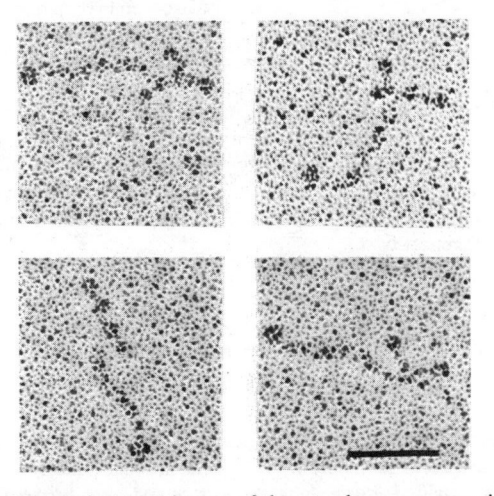

FIGURE 4. Selected rotary shadowed images of the rat schwannoma neurite-promoting-factor preparation. The NPF preparation was dialyzed into 0.2 M ammonium acetate and prepared further for rotary shadowing electron microscopy as described.[25,30] Four cross-shaped images are shown which resemble published images of laminin.[30] Bar equals 50 nm.

addition, NPF activities from rat PC12 pheochromocytoma, mouse C2 myoblast, and PF HR-9 embryonal carcinoma conditioned medium could be removed from solution using antilaminin antibodies.[24] This list can be extended further since NPF activities from rat astroglial conditioned medium as well as from an *in vivo* nerve regeneration chamber fluid collected four weeks after chamber implantation can be immuno-sequestered with immobilized antilaminin antibodies (Davis, unpublished observations). TABLE 2 lists the currently known NPFs that are believed to contain laminin as a component.

Although there is no direct evidence that laminin is a neurite-promoting factor *in vivo,* several studies suggest such a role. Schwann cells *in vivo* are known to express laminin on their cell surface as well as in their adjacent basement membranes.[35] Both of these substrata have been strongly implicated as permissive surfaces for regenerating axons.[36,37] In one study, regenerating axons (visualized by antineurofilament antibody staining) were found to colocalize with laminin antigens expressed on Schwann cell surfaces.[38] In another study, laminin antigens were expressed by migrating cells in a silicone chamber matrix and the appearance of these laminin-producing cells correlated temporally with the elongating front of axons.[27] Also, the NPF activity (measured *in vitro*) present in the chamber fluid increased and reached very high levels over the

TABLE 2. Neurite-Promoting-Factor Activities from "Conditioned Media" that Contain Laminin as a Component

Species	Source
Rat	RN22 schwannoma
	Astroglia
	PC12 pheochromocytoma
	In vivo nerve chamber fluid
Mouse	C2 myoblast
	PFHR-9 embryonal carcinoma
Bovine	Corneal endothelial

same time period during which axonal regeneration took place. As mentioned above, this NPF activity was found to contain laminin by immunosequestration experiments. The results of this chamber model study encourage the view that these laminin-containing NPFs are produced *in vivo* and are probably a very important component in the favorable substratum provided by Schwann cell surfaces and basement membranes for axonal regeneration.

RAT SCIATIC NERVE CILIARY NEURONOTROPHIC FACTOR

We have recently completed the purification of two CNTFs, one from the E 15 chick eye[15] and the other from adult rat sciatic nerve extracts.[16] The chick and rat CNTFs were both purified from their respective extracts by sequential DE52 ion-exchange chromatography, sucrose density gradient centrifugation, and preparative SDS-PAGE. Currently, the two factors can only be distinguished by their slight differences in molecular weight and in isoelectric point (see TABLE 1). Both of these factors can be distinguished from NGF and BDNF by their differences in size, charge, neuronal target specificity (see TABLE 1), and lack of reactivity with anti-NGF antibodies. It should also be noted that the two tissue sources containing the highest CNTF specific activity (trophic units/mg protein) in either the adult chicken or rat are peripheral nerve and the eye.[47] The level of CNTF in rat sciatic nerve extracts can be estimated (based on the specific activity of purified nerve CNTF and the amount of trophic activity per wet weight of nerve) to be about 25 μg/g tissue, an 8000-fold higher concentration than the 3 ng/g tissue of NGF reported to be present in normal sciatic nerve.[39] The functional significance of the CNTF and its high levels in nerve is unclear at present.

One interesting question here is the cellular source of the rat CNTF in peripheral nerve. Several lines of evidence suggest a glial cell origin, although more extensive studies will be necessary to prove this point. The amount of CNTF in different nerve extracts from pure sensory, motor, and mixed nerves is roughly similar,[40] suggesting that common cellular elements within these nerves are likely responsible for the activity. Also, isolated glial cells, such as Schwann cells and astroglia, produce a CNTF activity in culture.[41,42]

Recently we have developed a novel method for the identification of active CNTF polypeptides from crude sources.[43,47] The source materials, containing many different proteins, are submitted to SDS-PAGE and the separated proteins transferred to nitrocellulose paper. These nitrocellulose blots are then seeded with purified ciliary ganglion neurons. The neurons can be shown to attach uniformly to the paper but will only survive when they are in contact with CNTF. Hence, the neurons survive only over the region of the CNTF band and their presence can be detected by the appearance of a band of cells on the nitrocellulose blot after the addition of the vital dye MTT [13-(4,5-dimethyltheozol-2-yl)-2,5-diphenyl tetrazolium bromide]. FIGURE 5 shows such a "cell blot" and illustrates the survival of ciliary neurons on 24 and 19 kD CNTF bands from rat sciatic nerve extracts. In addition to its obvious applications toward the identification of CNTFs from different sources and species, the nitrocellulose blot method may also be directly applicable to other NTFs and other neuronal target cells.

These results also have implications concerning the way NTFs may be presented to neurons *in vivo*. Classically, the NTFs have been described as humoral or soluble factors, but as illustrated above, the CNTF appears to exert its survival influence on the nitrocellulose paper in a substratum-bound form. In addition, a recent report illustrates that substratum-bound NGF can influence neuritic guidance from explanted dorsal root ganglia.[44] Future experiments should better define the role of NTFs *in vivo* and how they are presented to developing and regenerating neurons.

CONCLUSIONS

What is the possible significance of factors such as laminin and CNTF for neurofibromatosis? If the disease has its roots in some abnormality in neuronal-Schwann cell interactions, then they may indeed have a role. If the Schwann cells, for example, were to abnormally produce increased amounts of CNTF or laminin, axons might be induced to sprout and this might in turn influence Schwann cell behaviors such as increased proliferation. Neurites are known to express cell surface mitogens for Schwann cells,[45,46] and any increase in neurite surface area might be expected to result

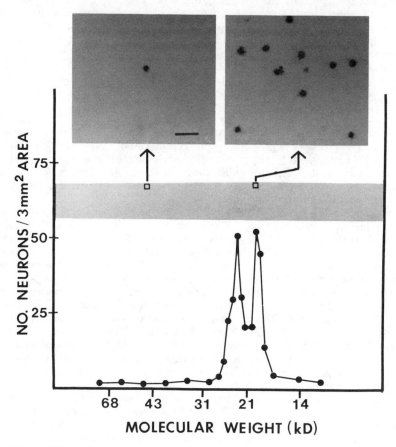

FIGURE 5. Nitrocellulose blot method for the identification of ciliary neuronotrophic factor (CNTF) bands from rat sciatic nerve extracts. Twenty-five microliters of sciatic nerve extract (4% extract w:v) was loaded into a lane and run on an SDS, 7.5-20% polyacrylamide gradient gel as described.[43,47] The proteins were then electrophoretically transferred to nitrocellulose paper, the blot blocked with 1% ovalbumin in buffered saline, and then seeded with purified ciliary ganglion neurons. After 24 hours of culture time, the vital dye MTT (see text for technical name) was added for 3 hours at 37°C and the blot culture was fixed with glutaraldehyde. The lane was then photographed at low power (lower panel) and at higher power in an area away from the CNTF bands (upper left panel) and an area within one of the CNTF bands (upper right panel). The surviving neurons accumulate the dye and form a blue formazan reaction product and hence appear as round blue cells when visualized under the microscope. The number of surviving neurons was also quantitated (3 mm² of area) along the length of the lane by direct counts using light microscopy. Molecular weight standards are indicated along the horizontal axis. Bar in upper left panel is 50 μm.

in an increase in Schwann cell numbers. In a cascade fashion, this might cause more laminin or CNTF production, more axonal growth, and more Schwann cell proliferation and hence eventually could result in the development of a peripheral nerve tumor. Alternatively, such factors as CNTF and laminin may not be directly involved in the basic defect in neurofibromatosis, but may be important in the expression of the disease because of their dramatic influences on neuronal and glial cell behaviors. In any case, further studies should address whether such identified proteins play any role in neurofibromatosis.

ACKNOWLEDGMENTS

The authors would like to thank Drs. Eva Engvall and Erkki Ruoslahti for the purified rat laminin and antisera against laminin as well as advice and assistance at various stages of this work. We would also like to thank Eleanore Hewitt for excellent technical assistance, Drs. Thomas Carnow and John Rudge for assistance with the "cell blot" technique, and George Klier for excellent technical assistance with the rotary shadowing electron microscopy.

REFERENCES

1. LE DOUARIN, N. M. 1982. The Neural Crest. Cambridge University Press. Cambridge, England.
2. WESTON, J. A. 1981. The regulation of normal and abnormal neural crest cell development. Adv. Neurol. **29:** 77-95.
3. LE DOUARIN, M. M. 1984. Cell migrations in embryos. Cell **38:** 353-360.
4. ROVASIO, R. A., A. DELOUVEE, K. M. YAMADA, R. TIMPL & J. P. THIERY. 1983. Neural crest cell migration: requirements for exogenous fibronectin and high cell density. J. Cell Biol. **96:** 462-473.
5. EDELMAN, G. M. 1983. Cell adhesion molecules. Science **219:** 450-457.
6. SANES, J. R. 1983. Roles of extracellular matrix in neural development. Annu. Rev. Physiol. **45:** 581-600.
7. RICCARDI, V. M. 1981. Von Recklinghausen neurofibromatosis. N. Engl. J. Med. **305:** 1617-1627.
8. RUSSELL, D. S. & L. J. RUBINSTEIN. 1977. Pathology of Tumors of the Nervous System: 389-397. Williams and Wilkins. Baltimore, Md.
9. LOTT, I. T. & E. P. RICHARDSON. 1981. Neuropathological findings and the biology of neurofibromatosis. Adv. Neurol. **29:** 23-32.
10. VARON, S. & G. SOMJEN. 1979. Neuron-glia interactions. Neurosci. Res. Prog. Bull. **17:** 1-239.
11. VARON, S. & M. MANTHORPE. 1982. Schwann cells: an in vitro perspective. Adv. Cell. Neurobiol. **3:** 35-95.
12. MANTHORPE, M., J. S. RUDGE & S. VARON. Astroglial cell contributions to neuronal survival and neuritic growth. *In* Astrocytes, **2.** Academic Press, Inc. New York, N.Y. (In press.)
13. GREENE, L. A. & E. M. SHOOTER. 1980. The nerve growth factor: biochemistry, synthesis and mechanism of action. Annu. Rev. Neurosci. **3:** 353-402.
14. BARDE, Y. A., D. EDGAR & H. THOENEN. 1982. Purification of a new neuronotrophic factor from mammalian brain. EMBO J. **1:** 549-553.

15. BARBIN, G., M. MANTHORPE & S. VARON. 1984. Purification of the chick eye ciliary neuronotrophic factor (CNTF). J. Neurochem. **43:** 1468-1478.
16. MANTHORPE, M., S. D. SKAPER, L. R. WILLIAMS & S. VARON. 1986. Purification of rat nerve ciliary neuronotrophic factor. Brain Res. **367:** 282-286.
17. COLLINS, F. 1978. Induction of neurite outgrowth by a conditioned medium factor bound to culture substratum. Proc. Nat. Acad. Sci. USA **75:** 5210-5213.
18. ADLER, R. & S. VARON. 1980. Cholinergic neuronotrophic factors. V. Segregation of survival- and neurite-promoting activities in heart conditioned media. Brain Res. **188:** 437-448.
19. ADLER, R., M. MANTHORPE, S. D. SKAPER & S. VARON. 1981. Polyornithine-attached neurite promoting factors (PNPFs). Culture sources and responsive neurons. Brain Res. **206:** 129-144.
20. BARON VAN EVERCOOREN, A., H. K. KLEINMAN, S. OHNO, P. MARANGOS, J. P. SCHWARTZ & M. E. DUBOIS-DALCQ. 1982. Nerve growth factor, laminin and fibronectin promote neurite growth in human fetal sensory ganglia cultures. J. Neurosci. Res. **8:** 179-194.
21. ROGERS, S. L., P. C. LETOURNEAU, S. L. PALM, J. MCCARTHY & L. T. FURCHT. 1983. Neurite extension by peripheral and central nervous system neurons in response to substratum-bound fibronectin and laminin. Dev. Biol. **98:** 212-220.
22. MANTHORPE, M., E. ENGVALL, E. RUOSLAHTI, F. M. LONGO, G. E. DAVIS & S. VARON. 1983. Laminin promotes neuritic regeneration from cultured peripheral and central neurons. J. Cell Biol. **97:** 1882-1890.
23. WEWER, U., R. ALBRECHTSEN, M. MANTHORPE, S. VARON, E. ENGVALL & E. RUOSLAHTI. 1983. Human laminin isolated in a nearly intact, biologically active form from placenta by limited proteolysis. J. Biol. Chem. **250:** 12654-12660.
24. LANDER, A. D., D. K. FUJII & L. F. REICHARDT. 1985. Laminin is associated with the "neurite outgrowth promoting factors" found in conditioned media. Proc. Nat. Acad. Sci. USA **82:** 2183-2189.
25. DAVIS, G. E., M. MANTHORPE, E. ENGVALL & S. VARON. 1985. Isolation and characterization of rat schwannoma neurite promoting factor: evidence that the factor contains laminin. J. Neurosci. **5:** 2662-2671.
26. DAVIS, G. E., S. VARON & M. MANTHORPE. 1985. Substratum-binding neurite promoting factors: relationships to laminin. Trends Neurosci. **8:** 528-532.
27. LONGO, F. M., E. G. HAYMAN, G. E. DAVIS, E. RUOSLAHTI, E. ENGVALL, M. MANTHORPE & S. VARON. 1984. Neurite promoting factors and extracellular matrix components accumulating *in vivo* within nerve regeneration chambers. Brain Res. **309:** 105-117.
28. PFEIFFER, S. E. & W. WECHSLER. 1972. A biochemically differentiated line of Schwann cells. Proc. Nat. Acad. Sci. USA **69:** 2885-2889.
29. DAVIS, G. E., M. MANTHORPE & S. VARON. 1985. Parameters of neuritic growth from ciliary ganglion neurons in vitro: influence of laminin, schwannoma polyornithine-binding neurite promoting factor and ciliary neuronotrophic factor. Dev. Brain Res. **17:** 75-84.
30. ENGEL, J., E. ODERMATT, A. ENGEL, J. A. MADRI, H. FURTHMAYR, H. ROHDE & R. TIMPL. 1981. Shapes, domain organizations and flexibility of laminin and fibronectin, two multifunctional proteins of the extracellular matrix. J. Mol. Biol. **150:** 97-120.
31. RAO, C. N., I. M. K. MARGULIES, T. S. TRALKA, V. P. TERRANOVA, J. A. MADRI & L. A. LIOTTA. 1982. Isolation of a subunit of laminin and its role in molecular structure and tumor cell attachment. J. Biol. Chem. **257:** 9740-9744.
32. TIMPL, R., S. JOHANSSON, V. VAN DELDEN, I. OBERBAUMER & M. HOOK. 1983. Characterization of protease-resistant fragments of laminin mediating attachment and spreading of rat hepatocytes. J. Biol. Chem. **258:** 8922-8927.
33. EDGAR, D., R. TIMPL & H. THOENEN. 1984. The heparin-binding domain of laminin is responsible for its effects on neurite outgrowth and neuronal survival. EMBO J. **3:** 1463-1468.
34. FUJIWARA, S., H. WIEDEMANN, R. TIMPL, A. LUSTIG & J. ENGEL. 1984. Structure and interactions of heparan sulfate proteoglycans from a mouse tumor basement membrane. Eur. J. Biochem. **143:** 145-157.

35. CORNBROOKS, C. J., D. J. CAREY, J. A. MCDONALD, R. TIMPL & R. P. BUNGE. 1983. *In vivo* and *in vitro* observations on laminin production by Schwann cells. Proc. Nat. Acad. Sci. USA **80:** 3850-3854.
36. THOMAS, P. K. 1966. The cellular response to nerve injury. I. The cellular outgrowth from the distal stump of transected nerve. J. Anat. **100:** 287-303.
37. IDE, C., K. TOHYAMA, R. YOKOTO, T. NITATORI & S. ONODERA. 1983. Schwann cell basal lamina and nerve regeneration. Brain Res. **288:** 61-75.
38. BIGNAMI, A., N. H. CHI & D. DAHL. 1984. Laminin in rat sciatic nerve undergoing Wallerian degeneration—immunofluorescence study with laminin and neurofilament antisera. J. Neuropathol. Exp. Neurol. **43:** 94-103.
39. KORSCHING, S. & H. THOENEN. 1983. Quantitative demonstration of the retrograde transport of endogenous nerve growth factor. Neurosci. Lett. **39:** 1-4.
40. WILLIAMS, L. R., M. MANTHORPE, M. NIETO-SAMPEDRO, C. W. COTMAN & S. VARON. 1984. High ciliary neuronotrophic specific activity in rat peripheral nerve. Int. J. Dev. Neurobiol. **2:** 177-180.
41. VARON, S. & M. MANTHORPE. 1985. In vitro models for neuroplasticity and repair. *In* Central Nervous System Plasticity and Repair. A. Bignami, F. E. Bloom, C. L. Bolis & A. Adeloye, Eds.: 13-23. Raven Press. New York, N.Y.
42. RUDGE, J. S., M. MANTHORPE & S. VARON. 1985. The output of neuronotrophic and neurite-promoting agents from rat brain astroglial cells: a microculture method for screening potential regulatory molecules. Dev. Brain Res. **19:** 161-172.
43. CARNOW, T. B., M. MANTHORPE, G. E. DAVIS & S. VARON. 1985. Localized survival of ciliary ganglionic neurons identifies neuronotrophic factor bands on nitrocellulose blots. J. Neurosci. **5:** 1965-1971.
44. GUNDERSON, R. W. 1985. Sensory neurite growth cone guidance by substrate adsorbed nerve growth factor. J. Neurosci. Res. **13:** 199-212.
45. WOOD, P. M. & R. P. BUNGE. 1975. Evidence that sensory axons are mitogenic for Schwann cells. Nature **256:** 662-664.
46. SALZER, J. L., R. P. BUNGE & L. GLASER. 1980. Studies of Schwann cell proliferation. III. Evidence for the surface localization of the neurite mitogen. J. Cell Biol. **84:** 767-778.
47. RUDGE, J. S., G. E. DAVIS, M. MANTHORPE & S. VARON. An examination of ciliary neuronotrophic factors from avian and rodent tissue extracts using a blot and culture technique. Dev. Brain Res. (Submitted.)

Growth-Promoting Factors in Neurofibroma Crude Extracts[a]

VINCENT M. RICCARDI

Neurofibromatosis Program
Baylor College of Medicine
1 Baylor Plaza
Houston, Texas 77030

INTRODUCTION

Neurofibromatosis (NF) is primarily a disorder of growth. Except for the pigmentation defects (e.g., café-au-lait spots, freckling), all of the primary features of NF appear to represent an abnormal proliferation of cells, manifest either as dysplasias (e.g., tibial pseudarthrosis), benign tumors (e.g., astrocytomas, neurofibromas), or malignant tumors (e.g., neurofibrosarcomas); and even the pigmented lesions may eventually be shown to represent an abnormal clonal proliferation. While the malignant tumors are likely to result from a somatic mutational event in affected cells, endowing them with an intrinsic ability to proliferate abnormally, there is no a priori reason to presume that the other disturbances of cell proliferation characterizing NF, particularly the neurofibromas and central nervous system (CNS) tumors, will be explained solely in terms of the NF mutation per se.[12,15] To the contrary, there are compelling reasons to consider that the growth abnormalities of NF are mediated by the abnormal availability or effect of extrinsic factors that act in an autocrine or paracrine manner. The putative role of neural crest derivatives in NF pathogenesis[1,9] may suggest or account for specific factors, for example, nerve growth factor (NGF), ultimately found to be involved.

Previous work addressing a potential aberration of hormones, growth factors, or receptor sites in NF has been uneven and sparse until very recently, the change being exemplified by this symposium. Most of the work to date has focused on epidermal growth factor (EGF) and its receptor site in cultured NF skin cells;[21,22] NGF in the blood of NF patients[18] and in the native tumors, cultured tumor cells, and their conditioned medium (Riopelle, R. J. and Riccardi, V. M., unpublished data); glial growth factor;[6] and axolemmal-membrane-derived substances.[8]

Parenthetically, the high likelihood that different forms of NF will show different levels of and/or responses to specific growth factors would emphasize what the author has been stressing from the clinical standpoint,[13] namely, the importance of NF heterogeneity. The results of cell biology investigations, including those relating to growth factor production, availability, activity, and kinetics, may well be different for

[a] This work was supported in part by the Texas NF Foundation, The Neurofibromatosis Institute, Inc., the Lyle S. Thompson Memorial Fund, and National Institutes of Health Grant CA 32064.

different forms or types of the disease. Thus, in the study presented here, the patient material will all have been derived from patients with von Recklinghausen NF[11] (or NF-I, as defined in Reference 13), unless otherwise stated.

The main purpose of the present study was to determine whether crude extracts of intact neurofibromas could augment the proliferation of one or more cell types in monolayer cultures, particularly cells derived from neurofibromas. Additional background data relating to culture medium supplementation, other culture conditions, and intracellular nucleotides will also be discussed.

MATERIALS AND METHODS

All NF patients supplying skin and/or tumor specimens were or are participants in the Baylor NF Program, and are considered to have NF-I.[11,13] Each specimen was obtained incidental to therapeutic surgery, except in one instance when large amounts of skin and tumor were obtained at autopsy. Specimens were processed directly or frozen at −80°C.

Crude extracts of neurofibromas were prepared from 14 to 44 g of frozen tumor, 10-20 months after it was originally obtained. Each specimen was thawed, then cut with scissors or a knife blade down to pieces 3-4 mm in diameter (on ice). The minced tumor was then homogenized with high-speed revolving blades (Polytron) in two to four 30-second pulses, all the while kept on ice. The homogenized tumor was decanted into a 50 ml conical tube and centrifuged at 19,500 rpm at 4°C for 1.5 hours. At that time the supernatant cell sap, representing about 25% of the specimen volume, was filtered through a 0.2 μ filter (Millipore) and frozen (−80°C or liquid nitrogen) in 0.5 ml aliquots for later use. At no time were solvents or buffers used in the preparation or storage of the extract. When ready for use, each aliquot was thawed and added directly to the culture medium in each individual culture vessel. Once thawed, the extract was kept at 4°C until it was used up, usually within 2 weeks.

Extract 1 was derived from a tumor from patient NF82-315-1, a 23-year-old white woman. The tumor was a diffuse plexiform neurofibroma from the retroperitoneal region, and it was obtained at the time of therapeutic surgery. Extracts 2 through 5 were derived from different portions of a diffuse plexiform neurofibroma from the nuchal region of a 14-year-old black girl (patient NF78-15-2; see Reference 10, Figure 6) at the time of her autopsy. Each extract was more or less comparable to the others in terms of in vitro experimental data, both by direct comparisons and overall results.

Routine culture medium, hereafter referred to as "regular medium," was Eagle's minimal essential medium, with Earle's salts, supplemented with glutamine, sodium bicarbonate, penicillin/streptomycin, and 10% fetal bovine serum (FBS). Other sera used were pooled normal human serum (HUS), either obtained commercially (Gibco or Hazleton) or from laboratory personnel, and pooled serum from six adult NF-I patient (NFS). A serum substitute product, Nu-serum (Collaborative Research), was also used as designated. Routine culture conditions, which obtained for all experiments described here except as noted otherwise, included a temperature of 37°C, and humidified air containing 5% carbon dioxide. Culture vessels were plastic (Falcon), either 25 cm² T-flasks, 60 mm petri dishes, or 35 mm petri dishes. Ordinarily, medium was replenished twice weekly.

Explant cultures were established under sterile conditions by mincing each specimen with no. 15 surgical blades into 1-2 mm pieces and scratching (scoring) each piece into the surface of a 60 mm plastic petri dish, 3-5 pieces per petri dish. After 10-20 days the cells were released from the petri dish surface by the action of a dilute (0.25%) trypsin solution (Gibco), and either dispersed over the surface of the original dish, or split into two or three petri dishes or flasks.

A total of 13 specimens gave cultured cells that were tested for an effect of neurofibroma extract as reported here. Included were 8 neurofibromas (1 with matching skin fibroblasts), 1 tibial pseudarthrosis (with matching skin fibroblasts), 1 NF patient's normal skin (and no associated neurofibroma), and 1 normal subject's skin fibroblasts.

For some experiments, using phase microscopy, the cell number in a culture vessel was roughly estimated, the cells suspended (by trypsinization) and diluted to give a final concentration of 500-1000 cells per ml, and 5 ml of the suspension inoculated into each of the respective experiment's culture vessels. In other instances, a hemocytometer cell count of the original trypsin-treated suspension was performed and subsequent petri inoculations were based on specific predetermined cell numbers, ranging from 100 cells to 50,000 cells per petri dish, depending on the specific experiment.

For radionuclide studies, [^{3}]H-thymidine (19.3 mCi/mmol; New England Nuclear) was used. For each experiment the original material was diluted in regular medium to a final concentration of 10 μCi/ml. Quantification of uptake utilized scintillation counting. Spent radioactive medium was aspirated from each 35 mm plastic petri dish, the cells washed three times with fresh medium, fixed with 10% trichloroacetic acid for 30 minutes at 4°C, air dried, and finally the petri dish was dissolved in scintillation fluid in its own vial. Scintillation counting was performed with a Beckman LS 2800.

Live fertilized eggs and unhatched embryos of the bicolor damselfish *(Pomacentrus*

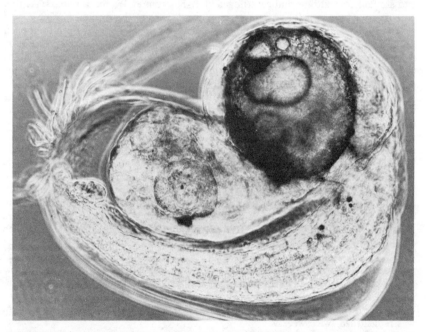

FIGURE 1. A bicolor damselfish embryo being removed from its egg case; the head is already out, but most of the body and yolk sac are still inside the egg case.

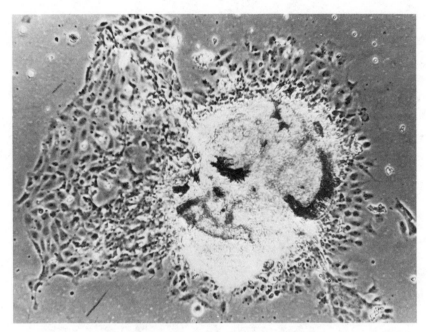

FIGURE 2. The appearance of a bicolor damselfish embryo explant culture after about 10 days under baseline conditions; the predominant cell outgrowth consists of small, shortened fibroblasts.

partitus) at risk for neurofibromatosis[19] were provided by M. Schmale, Ph.D. After treating their seawater with Furizone Light (nitrofuran, furadolazone, and methylene blue) for 1 hour, individual live embryos were identified with the aid of a dissecting microscope, and, under sterile conditions, one live embryo was placed in each of many 35 mm plastic petri dishes. The embryo was removed from its egg case (FIGURE 1) and explanted by scoring it into the petri dish surface. The attached specimen was then bathed with marine teleost culture medium, which consisted of regular medium with NaCl supplementation to a final concentration of 11.5 g/L.[20] Cell culture was then carried out at 27°C in humidified air containing 2% carbon dioxide, with replenishment of the culture medium weekly or biweekly. In two instances, after substantial cellular explant outgrowth had been established (FIGURE 2), the culture medium was supplemented with neurofibroma Extract 1 (25 μl/ml).

RESULTS

General Growth Properties of Cultured NF Specimens

In *Experiment 83-4,* 83-391T (neurofibroma) cells showed the following cloning efficiencies: 10.1% in 10% FBS, 0% in 10% normal human serum (HUS; Gibco),

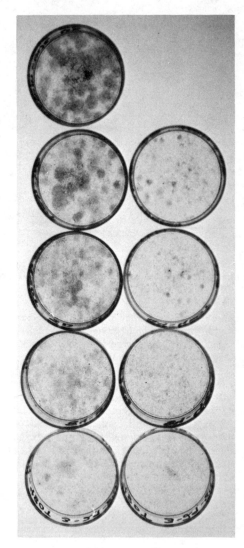

FIGURE 3. Comparison of petri dishes with 84-480T Giemsa-stained cells after 6, 8, and 11 days in Extract 1 (25 μl/ml; top row) or in its absence.

and 16.8% in NF human serum (NFS). In *Experiment 83-5,* 83-391T cells showed the following cloning efficiencies: 19.5% in 10% FBS and 16.9% in 10% NFS. In *Experiment 84-2,* 83-450T (neurofibroma) cells showed a cloning efficiency of 6% in 10% FBS. The mean average cloning efficiencies for these three experiments are 11.9% for 10% FBS and 16.8% for 10% NFS. In *Experiment 85-6,* 85-569T2 (neurofibroma) and 85-569s (NF skin fibroblast) cells showed growth in 10% HUS (Hazleton) that was at least equivalent to growth in 10% FBS. Similar results in *Experiment 85-4*

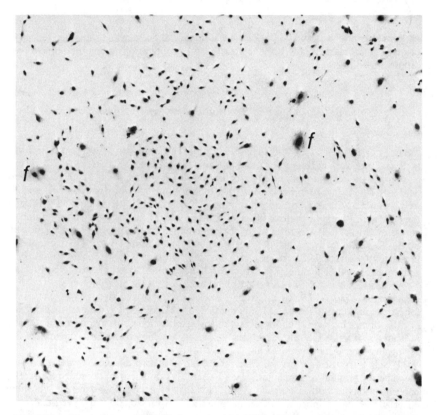

FIGURE 4. Photomicrograph of Giemsa-stained 84-480T cells after eight days in the presence of Extract 1. The smaller spindle-shaped cells are seen to predominate, and an occasional ordinary fibroblast (f) is seen.

were obtained for 85-575s (NF skin fibroblast) cells, comparing 10% HUS (Hazleton) with 10% FBS. In *Experiment 85-7,* 84-469T (neurofibroma) cells showed a 2.58-fold increase in number in regular medium over 48 hours (triplicate cell counts at 24 and 72 hours after inoculation of 35 mm petri dishes). In *Experiment 84-8,* 84-469T cells in regular medium showed a 3.48-fold increase in number over 48 hours, and 2.33-fold and 1.55-fold increases over each of the two intervening 24-hour periods, respectively (triplicate cell counts at 24, 48, and 72 hours after inoculation of 35 mm petri dishes). The mean average 24-hour increase was 1.94-fold, and the mean average

TABLE 1. Proliferation Response of Cultured Neurofibroma-Derived Cells (84-493T) after 5 Days in the Presence of Neurofibroma Extract 3[a]

	Extract 3 (μl/ml)				
	0	5	15	25	50
cpm	2.8	12.8	17.4	23.0	31.4

[a][3]H-Thymidine counts per minute (cpm), mean averages of triplicate samples × 1000.

48-hour increase was thus 3.03-fold. In summary then, neurofibroma-derived cells, primarily fibroblasts, show normal growth and proliferation under the culture conditions noted here.

Responses of Tumor and Skin Cultures to Neurofibroma Extracts

In *Experiment 84-16*, 84-480T (neurofibroma) cells, following 3 weeks prior growth in Extract 1, were cultured with and without the presence of Extract 2 (25 μl/ml) and showed a definite positive effect of Extract 2 (FIGURES 3 and 4). In *Experiment 84-17*, 84-493T (neurofibroma) cells, this time following prior growth in Extract 2, were cultured with and without the continued presence of Extract 2 (25 μl/ml) and they showed a definite positive effect of Extract 2, both in terms of colony numbers and sizes (FIGURE 5) and in terms of the preferential growth of spindle cells (FIGURE 6). In *Experiment 84-18*, 84-493T cells were again cultured with and without the presence of Extract 2 (25 μl/ml), but this time without prior exposure to any neurofibroma extract. The differential growth enhancement afforded by Extract 2 (FIGURE 7) was thus shown not to depend on pretreatment with the neurofibroma extract. In *Experiment 84-20*, 84-493T cells, after 2 weeks of growth in Extract 3, were cultured for 5 days in doses of Extract 2 including 0, 5, 15, 25, and 50 μl/ml, and their uptake of ^{3}H-thymidine over 4 hours measured (by scintillation counting, in triplicate). As indicated in TABLE 1, a dose-dependent response was documented. In *Experiment 84-25*, again using ^{3}H-thymidine uptake over 4 hours as an index of proliferation, 84-493T cells were used to test the effect of Extract 3 at two dosages, as well as to test the effect of original cell inoculum size (TABLE 2). Compared to no added Extract 3, concentrations of both 5 and 25 μl/ml showed a clear-cut dose-dependent positive effect at the higher inocula (with a maximum effect for 20,000 cells/petri dish, and

TABLE 2. Proliferation Response of Neurofibroma-Derived Cells (84-493T) in Culture, after 2 Days in the Presence of Neurofibroma Extract 3, for 3 Different Original Cell Inocula[a]

	Extract 3 (μl/ml)		
Inoculum	0	5	25
2,000	3.87	3.31	4.38
10,000	17.57	20.01	52.63
20,000	76.15	111.22	173.32

[a][3]H-Thymidine cpm, averages of duplicate samples × 1000.

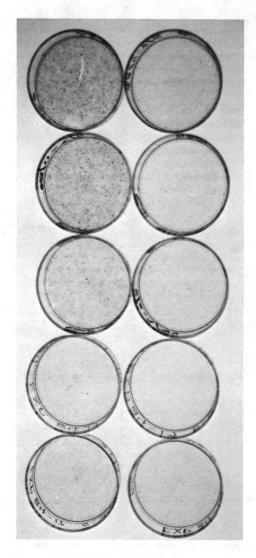

FIGURE 5. Comparison of Giemsa-stained petri dishes of Experiment 84-17, showing the effect of the presence of 25 µl/ml of Extract 2 (top row) versus no extract (bottom row).

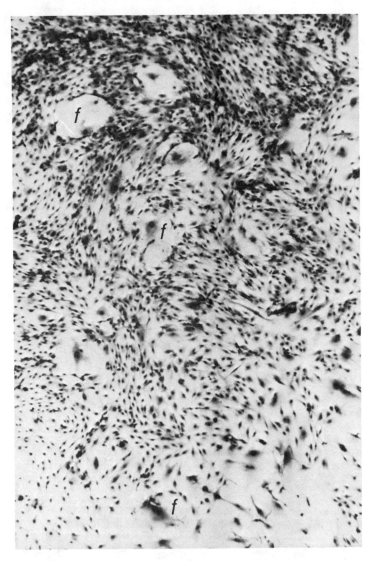

FIGURE 6. Photomicrograph of Giemsa-stained cells from Experiment 84-17 after 10 days in the presence of Extract 2. Again, the small spindle-shaped cells predominate and an occasional ordinary fibroblast (f) is seen.

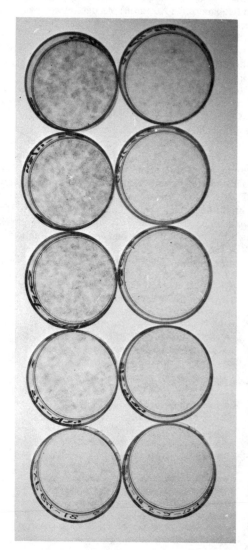

FIGURE 7. Comparison of Giemsa-stained petri dishes of Experiment 84-18, showing the effect of the presence of 25 μl/ml of Extract 2 (top row) versus no extract (bottom row).

a moderate effect at 10,000 cells/petri dish), but a much more modest effect with an initial inoculum of 2000 cells/petri dish.

In *Experiment 84-19*, 84-493T cells, previously grown in Extract 2, were cultured with or without the continued presence of Extract 2 (25 μl/ml), and in either case in the presence of either 10% FBS or a 10% concentration of a commercial serum substitute, Nu-serum (Collaborative Research). As determined by the Giemsa-staining density of petri dishes, in the presence of FBS there was the expected positive effect of Extract 2. However, Nu-serum was associated with a much lower degree of cell proliferation, which was not significantly influenced by the presence of Extract 2. That is, neither the components of Nu-serum nor of Extract 2 were able to substitute for some crucial factor in FBS under these culture conditions.

In *Experiment 84-33* a new cell strain, 84-552T (neurofibroma), and a new neurofibroma extract (Extract 5) were tested, both to demonstrate the extract's immediate positive effect and to consider the effect of 2 weeks pretreatment. Using petri dish staining density as a cell proliferation index, a positive effect of Extract 5 was shown, with a slight, but definite, positive effect of pretreatment (FIGURE 8). In *Experiment 84-35*, 84-552T cells were plated at 100 cells/petri dish and colony counts carried out after Giemsa-staining at 10 days of culture. Colony counts (average of duplicate or triplicate petri dishes) for the various Extract 5 doses were as follows: 0 μl/ml = 4; 1.5 μl/ml = 22.5; 2 μl/ml = 24.0; 5 μl/ml = 27.0; 10 μl/ml = 23.5; and 15 μl/ml = 23.0. By bright-field microscopy, Giemsa-stained cells failed to show the overwhelming preponderance of spindle cells as noted in previous experiments. Whether this reflects differences in extracts and/or in cell strains is uncertain.

In *Experiment 84-36*, 84-552T cells at low density (100 cells per 35 mm petri dish) grew poorly in serum-free medium, with an equivocally positive effect of Extract 5

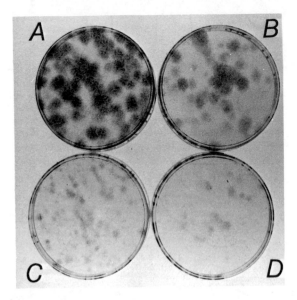

FIGURE 8. Giemsa-stained petri dishes from Experiment 84-33, showing the effect of 10 days exposure to 25 μl/ml of Extract 5 (A and B), with prior (A and C) and no prior (B and D) growth in the presence of Extract 5.

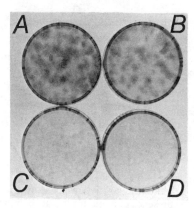

FIGURE 9. Giemsa-stained petri dishes from Experiment 84-43, showing the effect of 10 days exposure to 5 μl/ml of Extract 5 (A and B), both at 37°C (A and C) and at 38.5°C (B and D).

at 5 μl/ml (but no response at all at 2 and 15 μl/ml). In *Experiment 84-42* and in *Experiment 84-44,* again there was even less of an apparent ability of Extract 5 to enhance the growth of 84-552T cells in serum-free medium, though in the presence of 10% FBS the expected positive effect of 5 μl/ml was seen.

Experiment 84-43 was the first of several experiments designed to examine the effect of elevated cell culture incubation temperatures, with and without the presence of 5 μl/ml of Extract 5. In this experiment, using 84-552T cells, there was a positive effect of Extract 5 at both 37°C and 38.5°C, and an enhancement of growth (as determined by petri dish Giemsa stain density at 10 days of culture) at 38.5°C, with and without Extract 5 added (FIGURE 9). In *Experiment 84-46,* 84-356TR (neurofibroma) cells showed comparable excellent growth at 37°C and 39.5°C (after 10 days), but the high original inoculum did not allow demonstration of a clear positive effect of Extract 5 (5 μl/ml) at either temperature. In *Experiment 85-1,* 84-356TR cells, during 7 days in culture, showed a low-grade, but definite clonal proliferation, at 40.5°C, but much less than at 37°C, with a typical positive effect of Extract 5 at 37°C and a possible positive effect of Extract 5 at 40.5°C. MB cells (skin fibroblast cells from a normal young adult) showed no effect of Extract 5 at either 37°C or 40.5°C, and MB cells, in contrast to 84-356TR cells, showed only survival, but no significant proliferation, at 40.5°C.

In *Experiment 85-2,* 85-569T2 (neurofibroma) cells and 85-569s (skin fibroblast) cells, using Giemsa-staining density of petri dishes at 7 days culture, both showed a positive effect of Extract 5 (5 μl/ml), though somewhat more for the neurofibroma-derived cells than for the skin fibroblasts. In *Experiment 85-5,* a repeat of Experiment 85-2, 85-569T2 and 85-569s cells showed equivalent positive effects of Extract 5. In contrast, in *Experiment 85-9,* both Extract 3 and Extract 5 (each at 5 μl/ml) showed a proliferation enhancement (i.e., positive) effect on 85-569s cells, but no apparent effect on the MB (normal skin fibroblast) cells.

In *Experiment 85-7,* 85-576T (NF tibial pseudarthrosis) and 85-576s (NF skin fibroblast) cells showed equivalent growth-enhancement effects of Extract 5, measured at 8 days by Giemsa stain density of petri dishes. That is, both the NF lesion and ostensibly uninvolved skin provided cells with comparable response to crude neurofibroma extract.

Bicolor Damselfish Embryo Cell Cultures

Treatment of two bicolor damselfish embryo explant cultures with neurofibroma extract led to no response in one instance, and in the other instance to a very vigorous proliferation of cells very reminiscent of the spindle cell outgrowth of human neurofibroma described above (FIGURE 10). However, after the initial surge of growth, which lasted for approximately 1 week, in the continued presence of Extract 1 the culture became quiescent and remained so for many weeks thereafter until it was discarded. [Although we had previously established bicolor damselfish neurofibromas in explant culture (as described for human tumors, but with the use of marine teleost cell culture conditions described above), no such culture material was subsequently available for direct testing of the human neurofibroma extract on the fish tumor culture cells.] It is unknown as to whether the positive response of the one bicolor damselfish embryo explant reflected the presence of a mutant NF gene in that fish or a nonspecific response of one or more cell types available in the explant culture at the time the extract was added.

DISCUSSION

Background

Explant cell culture of neurofibromas and other NF-derived tissues has been a major undertaking of the Baylor NF Program since its inception in March 1978. Our earliest efforts gave us several insights[16,17] that are worth reviewing here. First, cells that derive from neurofibromas under routine culture conditions are heterogeneous in terms of morphology, growth rate, and overall behavior. This heterogeneity is in part a function of the time in culture. Initially (Phase I), there is a melange of five types of cells (FIGURE 11): (1) motile macrophages, which involute and fail to divide; (2) small stellate cells, often with one or more very long cytoplasmic extensions—these cells also appear not to divide; (3) small, discoid epithelial cells, presumably of endothelial origin; (4) small spindle-shaped bipolar cells; (5) larger fusiform or flattened fibroblasts (i.e., essentially indistinguishable from skin-derived fibroblasts). In the next stage (Phase II) there is some modest, but definite, proliferation of the putative endothelial cells, of the spindle cells, and, to a greater degree, of the fibroblasts, over a period lasting from about the 7th to the 20th day in culture. Subsequently (i.e., in Phase III), the fibroblasts become the overwhelmingly preponderant cell type because of an enhanced proliferation rate compared to the other two cell types and because the latter are relatively resistant to the action of trypsin used for passaging of the cells. The fibroblasts that derive from any one neurofibroma are usually the same from one petri dish to another, although in any one tumor the fibroblasts may be somewhat different in that they are less fusiform, flatter, and much more slowly growing. Other than these unusual "fibroblast-like" cells, with their slower growth rate, neurofibroma-derived fibroblasts generally have a proliferation ability comparable to NF-patient skin fibroblasts and control (i.e., normal) subject skin fibroblasts, as determined by serial cell-count experiments.

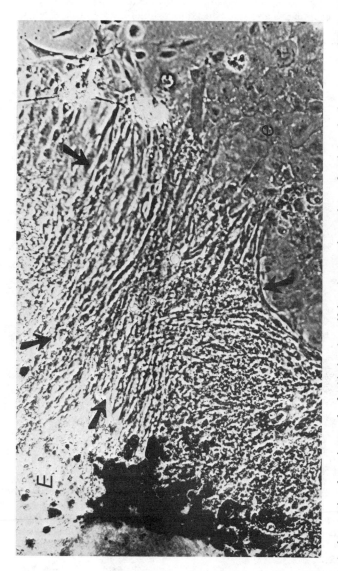

FIGURE 10. A phase optics photomicrograph of a bicolor damselfish embryo explant culture after 6 days in the presence of Extract 1, showing a cluster of spindle-shaped cells (arrows) emanating from the bulk of the embryo (E), and superimposed on the more ordinary epithelial cells (e).

In contrast, if proliferation ability is measured by scintillation counting of ^{3}H-thymidine pulse labeling of NF-derived cells, the NF-cell proliferation rate may appear to be low compared to non-NF cells,[21] though the proportion of cells showing S-phase DNA synthesis is the same for both NF-derived and normal control cells.[17] Moreover, the apparent decrease in the uptake of ^{3}H-thymidine in NF cells, as determined by scintillation counting, is also seen when other tritium-labeled nucleosides, specifically cytosine, guanosine, and adenosine, are used to measure DNA synthesis and cell proliferation rates (data not shown). The sum of our data indicates that fibroblasts

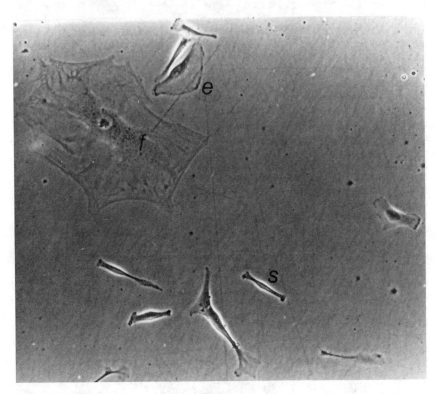

FIGURE 11. Phase-contrast photomicrograph showing early Phase II cells: e = presumed endothelial cell; f = fibroblast; s = spindle cell.

derived from NF skin or NF neurofibromas proliferate at a normal rate, and that efforts to quantify proliferation using a riboside uptake into DNA may have to consider a number of confounding factors, for example, altered intracellular riboside and ribotide pools.

As alluded to above, by routine phase and bright-field microscopy, NF skin and neurofibroma-derived fibroblasts are ordinarily indistinguishable from normal skin fibroblasts. Likewise, we have found no significant differences by transmission and scanning electron microscopy (Reference 17 and A. Martinez-Palomo and V. M. Riccardi, unpublished observations).

In several instances, S-100 protein positive staining of Phase II spindle cells was demonstrated in NF neurofibroma explant cultures (B. Clark and V. M. Riccardi, unpublished data). These data, plus transmission electron microscopy studies of similar cells from Phase II and Phase III neurofibroma cultures (A. Martinez-Palomo and V. M. Riccardi, unpublished observations) combined to suggest that the neurofibroma-derived spindle cells are putatively Schwann cells, and thus of special interest for studying the NF mutation *in vitro* (see also Reference 5). However, their slow growth and poor ability to be passaged using trypsin solutions would lead quickly to their being overgrown by the fibroblasts described above. Thus, we sought to enhance the growth potential of these spindle cells.

As a first clue, we respected the fact that the most intense spindle cell growth was adjacent to the edges of the explant piece itself (FIGURE 12), perhaps indicating a critical locally available factor. One way of testing this was to place a segment of mongrel dog femoral nerve on a petri dish surface already shown to have spindle cells present in low numbers. Indeed, these femoral nerve segments, whether transferred directly to the petri or frozen at −80°C overnight first, led to a significant increase in the number of adjacent spindle cells (FIGURE 13). [It should be noted here, however, that we did not distinguish between preferential proliferation, preferential migration, and/or metaplasia (e.g., from fibroblast to spindle cell) as explanations for these findings.]

We then proceeded to determine whether neurofibromas could have a similar positive effect on spindle cell growth. In collaboration with R. J. Riopelle (unpublished observations), we had already shown that intact portions of previously frozen NF neurofibromas could give positive results in an *in vitro* NGF assay system. However, rather than use intact neurofibroma segments, we elected to proceed directly to cell-free crude extracts to test for factors that would enhance the growth of neurofibroma-derived cells, especially spindle cells.

Although the results of some studies have suggested an excess of NGF in the serum of NF patients,[3,4] the data of Riopelle *et al.* indicate no such abnormalities among NF-I patients,[18] specifically. In addition, Darby *et al.* have excluded linkage between the beta-NGF gene locus and NF-I.[23] On the other hand, the data of Riopelle *et al.* suggest the presence of some, yet undefined, growth factor in NF-I patient serum that is detectable in their *in vitro* NGF assay.[18] For this reason, plus the ultimate need to study the cell culture effect of serum from NF patients, we specifically tested the ability of neurofibroma-derived fibroblasts to grow in the absence of fetal bovine serum, but in the alternative presence of four types of human serum as described above (Materials and Methods).

NF-I Neurofibroma Extracts

The ability of human NF-I neurofibroma-derived fibroblasts (or fibroblast-like cells) to grow more or less normally is now reasonably well established.[5,17] The present work confirms this, and emphasizes the already well-known importance of the type of serum used in the culture medium. It is of some interest in this regard that human serum from both NF patients (NFS) and non-NF persons (HUS) supported growth essentially the same as did FBS. Similarly, the morphology of cells in Giemsa-stained petri dishes was the same, regardless of human serum source.

It is also of interest that neurofibroma-derived cells are able to proliferate at 40.5°C, in contrast to normal skin fibroblasts. In particular, the possibility that the NF-I

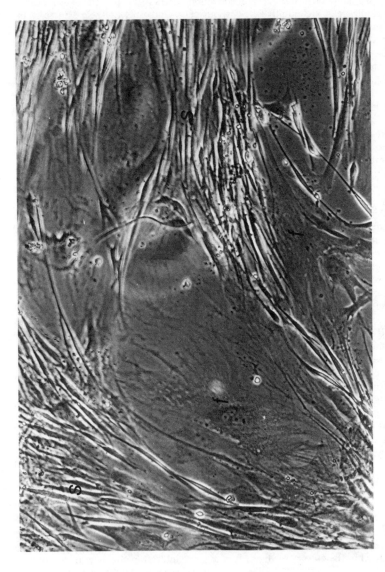

FIGURE 12. Phase-contrast photomicrograph showing the typical parallel arrays of spindle cells (s) emanating from a neurofibroma explant (to the left and below), and superimposed on ordinary fibroblasts (f).

mutation is temperature sensitive has been suggested[14] as an explanation for both the development of freckling at skin folds and sites of friction and the virtual sparing of the shins from neurofibroma development. The data presented here, while still preliminary, certainly suggest the need to investigate further the influence of temperatures above and below 37°C on the expression of NF mutations.

These and other experiments still leave unanswered the question as to which type of cell in neurofibroma-derived cultures should be used to draw conclusions about the pathogenesis of NF and the nature of the NF mutation(s). While intuitively it seems appropriate to utilize cells other than fibroblasts, particularly neural crest derivatives such as Schwann cells, which characterize these tumors, technical problems seem to

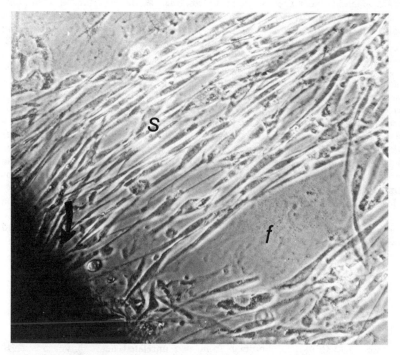

FIGURE 13. Phase-contrast photomicrograph of neurofibroma-explant spindle cells (s) that have accumulated in tight parallel arrays in regions adjacent to a segment of canine femoral nerve (arrow). An ordinary fibroblast is designated by f.

have detracted from this approach. In this context, the possibility of a growth-promoting factor active in the *in vivo* neurofibromas assumes another level of importance: not only may it explain certain elements of NF pathogenesis, it will also afford a more direct *in vitro* assessment of this pathogenesis, both in terms of characterizing the factor itself and in terms of enhancing the growth (and quantities) of its target cells.

The results presented here make it clear that one or more factors in NF-I neurofibromas can apparently enhance the growth of neurofibroma-derived cells in culture, and that the morphology of the responding cells is largely, but not always, distinct from ordinary cultured fibroblasts. Moreover, these spindle cells, by virtue of their S-

100-positive staining, general morphology, and electron microscopic appearance, are likely to be of greater interest than ordinary fibroblasts for studying NF *in vitro*. The consistency of the response by multiple cell strains to fixed doses of extract from two different patients is strong evidence for the active principle reflecting the pathogenesis of a neurofibroma as such, though it leaves open the question as to whether non-NF neurofibromas have similar properties. That is, it is not yet clear whether such a factor is instructive about both neurofibromas in general and NF mutations in particular.

The fact that in at least some instances NF skin-derived cultures appeared to respond as did neurofibroma-derived cultures suggests either that the response merely reflects the NF mutation (a non-NF skin-derived culture failed to respond) or that ostensibly normal skin from NF patients may harbor neurofibroma elements that only become apparent under special circumstances, such as the experimental conditions described here. While these and many other cogent questions remain unanswered, certainly the data presented here clarify the need to elucidate further the identity and properties of the substance or substances mediating the cell culture responses to NF neurofibroma extracts.

On the one hand, the substance(s) will be of great interest on its own. On the other hand, such an approach is also important to the extent that it emphasizes tumor growth as a function of intercellular cooperation (e.g., in terms of autocrine and/or paracrine factors). While the idea that NF neurofibromas result from disturbed cellular interaction has been around for some time,[9,10,13] recently there is an increasing tendency to presume that tumors (benign or malignant) result exclusively from an intracellular genetic aberration (i.e., somatic mutation), with a consequent clonal proliferation. The recent demonstration of gene loss to explain the origin of retinoblastomas[2] and Wilms tumors[7] has prompted the application of this approach to many genetic conditions characterized by tumors. However, the hamartomatous nature of NF neurofibromas, the histologic constancy of an individual neurofibroma over time and from one portion to another, plus the cogency of the cellular interaction proposals to explain NF lesions,[9,12] all add to detract from a simple clonal theory to explain the origin and growth of these tumors. The demonstration of a factor (or factors) in NF neurofibromas, as demonstrated here, both adds to this argument and is nurtured by it.

SUMMARY

Crude extracts of neurofibromas from two unrelated neurofibromatosis (NF) patients were prepared by mincing, homogenizing, and ultracentrifugation in the absence of added solvents. Explant cultures of neurofibromas from other NF patients were grown at low density in culture medium with and without neurofibroma extract supplementation. Differences in growth were monitored by comparing monolayer densities, colony counts, or uptake of ^{3}H-thymidine. A consistent enhancement of growth rate was demonstrated, and titration curves showed an increasing effect with increasing dosage (ranging from 1.5 $\mu l/ml$ to 25 $\mu l/ml$). However, the extract could not substitute for fetal bovine serum. As determined by microscopic examination of Giemsa-stained petri dishes, small spindle-shaped cells, distinct in morphology from ordinary fibroblasts, were the overwhelmingly predominant cell type in most extract-treated cultures. While the specific identity of the growth factor(s) involved is unknown, the following may be stated: (1) The presence of one or more growth factors that may act in an autocrine or paracrine manner in neurofibromas *in vivo* is demonstrated. (2) There is a preferential effect of such a factor on spindle-shaped cells (presumably

Schwann cells), allowing for the selective enrichment of these cells *in vitro*. (3) There is an enhanced yield of clones derived from single cells, allowing further analysis of the cellular heterogeneity of neurofibromas at the biochemical and molecular levels. These considerations should help to distinguish between those models for neurofibroma growth that emphasize secondary somatic mutations (including allelic exclusion) on the one hand, and cellular interaction on the other hand.

ACKNOWLEDGMENTS

Thanks to Mr. D. W. Elder and Ms. Wendy Carle for expert technical assistance and to Ms. Stephanie Powell for assistance in manuscript preparation.

REFERENCES

1. BOLANDE, R. P. 1981. Neurofibromatosis—the quintessential neurocristopathy: pathogenetic concepts and relationships. Adv. Neurol. **29**: 67-75.
2. DRYJA, T. P., W. CAVANEE, R. WHITE, J. M. RAPAPORT, R. PETERSEN, D. M. ALBERT & G. A. BRUNS. 1984. Homocygosity of chromosome 13 in retinoblastoma. N. Engl. J. Med. **310**: 550-553.
3. FABRICANT, R. N. & G. J. TODARO. 1981. Increased serum levels of nerve growth factor in von Recklinghausen's disease. Arch. Neurol. **38**: 401-405.
4. FABRICANT, R. N., G. J. TODARO & R. ELDRIDGE. 1979. Increased levels of a nerve-growth-factor cross-reacting protein in "central" neurofibromatosis. Lancet **1**: 4-7.
5. KRONE, W., G. JIRIKOWSKI, O. MUHLECK, H. KLING & H. GALL. 1983. Cell culture studies on neurofibromatosis (von Recklinghausen). II. Occurrence of glial cells in primary cultures of peripheral neurofibromas. Hum. Genet. **63**: 247-251.
6. LEMKE, G. E. & J. P. BROCKES. 1983. Glial growth factor: a mitogenic polypeptide of the brain and pituitary. Fed. Proc. **42**: 2627-2629.
7. ORKIN, S. H., D. S. GOLDMAN & S. E. SALLAN. 1984. Development of homozygosity for chromosome 11p markers in Wilms' tumor. Nature **309**: 172-174.
8. PLEASURE, D., G. SOBUE, K. H. SONNENFELD & A. E. RUBENSTEIN. 1986. Effect of mitogens on the proliferation of Schwann cells from neurofibromas. Ann. N.Y. Acad. Sci. (This volume.)
9. RICCARDI, V. M. 1979. Cell-cell interaction as an epigenetic determinant in the expression of mutant neural crest cells. Birth Defects **15**(8): 89-98.
10. RICCARDI, V. M. 1980. The pathophysiology of neurofibromatosis. IV. Dermatologic insights into heterogeneity and pathogenesis. J. Am. Acad. Dermatol. **3**: 157-166.
11. RICCARDI, V. M. 1981. Neurofibromatosis (von Recklinghausen disease). N. Engl. J. Med. **305**: 1617-1627.
12. RICCARDI, V. M. 1981. Cutaneous manifestations of neurofibromatosis: cellular interaction, pigmentation and mast cells. Birth Defects **17**(1): 129-145.
13. RICCARDI, V. M. 1982. Neurofibromatosis: clinical heterogeneity. Curr. Prob. Cancer **7**(2): 1-35.
14. RICCARDI, V. M. & J. E. EICHNER. 1986. Neurofibromatosis: Phenotype, Natural History, and Pathogenesis. Johns Hopkins University Press. Baltimore, Md.
15. RICCARDI, V. M., B. KLEINER & M. L. LUBS. 1979. Neurofibromatosis: variable expression is not intrinsic to the mutant gene. Birth Defects **15**(5B): 283-289.
16. RICCARDI, V. M. & V. A. MARAGOS. 1980. The pathophysiology of neurofibromatosis. I. Resistance in vitro to 3-nitrotyrosine as an expression of the mutation. In Vitro **16**: 706-714.

17. RICCARDI, V. M. & V. A. MARAGOS. 1981. Characteristics of skin and tumor fibroblasts from neurofibromatosis patients. Adv. Neurol. **29:** 191-198.
18. RIOPELLE, R. J., V. M. RICCARDI, S. FAULKNER & M. C. MARTIN. 1984. Serum neuronal growth factors in von Recklinghausen neurofibromatosis. Ann. Neurol. **16:** 54-59.
19. SCHMALE, M. C., G. HENSLEY & L. R. UDEY. 1983. Multiple schwannomas in the bicolor damselfish, *Pomacentrus partitus,* a possible model of von Recklinghausen neurofibromatosis. Am. J. Pathol. **112:** 238-241.
20. WOLF, K. & M. C. QUIMBY. 1969. Fish cell and tissue culture. *In* Fish Physiology. W. S. Hoar & D. J. Randall, Eds.: 253-305. Academic Press. New York, N.Y.
21. ZELKOWITZ, M. 1981. Neurofibromatosis fibroblasts: abnormal growth and binding to epidermal growth factor. Adv. Neurol. **29:** 173-189.
22. ZELKOWITZ, M. & J. STAMBOULY. 1981. Neurofibromatosis fibroblasts: slow growth and abnormal morphology. Pediatr. Res. **15:** 290-293.
23. DARBY, J. K., J. FEDER, M. SELBY, V. M. RICCARDI, R. FERRELL, D. SIAO, K. GOSLIN, W. RUTTER, E. M. SHOOTER & L. L. CAVALLI-SFORZA. 1985. A discordant sibship analysis between beta-NGF and neurofibromatosis. Am. J. Hum. Genet. **37:** 52-59.

Schwann-Like Cells Cultured from Human Dermal Neurofibromas[a]

Immunohistological Identification and Response to Schwann Cell Mitogens

DAVID PLEASURE,[b] BARBARA KREIDER,[b]
GEN SOBUE,[b] ALONZO H. ROSS,[c] HILARY
KOPROWSKI,[c] KENNETH H. SONNENFELD,[d]
AND ALLAN E. RUBENSTEIN[d]

[b]*Department of Neurology*
Children's Hospital of Philadelphia
Thirty-fourth and Civic Center Boulevard
Philadelphia, Pennsylvania 19104

[c]*The Wistar Institute of Anatomy and Biology*
Thirty-sixth Street at Spruce
Philadelphia, Pennsylvania 19104

[d]*Department of Neurology*
Mount Sinai School of Medicine
1 Gustave Levy Place
New York, New York 10029

Neurofibromatosis is a common, dominantly inherited neurological disorder which is characterized by tumors containing elongated, spindle-shaped Schwann-like cells (SLC) and pleomorphic fibroblast-like cells (FLC), with lesser numbers of other cell types (mast cells, endothelial cells, axonal twigs).[1-5] Present knowledge is insufficient to permit choice between two alternate mechanisms leading to SLC hyperplasia in patients with neurofibromatosis:

1. SLC are normal Schwann cells, and a mitogen for Schwann cells, present in greater than normal activity, induces these Schwann cells to proliferate excessively. If this is true, the rate of mitosis of neurofibroma SLC maintained in tissue culture should be similar to that of normal human Schwann cells maintained in the same medium.

[a]Supported by funds from the National Neurofibromatosis Society, Muscular Dystrophy Association, and National Institutes of Health (NS07245, NS08075, CA25874, HD08536 and NS11037). Barbara Kreider Ph.D. was an NIH Research Postdoctoral Fellow and Gen Sobue M.D. was a Muscular Dystrophy Association Research Postdoctoral Fellow.

227

2. Neurofibroma SLC differ from normal Schwann cells in capacity to proliferate, due either to an entirely autogenous change in cell cycle regulation or to hyperresponsiveness to normal concentrations of one or more normal Schwann cell mitogens. If this is true, cultured neurofibroma Schwann-like cells might exhibit an excessive baseline rate of mitosis or an exaggerated response to some or all Schwann cell mitogens.

To pursue this issue, we have developed methods for isolation and culture of neurofibroma cells. The yield of neurofibroma cells was dramatically improved by dissociating the tumor with a combination of Dispase, collagenase, and hyaluronidase. These cultures contain both elongated, bipolar or multipolar SLC and flat, pleomorphic FLC. Viable SLC were purified from the mixed SLC/FLC cultures by preparative cytofluorography using a monoclonal antibody against human nerve growth factor receptors (anti-NGFR)[6,7] which binds to the surface of SLC but not FLC. Using tritiated thymidine radioautography, we have examined the response of SLC in mixed SLC/FLC cultures to three known Schwann cell mitogens: axolemmal fragments,[8-12] analogues of cyclic adenosine 3',5'-monophosphate (cAMP),[13-15] and glial growth factor,[16-19] and also the response of cultures enriched in SLC to glial growth factor; results of these studies, some of which have been reported previously,[20] are reviewed in the present paper.

METHODS

Dissociation and Culture of Neurofibroma Cells

Neurofibromas were minced in Hank's balanced salt solution with 1 mM EDTA and without magnesium or calcium, then transferred to RPMI 1640 medium containing 15% (v/v) fetal calf serum, 25 mM HEPES, 1.25 units/mL Dispase (crude, Behringer), 0.05% (w/v) collagenase (Worthington), 0.1% (w/v) hyaluronidase (Sigma H-3884), and incubated overnight at 37°C in 5% CO_2/95% air. The next day the medium was removed and replaced with RPMI 1640 without serum containing 1.25 units/mL Dispase and 0.05% collagenase. After 30 minutes of incubation at 37°C, the suspension was pipetted vigorously, then spun down and the pellet washed three times with RPMI 1640 medium containing 15% (v/v) fetal calf serum. The cells were seeded on poly-L-lysine (Sigma) coated glass coverslips which were maintained in 24 multiwell plates (for immunohistological and radioautographic study) or in poly-L-lysine coated plastic flasks (until cytofluorography).

Indirect Immunofluorescence Light Microscopy

Coverslips bearing the unfixed cells were overlaid with antiserum against laminin [from Dr. Rupert Timpl, Max-Plank-Institut fur Biochemie, Munich, or from Bethesda Research Laboratories, diluted 1/50 or 1/100 in Eagle's minimum essential medium (MEM)] or against fibronectin (from Bethesda Research Laboratories, diluted 1/50 in MEM) or a monoclonal antibody (ME20.4) against NGFR (culture supernatant, undiluted). The coverslips were then washed with MEM and overlaid with rhodamine-conjugated goat antirabbit immunoglobulin or rhodamine-conjugated rabbit antimouse immunoglobulin (Cappel). After washing with MEM, the cells were fixed in ice-cold 5% acetic acid (v/v) in ethanol, then washed five times with MEM and once with water. The coverslips, mounted in glycerol/phosphate-buffered saline (PBS) (1/1, v/v), were observed using a Leitz microscope fitted for epifluorescence with 63× and 50× phase-fluorescence objectives.

Analytical and Preparative Cytofluorography

Cells were harvested from the flasks by brief incubation at 37°C in RPMI 1640 medium containing Dispase (1.25 units/mL) and collagenase (0.05%), washed once with PBS, then resuspended in 0.1 mL of anti-NGFR (ME20.4 culture supernatant) or 0.1 mL of a nonspecific control monoclonal antibody (P3, culture supernatant of clone MOPC21) for 1 hour on ice; then the volume was brought to 2 mL with PBS and the cells were pelleted by centrifugation. The cell pellets were resuspended in 0.1 mL of fluorescein-conjugated rabbit antimouse immunoglobulin at 60 μg/mL and incubated for 1 hour on ice, then washed as above and resuspended in 1 mL of PBS. Analytical cytofluorography was with an Ortho Cytofluorograf 50HH with a linear fluorescence output divided into 200 channels; generally 3000 cells were counted per assay. A Becton-Dickinson FACS-IV was used for preparative cytofluorography. Cells exhibiting highest fluorescence (and therefore most surface NGFR) were collected in a tube containing RPMI 1640 medium with 20% fetal calf serum, then plated on polylysine-coated glass coverslips and maintained in 24 multiwell plates as above.

Schwann Cell Mitogens

Axolemmal fragments were isolated from the brain stems and cerebral white matter of adult female Sprague-Dawley rats by sucrose gradient ultracentrifugation.[21,22] Glial growth factor (GGF) was partially purified from bovine pituitary glands by ammonium sulfate precipitation followed by CM cellulose and phosphocellulose column chromatography.[17] Half-maximal mitogenic effect of this glial growth factor preparation for neonatal rat astroglia in a serum-free defined medium[23] was 0.1 μg/mL.

Tritiated Thymidine Radioautography

To measure effects of axolemmal fragments or cAMP analogues on proliferation of SLC, neurofibroma coverslip cultures were transferred from the RPMI medium to MEM containing 10% (v/v) calf serum. Twenty-four hours later, a preparation of rat central nervous system (CNS) axolemmal fragments suspended in MEM and equivalent to 65 to 130 μg of axolemmal fragment protein/well or a cAMP analogue (either 0.1 mM 8-bromo cAMP or 0.1 mM dibutyryl cAMP) dissolved in MEM was added to some of the wells and an equivalent volume of MEM without mitogen was added to control wells; after these additions, each well contained 0.5 mL of medium. Twenty-four hours later, 0.5 μCi of tritiated thymidine (specific activity 20 Ci/mmol, New England Nuclear) was added to each well; and, after an additional 24 hours, the coverslips were washed with PBS, fixed in ice-cold 3% glutaraldehyde (v/v) in PBS, washed five times with PBS and once with water, dipped in NTB-2 emulsion (Eastman Kodak), exposed at 5°C for 7 days in a light-tight box, developed, and stained with 0.3% toluidine blue (w/v) in PBS (pH adjusted to 6.2). Under the conditions of this assay, nuclei were either completely blackened by confluent silver grains (scored "positive") or were overlaid with only a few scattered silver grains (scored "negative"). At least 200 SLC were scored on each coverslip by at least two independent observers. The percent labeling index was calculated as the ratio of labeled to total SLC $\times$ 100. The stimulation index was then calculated as the ratio of percent labeling index in treated cultures to that in the simultaneous control cultures. Experiments to determine the effects of glial growth factor on SLC proliferation were carried out in the same fashion, except that the tissue culture medium was RPMI 1640 containing 15% fetal calf serum.

RESULTS AND DISCUSSION

Culture Morphology

Judged by phase contrast microscopy and inspection after fixation and toluidine blue staining, cultures prepared from dissociated dermal neurofibromas contained two cell types: elongated, bipolar or multipolar cells with an oval nucleus (SLC); and flat, polymorphic cells with a round nucleus (FLC) (FIGURES 1 and 2). By indirect immunofluorescence microscopy, unfixed SLC bound antibodies against laminin and NGFR to their surface, but did not bind antibodies against fibronectin. All cells that had the phase contrast microscopic appearance of SLC showed immunofluorescence with anti-NGFR and with antilaminin. Unfixed FLC bound antibodies against fibronectin but not against laminin or NGFR (FIGURES 1 and 2). Dissociated cultures prepared from two plexiform neurofibromas (one from a patient's flank, one mediastinal) and an acoustic neurofibroma (TABLE 1) were indistinguishable from those derived from the dermal neurofibromas (not shown). Traumatic neuromas were obtained from the distal stumps of severed mixed motor-sensory nerves from two young adults undergoing secondary nerve repair (1 and 2 months postinjury), and dissociated cultures were prepared and maintained just as with the neurofibromas. These cultures were made up of Schwann cells, which resembled SLC in morphology and immunohistological properties (TABLE 2), and fibroblasts, which resembled FLC in morphology and immunohistological properties (FIGURE 3).

Analytical and Preparative Cytofluorography

Analytical cytofluorography using anti-human NGFR[6,7] contained in the supernatant of cultures of the hybridoma clone ME20.4 as first antibody, followed by

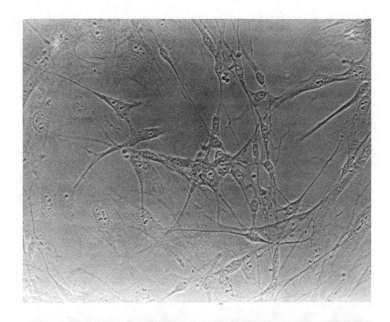

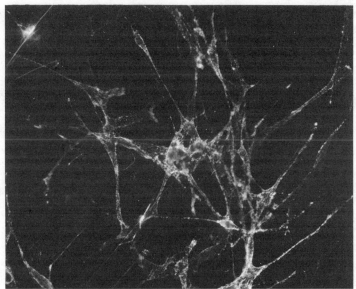

FIGURE 1. Phase contrast and indirect immunofluorescence (anti-human nerve growth factor receptor) appearance of culture derived from a dermal neurofibroma. The culture was maintained in RPMI medium with 15% (v/v) fetal calf serum for 5 days. Elongated bipolar or multipolar Schwann-like cells (SLC) bind anti-NGFR to their surface, whereas flat, pleomorphic fibroblast-like cells (FLC) do not (approximate magnification × 500).

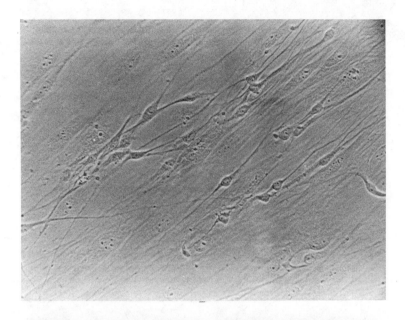

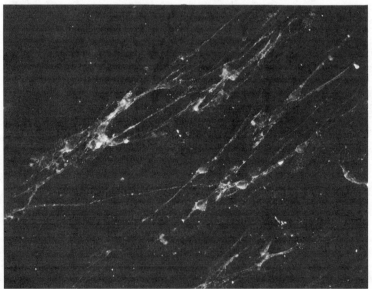

FIGURE 2. Phase contrast and indirect immunofluorescence (antilaminin) appearance of culture derived from a dermal neurofibroma. The culture, derived from dermal neurofibromas from patient 4 (TABLE 1), was maintained in RPMI medium with 15% (v/v) fetal calf serum for 7 days. The surface laminin-negative FLC have formed a confluent monolayer, upon which are scattered surface laminin-positive SLC (approximate magnification × 500).

fluorescein-conjugated rabbit antimouse immunoglobulin, were conducted with unfixed cell suspensions prepared by dissociation and short-term culture (6 hours to 5 days) of nine dermal neurofibromas (from eight patients). Two plexiform neurofibromas, an acoustic neurofibroma, and a traumatic neuroma were also studied (TABLE 1). The proportion of cells in the cultures derived from dermal neurofibromas binding anti-NGFR, calculated as the difference between the proportion binding ME20.4 anti-NGFR and the proportion binding P3, a nonspecific monoclonal antibody, varied between 10% and 67% (TABLE 1). The scans obtained with dermal neurofibromas from patient 4 (TABLE 1) are shown in FIGURE 4. Results with the two plexiform neurofibromas fell within the range observed with the dermal neurofibromas (TABLE 1).

Preparative cytofluorography was carried out with a cell suspension prepared from the two dermal neurofibromas from patient 4. The 15% of cells having greatest immunofluorescence with anti-NGFR were collected and cultured. Yield was 40% of that predicted by multiplying the number of cells applied by 0.15. When examined 4 days following preparative cytofluorography, greater than 95% of the cells had the phase contrast appearance of SLC and bound antilaminin antibodies (FIGURE 5). The 15% of cells having least immunofluorescence with anti-NGFR were also collected and cultured. Four days later, all of the cells in these cultures were flat and pleomorphic and none bound antilaminin antibodies (not shown).

Baseline Rates of Mitosis of Cultured Schwann-Like Cells and Fibroblast-Like Cells

Tritiated thymidine radioautography (24 hour radiolabeling period) indicated that, in MEM with 10% (v/v) calf serum, the percent labeling index of dermal neurofibroma SLC in mixed SLC/FLC cultures varied between 0.7% and 4.0% ($n = 6$), considerably less than the percent labeling index of FLC in the same cultures (6.5 to 26%, $n = 6$).[20] The more rapid proliferation of FLC than SLC in these cultures led to the formation of an FLC monolayer with scattered SLC adhering to its surface within 10 days after the cultures were established. The SLC percent labeling index rose to 20% ($n = 2$) when the mixed SLC/FLC cultures were maintained in RPMI 1640 medium containing 15% (v/v) fetal calf serum.

Response of Cultured Schwann-Like Cells to Axolemmal Fragments

Addition of rat CNS axolemmal fragments elicited a 10-fold or greater proliferative response from SLC in SLC/FLC mixed cultures prepared from three of seven dermal neurofibromas maintained in MEM with 10% (v/v) calf serum. Axolemmal fragments had no effect on SLC percent labeling index in cultures derived from the other four dermal neurofibromas. Human CNS axolemmal fragments were added to cultures derived from four dermal neurofibromas; a 20-fold stimulation index was obtained in one instance (a neurofibroma that had also demonstrated a mitogenic response to rat axolemmal fragments), and no effect on SLC percent labeling index was noted in the other three (each also unresponsive to rat CNS axolemmal fragments).[20] Axolemmal fragments (rat or human) had no effect on FLC nuclear labeling index in any instance.

TABLE 1. Cytofluorography of Neurofibroma Cells Employing a Monoclonal Antibody (ME20.4) against Human Nerve Growth Factor Receptors

Patient	Age, Sex	Neurofibroma Type	Percent + P3	Percent + ME20.4
1	40, F	Dermal	6	52
2	2, F	Dermal	1	17
3	26, F	Dermal	4	41
4	37, F			
		(a) Dermal	3	63
		(b) Dermal	3	70
5	21, M	Dermal	10	21
6	30, F	Dermal	3	37
7	31, F			
		(a) Dermal	5	29
		(b) Dermal	5	47
8	9, F			
		(a) Dermal	1	11
		(b) Plexiform acoustic	9	60
9	38, F	Plexiform mediastinal	3	20
10	18, F	Traumatic neuroma	30	52

Response of Cultured Schwann-Like Cells to Analogues of cAMP

We chose to test the effects on proliferation of 0.1 mM concentrations of the cAMP analogues 8-bromo cAMP and dibutyryl cAMP since previous studies with neonatal rat Schwann cells had established this to be optimal to elicit Schwann cell mitosis.[15] In all cultures treated with either of these cAMP analogues [in MEM with 10% (v/v) calf serum], SLC percent labeling index was slightly reduced by 8-bromo cAMP and not significantly changed from the control level by dibutyryl cAMP.

TABLE 2. Comparisons between Neurofibroma Schwann-Like Cells (SLC), Adult Human Schwann Cells, and Neonatal Rat Schwann Cells[a]

	SLC	Adult Human Schwann Cells	Neonatal Rat Schwann Cells
Elongated and bipolar or multipolar	Yes	Yes	Yes
Surface laminin	Yes	Yes	Yes
Surface nerve growth receptors	Yes	Yes	?
Surface fibronectin	No	No	No
Baseline proliferative rate in culture	Slow	Slow	Slow
Mitogenic response to axolemmal fragments	+++ or 0	+	+++
Mitogenic response to cyclic AMP analogues	Inhibitory	?	++
Mitogenic response to glial growth factor	++	++	++

[a]See Sonnenfeld et al., this volume.

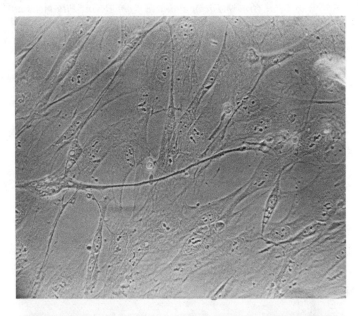

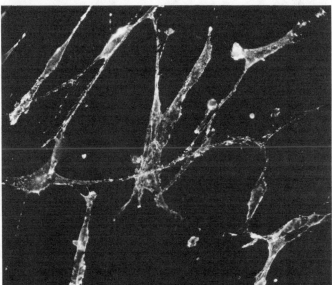

FIGURE 3. Phase contrast and indirect immunofluorescence (anti-NGFR) appearance of culture derived from the traumatic neuroma that formed on the distal stump of a severed nerve. The culture was maintained in RPMI medium with 15% (v/v) fetal calf serum for 7 days. Flat, pleomorphic fibroblasts, which do not bind anti-NGFR, have formed a monolayer, upon which lie surface anti-NGFR positive spindle-shaped bipolar and multipolar Schwann cells (approximate magnification × 500).

Effects of Glial Growth Factor Prepared from Bovine Pituitaries on Proliferation of Schwann-Like Cells in Mixed SLC/FLC Cultures and in Cultures of SLC Purified by Cytofluorography

A previous study had shown that the optimal response of neonatal rat sciatic nerve Schwann cells to glial growth factor is obtained in the presence of fetal calf serum;[18] hence the neurofibroma experiments were carried out in a medium containing 15% (v/v) fetal calf serum in RPMI 1640. Treatment of these cultures with 2 µg/mL of

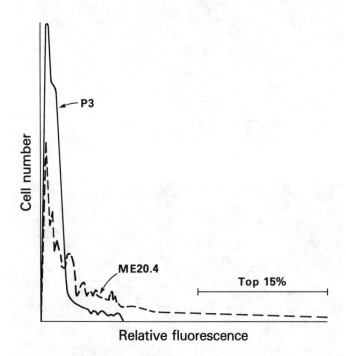

Relative fluorescence

FIGURE 4. Analytical cytofluorography using a nonspecific monoclonal antibody (P3) and anti-human nerve growth factor receptor (culture supernatant from clone ME20.4). Cells from two dermal neurofibromas from patient 4 (TABLE 1) were cultured for 4 days, then harvested. Methods for cytofluorography are described in the text.

glial growth factor (a concentration producing maximal mitogenic response of neonatal rat Schwann cells) elicited a 1.8- to 5-fold stimulation index ($n = 3$).

To determine whether the mitogenic effect of glial growth factor was exerted primarily on SLC or only as a result of some GGF-elicited alteration in the metabolism of FLC, we tested the effects of GGF on cultures of SLC purified from dermal neurofibromas from patient 4 by cytofluorography. In RPMI 1640 medium containing 15% fetal calf serum, the baseline SLC percent labeling index was 5.8%, and was increased to 33.7% (a 5.8-fold stimulation index) by 2 µg/mL of GGF.

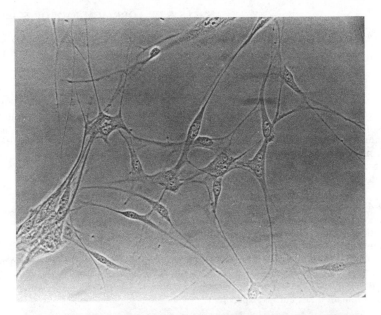

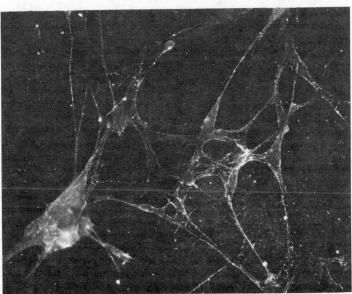

FIGURE 5. Phase contrast and indirect immunofluorescence (antilaminin) appearance of neurofibroma cells cultured after preparative cytofluorography. Cells from two dermal neurofibromas from patient 4 (see TABLE 1) were cultured for 4 days, then harvested and a small aliquot of the cell suspension was examined by analytical cytofluorography (see FIGURE 4). The remainder of the cell suspension was subjected to preparative cytofluorography, and the 15% of cells that were most intensely fluorescent were collected, cultured for an additional 3 days (total time *in vitro* 7 days), then examined. Appearance should be compared with that of cultures derived from the same neurofibromas and maintained for 7 days *in vitro* without cytofluorography (FIGURE 2) (approximate magnification × 500).

Comparisons between Responses to Mitogens of Normal Human Schwann
Cells and Neurofibroma Schwann-Like Cells (TABLE 2)

CNS axolemmal fragments elicited an SLC mitogenic response equivalent in magnitude to that observed with neonatal rat Schwann cells[10] in cultures from some neurofibromas, no detectable response from others. No comparable data on normal human Schwann cells are available. However, Schwann cells cultured by the explantation reexplantation technique[24] from human sural nerve biopsy specimens or from autopsied human nerve roots demonstrated a relatively small but consistent mitogenic response to treatment with rat CNS axolemmal fragments.[11]

Whereas neonatal rat Schwann cells exhibit a brisk proliferative response to 0.1 mM concentrations of 8-bromo cAMP or dibutyryl cAMP,[14,15] these agents in this concentration caused marked inhibition of SLC mitosis.[20] Effects of various concentrations of the cAMP analogues on survival and proliferation of normal human Schwann cells have not yet been tested.

Cultured SLC, both in SLC/FLC mixed cultures and after purification, exhibited a mitogenic response to glial growth factor. This response quantitatively resembled that previously observed with Schwann cells obtained from both neonatal rats[16-18] and from human adult autopsy specimens.[19]

SUMMARY AND CONCLUSIONS

Primary cultures prepared from dermal and plexiform neurofibromas contain Schwann-like cells and fibroblast-like cells. SLC are elongated and bipolar or multipolar. By indirect immunofluorescence light microscopy, living SLC bind antibodies against laminin and against nerve growth factor receptor to their surface, but not antibodies against fibronectin. In these respects, cultured SLC are indistinguishable from cultured human adult Schwann cells. FLC are flat and pleomorphic. By indirect immunofluorescence light microscopy, living FLC bind antibodies against fibronectin but not against laminin or NGFR. In these respects, cultured FLC are indistinguishable from cultured human adult endoneurial fibroblasts. Considerable purification of viable SLC from SLC/FLC mixed cultures can be achieved by flow cytofluorometry using a monoclonal anti-NGFR antibody.

Tritiated thymidine radioautography indicated that mitosis of SLC in mixed SLC/FLC cultures prepared from dermal neurofibromas is infrequent in MEM with 10% calf serum, more frequent in RPMI 1640 medium with 15% fetal calf serum. Central nervous system axolemmal fragments (rat or human) elicited a greater than 10-fold SLC proliferative response in mixed SLC/FLC cultures from three of seven dermal neurofibromas (from six patients with neurofibromatosis), but had no effect on SLC mitosis in cultures from the other four dermal neurofibromas. SLC mitosis was inhibited by concentrations of cyclic adenosine 3',5'-monophosphate analogues known to stimulate proliferation of normal rat Schwann cells. Glial growth factor partially purified from bovine pituitaries stimulated SLC mitosis both in SLC/FLC mixed cultures and in cultures of purified SLC. The studies we have described indicate that neurofibroma SLC can be cultured, unequivocally identified in culture by morphological and immunohistological criteria, purified, and stimulated to proliferate by several Schwann cell mitogens. Further quantitative comparisons of the baseline and mitogen-stimulated rates of proliferation of SLC and age-matched control human Schwann cells are needed, however, to determine which of the two alternate pathogenetic mechanisms for formation of neurofibromas mentioned in the introduction is correct.

ACKNOWLEDGMENTS

We thank Donna Jackson, Geoffry Faust, and Janet Stern for their help in these experiments, and Angela Obringer and Dr. Lee Osterman for assistance in obtaining specimens.

REFERENCES

1. WAGGENER, J. D. 1966. Ultrastructure of benign peripheral nerve sheath tumors. Cancer **19:** 699-709.
2. WEISER, G. 1975. An electron microscope study of "Pacinian neurofibroma." Virchows Arch. Pathol. Anat. Histol. **366:** 331-340.
3. KAMATA, Y. 1978. Study on the ultrastructure and acetylcholinesterase activity in von Recklinghausen's neurofibromatosis. Acta Pathol. Jpn. **28:** 393-410.
4. GAY, R. E., S. GAY & R. E. JONES. 1983. Histological and immunological identification of collagens in basement membranes of Schwann cells of neurofibromas. Am J. Dermatol. **5:** 317-325.
5. KRONE, W., G. JIRIKOWSKI, O. MUHLECK, H. KLING & H. GALL. 1983. Cell culture studies on neurofibromatosis (von Recklinghausen). II. Occurrence of glial cells in primary cultures of peripheral neurofibromas. Hum. Genet. **63:** 247-251.
6. ROSS, A. H., P. GROB, M. BOTHWELL, D. E. ELDER, C. S. ERNST, N. MARANO, B. F. D. GHRIST, C. C. SCHLEMP, M. HERLYN, B. ATKINSON & H. KOPROWSKI. 1984. Characterization of nerve growth factor receptor in neural crest tumors using monoclonal antibodies. Proc. Nat. Acad. Sci. USA **81:** 6681-6685.
7. ROSS, A. H., M. HERLYN, G. G. MAUL, H. KOPROWSKI, M. BOTHWELL, M. CHAO, D. PLEASURE & K. SONNENFELD. The nerve growth factor receptor in normal and transformed neural crest cells. Ann. N.Y. Acad. Sci. (This volume.)
8. DEVRIES, G., J. SALZER & R. BUNGE. 1982. Axolemma-enriched fractions isolated from PNS and CNS are mitogenic for cultured Schwann cells. Dev. Brain Res. **3:** 295-299.
9. CASSEL, D., P. M. WOOD, R. P. BUNGE & L. GLASSER. 1982. Mitogenicity of brain axolemma membranes and soluble factors for dorsal root ganglion Schwann cells. J. Cell. Biochem. **18:** 433-445.
10. SOBUE, G., B. KREIDER, A. ASBURY & D. PLEASURE. 1983. Specific and potent mitogenic effect of axolemmal fraction on Schwann cells from rat sciatic nerves in serum-containing and defined media. Brain Res. **280:** 263-275.
11. SOBUE, G., B. KREIDER, A. K. ASBURY & D. PLEASURE. 1984. Axolemma is a mitogen for human Schwann cells. Ann. Neurol. **15:** 449-452.
12. MEADOW-WOODRUFF, J. H., B. L. LEWIS & G. H. DEVRIES. 1984. Cyclic AMP and calcium as potential mediators of stimulation of cultured Schwann cell proliferation by axolemma-enriched and myelin-enriched membrane fractions. Biochem. Biophys. Res. Commun. **122:** 373-380.
13. RAFF, M. C., A. HORNBY-SMITH & J. P. BROCKES. 1978. Cyclic AMP is a mitogenic signal for cultured rat Schwann cells. Nature London **273:** 672-673.
14. SOBUE, G. & D. PLEASURE. 1984. Schwann cell galactocerebroside is induced by derivatives of adenosine 3′,5′-cyclic monophosphate. Science **224:** 72-74.

15. SOBUE, G., S. SHUMAN & D. PLEASURE. 1986. Schwann cell responses to cyclic AMP: proliferation, change in shape, and appearance of surface galactocerebroside. Brain Res. **362:** 23-32.
16. RAFF, M. C., E. ABNEY, J. P. BROCKES & A. HORNBY-SMITH. 1978. Schwann cell growth factors. Cell **15:** 813-822.
17. LEMKE, G. E. & J. P. BROCKES. 1984. Identification and purification of glial growth factor. J. Neurosci. **4:** 75-83.
18. KREIDER, B., J. COREY-BLOOM, R. LISAK, H. DOAN & D. PLEASURE. 1982. Stimulation of mitosis of cultured rat Schwann cells isolated by differential adhesion. Brain Res. **237:** 238-243.
19. MORETTO, G., S. U. KIM, D. H. SHIN, D. E. PLEASURE & N. RIZZURO. 1984. Long-term cultures of human adult Schwann cells isolated from autopsy materials. Acta Neuropathol. Berlin **64:** 15-21.
20. SOBUE, G., K. SONNENFELD, A. E. RUBENSTEIN & D. PLEASURE. 1985. Tissue culture studies of neurofibromatosis: effects of axolemmal fragments and cyclic adenosine 3',5'-monophosphate analogues on proliferation of Schwann-like and fibroblast-like neurofibroma cells. Ann. Neurol. **18:** 68-73.
21. DEVRIES, G. H., M. G. ANDERSON & D. JOHNSON. 1983. Fractionation of isolated rat CNS myelinated axons by sucrose density gradient centrifugation in a zonal rotor. J. Neurochem. **40:** 1709-1717.
22. SOBUE, G. & D. PLEASURE. 1985. Adhesion of axolemmal fragments to Schwann cells: a signal- and target-specific process closely linked to axolemmal induction of Schwann cell mitosis. J. Neurosci. **5:** 379-387.
23. KIM, S. U., J. STERN, M. KIM & D. PLEASURE. 1983. Culture of purified rat astrocytes in serum free medium supplemented with mitogen. Brain Res. **274:** 79-84.
24. ASKANAS, V., W. K. ENGEL, M. C. DALAKAS & L. S. CARTER. 1980. Human Schwann cells in tissue culture. Histochemical and ultrastructural studies. Arch. Neurol. **37:** 329-337.

Linkage between Schwann Cell Extracellular Matrix Production and Ensheathment Function[a]

MARY BARTLETT BUNGE AND RICHARD P. BUNGE

Department of Anatomy and Neurobiology
Washington University School of Medicine
660 South Euclid Avenue
St. Louis, Missouri 63110

Culture techniques are now available to study cellular interactions that occur during peripheral nerve development. In the animal the interior of peripheral nerve, the endoneurium, contains chiefly nerve fibers, Schwann cells, and fibroblasts, plus associated extracellular matrix. Early in animal development, peripheral nerve consists of large fascicles of nerve fibers with Schwann cells located only at the circumference of each fascicle. During the ensuing developmental period there is a sudden spurt in Schwann cell division, such that in a relatively short period of time there are enough Schwann cells generated to ensheathe every peripheral nerve fiber with either cytoplasm or myelin (for review, see Reference 1). One Schwann cell myelinates a length of one nerve fiber, whereas a number of smaller-diameter unmyelinated nerve fibers lie in troughs of cytoplasm provided by one Schwann cell. Every neuron-related Schwann cell acquires basal lamina, and collagen fibrils fill much of the intervening intercellular space between the Schwann cell-nerve fiber units; these collagen fibrils are oriented parallel to the length of the nerve fibers. Fibroblasts are scattered throughout the endoneurium. Bordering the endoneurium is the perineurium, which consists of a series of closely applied layers of flattened cells interspersed with extracellular matrix, the most prominent components of which are basal lamina and collagen. These flattened cells are related to one another by means of junctions, some of these being tight junctions. Thus, perineurium forms a permeability barrier between epineurium (found outside the perineurium) and the innermost area of nerve, the endoneurium (for review, see Reference 2).

Some of the components of endoneurial extracellular matrix in peripheral nerve *in situ* have been identified (for review, see References 3 and 4). Typically *in vivo* the Schwann cell basal lamina contains components that are found in basal laminae of many other cell types.[5] These components include types IV and V collagen, laminin, and heparan sulfate proteoglycan. It is also known that types I and III collagen are found in the endoneurium; these components are found between the Schwann cell-nerve fiber units in the intercellular space but are not constituents of the Schwann cell basal lamina. Fibronectin is also found in the intercellular space in peripheral nerve *in vivo*. When immunostaining is performed to demonstrate the position of

[a]Work in the authors' laboratory is supported by National Institutes of Health Grant NS 09923.

241

laminin or type IV collagen in cross-sectioned nerve, the staining is in the form of ringlike configurations that correspond to the transversely sectioned sleeves of basal lamina that encircle the Schwann cell exterior.

In order to better study the cell interactions and extracellular matrix formation that occur during peripheral nerve development, we have utilized new types of tissue culture preparations developed by Dr. Patrick Wood (Reference 6, reviewed in Reference 3) in our laboratory. Sensory ganglia from 15-18 day fetal rats are grown on reconstituted rat tail collagen and fed medium containing human placental serum, chick embryo extract, and nerve growth factor. Wood found that by the judicious use of antimitotic agents, notably fluorodeoxyuridine, fibroblasts are eliminated from cultures deriving from these sensory ganglia. Some Schwann cells survive this treatment and subsequently repopulate the outgrowth, to provide, in time, preparations containing only neurons and Schwann cells. Outgrowth regions of most of these cultures are seen by careful light and electron microscopic examination to be essentially free of fibroblasts. In the case of the explant culture (as opposed to the dissociated ganglion culture), removal of the explant (where the neuronal somata reside) results in rapid degeneration of the neurites, leaving only Schwann cells. Thus, removal of the neuronal somata-containing explant is the way in which a culture of Schwann cells only is obtained. If a sensory ganglion placed in culture is treated with a more extensive antimitotic regimen, then both Schwann cells and fibroblasts are removed from the culture leaving a preparation that contains only nerve cells.

Our initial studies have utilized mainly nerve cell-Schwann cell cultures devoid of fibroblasts to investigate a number of questions about peripheral nerve development. This type of culture preparation exhibits many of the features of differentiation found in peripheral nerve *in vivo*. If a neuron-Schwann cell culture is preserved with osmium tetroxide and then stained with Sudan black, the presence of myelin internodes is easily demonstrated. But, with experience, myelin is detectable in the living culture without fixation or Sudan black staining, thus providing a convenient functional assay for monitoring the progression of Schwann cell function throughout the culture period. If one examines the neuron-Schwann cell culture by electron microscopy,[7] a number of additional features of differentiation similar to those found in peripheral nerve in the animal may be seen. One Schwann cell is associated with one myelinated fiber (the axon being 1 μm or more in diameter) or more than one unmyelinated fiber, each unmyelinated fiber being surrounded by Schwann cell cytoplasm. On the exterior of these Schwann cells is basal lamina, and external to the basal lamina are thin collagenous fibrils (averaging about 20 nm in diameter) situated parallel to the nerve fibers. Thus, basal lamina and thin collagenous fibrils are formed in the absence of fibroblasts. It has been determined from work referred to below that these substances are formed by the Schwann cell and not the neuron.

If immunostaining is utilized to detect the location of either laminin or type IV collagen in these neuron-Schwann cell cultures, the staining pattern is consistent with the presence of these components in the basal lamina of the Schwann cell. Looking at whole mount cultures of immunostained material, the staining is present as a sleeve of material found along the neuron-Schwann cell units. On the basis of immunostaining it has been concluded that the Schwann cell basal lamina contains types IV[8] and type V[4] collagen, laminin,[9] entactin,[4] and heparan sulfate proteoglycan.[4] (The antibodies used in detecting these components were generously contributed by Drs. Timpl, Madri, Chung, and Cornbrooks.) In comparable cultures, Mehta *et al.* find that Schwann cells synthesize two heparan sulfate proteoglycans,[10] one of which is associated with basal lamina. Thus, the content of the Schwann cell basal lamina formed de novo in culture resembles that of the basal lamina found on Schwann cells in animal endoneurium.

Our investigations indicate that the Schwann cell is a highly secretory cell. If a radioactive precursor such as tritiated leucine or ^{35}S methionine is added to the medium of a neuron-Schwann cell culture and then 18 hours later the medium is removed and evaluated by sodium dodecyl sulfate-polyacrylimide gel electrophoresis (SDS-PAGE), more than 25 bands of labeled polypeptides ranging in molecular weight from M_r 15,000 to more than 250,000 are present in the gel.[11] If tritiated proline is added to the medium of a neuron-Schwann cell culture and then the medium is removed 18 hours later and subjected to pepsin treatment before loading onto the gel, polypeptides corresponding in electrophoretic mobility to those of types I, III, IV, and V collagen are visualized by fluorography.[3,8] The identification of one of these collagenous polypeptides, type IV, has been more thorough. For example, the polypeptide is immunoprecipitated with anti-type IV procollagen antibody from Dr. Timpl.[8]

In some experiments the neuronal somata are removed from the culture just before introduction of the labeled precursor to assess more accurately Schwann cell synthesis and secretion. The resulting gel pattern after biosynthetic radiolabeling is similar whether the neurons are present or not, indicating that the labeled products are secreted by the Schwann cells.[11] If the neuronal somata are removed from the neuron-Schwann cell culture two weeks before biosynthetic labeling and evaluation by electrophoresis, there are certain differences in the gel pattern from that obtained with medium collected from a Schwann cell culture divested of neurons just before labeling. One difference is a diminution (by 6-9 times) in the amount of labeled type IV procollagen in the medium, as evaluated by SDS-PAGE.[8] Additional differences, the presence of two new bands and the absence of two additional bands, have been found but have not yet been studied in detail. Thus, we have found that if Schwann cells are divested of neurons two weeks before biosynthetic labeling, secreted type IV procollagen is reduced. We conclude, therefore, that the presence of neurons regulates the secretion of type IV procollagen in the Schwann cell-neuron culture.

These data obtained by gel analysis following biosynthetic radiolabeling fit with results from a preceding electron microscopic study which demonstrated that the presence of neurons is required for the formation of a morphologically visible basal lamina.[12] If neuronal somata are removed from a relatively young neuron-Schwann cell culture (about a month old), most of the surfaces of the Schwann cells in the outgrowth region are clear of basal lamina seven days later. Eight weeks later the Schwann cell surfaces remain devoid of basal lamina; no new lamina forms in the intervening seven weeks. If neurons are added back to these Schwann cell cultures, basal lamina reappears in due course. In other experiments basal lamina was removed by means of trypsin treatment from neuron-Schwann cell cultures or Schwann cell cultures divested of neurons just before the treatment. Electron micrographs revealed the basal lamina to be either completely absent or lifting off the Schwann cell surface. Comparison of nerve cell-Schwann cell and Schwann cell only cultures one month after the trypsin treatment shows that basal lamina is reformed only in the cultures containing both neurons and Schwann cells.[12] The lack of reappearance of morphologically visible basal lamina in Schwann cell only cultures may be related to the reduction in type IV procollagen release by Schwann cells in the absence of neurons as evaluated by biosynthetic radiolabeling, SDS-PAGE, and fluorography. That the presence of neurons is required for the generation of Schwann cell basal lamina has been noted by others employing either in vitro or in vivo material.[13-18]

The regulation of type IV collagen assembly by neurons is in contrast to laminin secretion. In a number of culture situations in which type IV procollagen is not assembled and is not visible by immunostaining techniques, laminin is seen to be present on the surface of Schwann cells.[9] The pattern of staining is not indicative of the presence of basal lamina because the staining in these situations is of a patchy rather than linear nature. Laminin staining serves as a useful marker to distinguish between Schwann cells and fibroblasts in our cultures, whether or not basal lamina has been formed.[9]

Schwann cell secretion and assembly of extracellular matrix materials have been studied in a number of culture situations in which secretion is perturbed. One such situation is the addition of an analogue of proline to the culture medium. This analogue, cis-hydroxyproline, is built into the collagen molecule and, because of the position of the hydroxyl residue, does not allow normal hydroxylation and also interferes with triple helix formation.[19] When normal hydroxylation is prevented, collagen secretion and assembly are not normal. In the Schwann cell-neuron system, cis-hydroxyproline (200 μg/ml) reduces the accumulation of secreted collagens by 57% (and also the accumulation of noncollagenous polypeptides by 34%).[20] When cis-hydroxyproline is added to the culture medium during formation of the outgrowth, Schwann cells do not ensheathe neurites in the normal way and at the same time there is deficient basal lamina formation and lack of intercellular collagen fibrils.[21] This combination of defects, deficient ensheathment and myelination and reduced extracellular matrix formation, has been seen in a number of situations. There appears to be a linkage between Schwann cell function, that is, ensheathment and myelination, and extracellular matrix formation, particularly the organization of basal lamina.

Another perturbation in which we have observed this linkage is with the use of a defined medium, N2, devised by Bottentein and Sato to maintain neuroblastoma cell lines.[22] We find that in this medium normal primary neurons and Schwann cells grow and divide respectively. The neurons grown with Schwann cells remain healthy for months in this medium and neurites extend to form a dense outgrowth. With the development of this neurite outgrowth Schwann cells divide because of the mitogenic signal on the axolemmal surface. Schwann cells continue to divide in N2, leading to a large accumulation of Schwann cells. When these cultures are examined electron microscopically, the Schwann cell surface is found to be largely devoid of basal lamina and collagen fibrils are not present.[23] From these Schwann cells emanate many meandering processes that do not ensheathe neurites even though there may be neurites located adjacent to the Schwann cell processes and myelin is not formed. Thus, a linkage between Schwann cell function and extracellular matrix formation is again observed. If a culture grown in N2 medium is subsequently given normal medium (containing serum and embryo extract), within a week myelin formation begins and ensheathment of unmyelinated nerve fibers is initiated. At the same time basal lamina appears and collagen fibrils are formed.[23]

What components may be added to the defined medium to foster normal Schwann cell function and extracellular matrix formation? Because of the known role of ascorbic acid in collagen synthesis,[24] we have tested the efficacy of adding this component to defined medium. If a neuron-Schwann cell culture in N2 medium is biosynthetically labeled with tritiated proline and the medium is subjected to pepsin treatment 18 hours later just before placing on a gel, it can be seen after SDS-PAGE that there is no triple helical collagenous material in the medium.[3,25] If ascorbic acid is added to N2 medium, however, some triple helical collagenous material is observed to be present in the medium assessed by SDS-PAGE.[25] There is at the same time a modest improvement in Schwann cell function; an occasional myelin sheath is found in such a culture.[26] But compared to the usual medium containing serum and embryo extract, triple helical collagen in the medium and ensheathment and myelination are at a minimal level when the neuron-Schwann cell culture is grown in ascorbate-containing N2 medium.[25,26]

Recently Charles Eldridge in our laboratory has found that Schwann cell function and extracellular matrix formation reach high levels by adding both serum and ascorbic acid to defined medium.[26] The amount of myelin formed in these cultures is very striking. He has performed a number of experiments in which embryo extract, human placental serum, and ascorbic acid have been tested and has quantitated the amount of myelin formed in these cultures. For example, he finds that in medium containing human placental serum and embryo extract, there may be 290 myelin segments per square millimeter in the outgrowth region of a neuron-Schwann cell culture.[26] If the defined medium contains serum plus ascorbic acid, at least as much myelin is formed. Nerve tissue culture work done over many years indicated that both human placental serum and embryo extract are needed to achieve myelination in sensory ganglion cultures. Mr. Eldridge finds that in some batches of serum the serum alone is adequate to promote myelination; in this case the embryo extract is not needed. If these batches of human placental serum are dialyzed before addition to the defined medium, however, the ability of this serum to foster myelination is eliminated. If ascorbate is added to this dialyzed serum, then ensheathment and myelination are once again achieved.[26] Within seven days, 50 μg/ml ascorbate and dialyzed serum added to N2 allow assembly of basal lamina containing laminin, type IV collagen, and heparan sulfate proteoglycan.[26] Thus, we conclude that some sera promote myelination independently of embryo extract; dialysis of such serum reduces its ability to promote myelination, but addition of ascorbic acid to such dialyzed serum restores the ability to foster myelination. For those sera requiring embryo extract to support myelination, ascorbic acid replaces the need for embryo extract.

The linkage of Schwann cell ensheathment and extracellular matrix formation is seen not only in culture systems but is also in the animal, notably the mutant dystrophic mouse (for a brief review, see Reference 4). In this mutant mouse some of the peripheral nerve roots are most severely affected. In certain foci of these roots there are fascicles in which the nerve fibers lie adjacent to one another, with no intervening Schwann cell cytoplasm. The Schwann cells are perched only on the circumference of the fascicle; they have not extended processes into the fascicle depth to ensheathe nerve fibers individually. Also, basal lamina on the surface of these Schwann cells is not normal but shows a patchy distribution. Ensheathment and basal lamina defects are also found in culture by utilizing sensory ganglia from the dystrophic mouse.[27,28]

CONCLUSION

Our work has demonstrated that the Schwann cell is a highly secretory cell. Among the products of the Schwann cell are types I, III, IV, and V collagen, laminin, entactin, and heparan sulfate proteoglycan. In medium with serum and embryo extract, all but types I and III collagen are organized into a basal lamina on the Schwann cell surface. The secretion and assembly of extracellular matrix products of the Schwann cell are modified by the removal of neurons, the addition of cis-hydroxyproline to the culture medium, or the use of defined medium without serum and embryo extract. Schwann cells in the absence of neurons do not organize a typical basal lamina; this appears to be due, at least in part, to neuronal regulation of type IV procollagen accumulation by the Schwann cell. A change in the secretion of Schwann cell products in the presence of neurons leads to deficient ensheathment and myelination, less basal lamina, and the absence of collagen fibrils. Ascorbic acid addition to defined medium modestly improves triple helical collagen accumulation, formation of basal lamina, and the assembly of collagen fibrils and at the same time leads to modest improvement in ensheathment and myelination. For full expression of Schwann cell ensheathment and myelination and extracellular matrix assembly, a component of serum is required in addition to ascorbate. One of the implications of our studies is that normal Schwann cell function (ensheathment and myelination) is linked to the ability of Schwann cells to organize extracellular matrix. We have elsewhere raised the question whether myelination by Schwann cells can be regulated by controlling basal lamina formation[3,4,29] because the Schwann cell, like other epithelial cells, requires polarization to reach full developmental potential.

ACKNOWLEDGMENTS

We gratefully acknowledge collaborators who shared in the work originating in our laboratory. These include Drs. Carey, Cornbrooks, Moya, and Wood, Mssrs. Copio and Eldridge, and Mrs. Ann Williams. We wish to thank Drs. Chung, Cornbrooks, Madri, and Timpl for antibodies to specific extracellular components used in our studies. We thank Susan Mantia for expert typing of the manuscript.

REFERENCES

1. WEBSTER, H. DE F. & T. J. FAVILLA. 1984. Development of peripheral nerve fibers. In Peripheral Neuropathy. P. J. Dyck, P. K. Thomas, E. H. Lambert & R. P. Bunge, Eds. 2nd edit.: 329-359. W.B. Saunders. Philadelphia, Pa.
2. THOMAS, P. K. & Y. OLSSON. 1984. Microscopic anatomy and function of the connective tissue components of peripheral nerve. In Peripheral Neuropathy. P. J. Dyck, P. K. Thomas, E. H. Lambert & R. P. Bunge, Eds. 2nd edit.: 97-120. W.B. Saunders. Philadelphia, Pa.
3. BUNGE, M. B., R. P. BUNGE, D. J. CAREY, C. J. CORNBROOKS, C. F. ELDRIDGE, A. K. WILLIAMS & P. M. WOOD. 1983. Axonal and non-axonal influences on Schwann cell development. In Developing and Regenerating Nervous Systems. P. W. Coates, R. R. Markwald & A. D. Kenny, Eds.: 71-105. Alan R. Liss. New York, N.Y.
4. BUNGE, R. P., M. B. BUNGE & C. F. ELDRIDGE. 1986. Linkage between axonal ensheathment and basal lamina production by Schwann cells. Annu. Rev. Neurosci. 9: 305-328.
5. TIMPL, R. & G. R. MARTIN. 1982. Components of basement membranes. In Immunochemistry of the Extracellular Matrix. H. Furthmayr, Ed. 2: 119-150. CRC Press, Boca Raton, Fla.
6. WOOD, P. M. 1976. Separation of functional Schwann cells and neurons from normal peripheral nerve tissue. Brain Res. 115: 361-375.
7. BUNGE, M. B., A. K. WILLIAMS, P. M. WOOD, J. UITTO & J. J. JEFFREY. 1980. Comparison of nerve cell and nerve cell plus Schwann cell cultures, with particular emphasis on basal lamina and collagen formation. J. Cell Biol. 84: 184-202.
8. CAREY, D. J., C. F. ELDRIDGE, C. J. CORNBROOKS, R. TIMPL & R. P. BUNGE. 1983. Biosynthesis of type IV collagen by cultured rat Schwann cells. J. Cell Biol. 97: 473-479.
9. CORNBROOKS, C. J., D. J. CAREY, J. A. McDONALD, R. TIMPL & R. P. BUNGE. 1983. In vivo and in vitro observations on laminin production by Schwann cells. Proc. Nat. Acad. Sci. USA 80: 3850-3854.
10. MEHTA, H., C. ORPHE, M. S. TODD, C. J. CORNBROOKS & D. J. CAREY. 1985. Synthesis by Schwann cells of basal lamina and membrane-associated heparan sulfate proteoglycan. J. Cell Biol. 101: 660-666.

11. CAREY, D. J. & R. P. BUNGE. 1981. Factors influencing the release of proteins by cultured Schwann cells. J. Cell Biol. **91:** 666-672.

12. BUNGE, M. B., A. K. WILLIAMS & P. M. WOOD. 1982. Neuron-Schwann cell interaction in basal lamina formation. Dev. Biol. **92:** 449-460.

13. ARMATI-GULSON, P. 1980. Schwann cells, basement lamina, and collagen in developing rat dorsal root ganglia in vitro. Dev. Biol. **77:** 213-217.

14. DUBOIS-DALCQ, M., B. RENTIER, A. BARON-VAN EVERCOOREN & B. W. BURGE. 1981. Structure and behavior of rat primary and secondary Schwann cells in vitro. Exp. Cell Res. **131:** 283-297.

15. FIELDS, K. L. & C. S. RAINE. 1982. Ultrastructure and immunocytochemistry of rat Schwann cells and fibroblasts in vitro. J. Neuroimmunol. **2:** 155-166.

16. MCGARVEY, J. L., A. BARON-VAN EVERCOOREN, H. K. KLEINMAN & M. DUBOIS-DALCQ. 1984. Synthesis and effects of basement membrane components in cultured rat Schwann cells. Dev. Biol. **105:** 18-28.

17. WEINBERG, H. J. & P. S. SPENCER. 1978. The fate of Schwann cells isolated from axonal contact. J. Neurocytol. **7:** 555-569.

18. PAYER, A. F. 1979. An ultrastructural study of Schwann cell response to axonal degeneration. J. Comp. Neurol. **183:** 365-384.

19. INOUYE, K., S. SAKAKIBARA & D. J. PROCKOP. 1976. Effects of the stereoconfiguration of the hydroxyl group in 4-hydroxyproline on the triple-helical structures formed by homogenous peptides resembling collagen. Biochim. Biophys. Acta **420:** 133-141.

20. ELDRIDGE, C. F., M. B. BUNGE & R. P. BUNGE. 1983. Biochemical effects of cis-4-hydroxy-L-proline on Schwann cells differentiating in vitro. J. Cell Biol. **97:** 244a.

21. COPIO, D. S. & M. B. BUNGE. 1980. Use of a proline analog to disrupt collagen synthesis prevents normal Schwann cell differentiation. J. Cell Biol. **87:** 114a.

22. BOTTENSTEIN, J. E. & G. H. SATO. 1979. Growth of a rat neuroblastoma cell line in serum-free supplemented media. Proc. Nat. Acad. Sci. USA **76:** 514-517.

23. MOYA, F., M. B. BUNGE & R. P. BUNGE. 1980. Schwann cells proliferate but fail to differentiate in defined medium. Proc. Nat. Acad. Sci. USA **77:** 6902-6906.

24. PROCKOP, D. J., R. A. BERG, K. I. KIVIRIKKO & J. JEFFREY. 1976. Intracellular steps in the biosynthesis of collagen. *In* Biochemistry of Collagen. G. N. Ramachandran & A. H. Reddi, Eds.: 163-273. Plenum Press. New York, N.Y.

25. ELDRIDGE, C. F., M. B. BUNGE & R. P. BUNGE. 1984. The effects of ascorbic acid on Schwann cell basal lamina assembly and myelination. J. Cell Biol. **99:** 404a.

26. ELDRIDGE, C. F., M. B. BUNGE & R. P. BUNGE. 1985. Serum ascorbic acid regulates myelin formation and basal lamina assembly by Schwann cells in vitro. Soc. Neurosci. Abstr. **11:** 956.

27. OKADA, E., R. P. BUNGE & M. B. BUNGE. 1980. Abnormalities expressed in long-term cultures of dorsal root ganglia from the dystrophic mouse. Brain Res. **194:** 455-470.

28. BUNGE, R. P., M. B. BUNGE, A. K. WILLIAMS & L. K. WARTELS. 1982. Does the dystrophic mouse nerve lesion result from an extracellular matrix abnormality? *In* Disorders of the Motor Unit. D.L. Schotland, Ed.: 23-34. John Wiley & Sons, Inc. New York, N.Y.

29. BUNGE, R. P. & M. B. BUNGE. 1983. Interrelationship between Schwann cell function and extracellular matrix production. Trends Neurosci. **6:** 499-505.

Basement Membrane Proteins Produced by Schwann Cells and in Neurofibromatosis[a]

MARIE DZIADEK,[b] DAVID EDGAR,[c]
MATS PAULSSON,[b] RUPERT TIMPL,[b]
AND RAUL FLEISCHMAJER[d]

[b]Department of Connective Tissue Research
Max Planck Institute for Biochemistry
D-8033 Martinsried, Federal Republic of Germany
[c]Department of Neurochemistry
Max Planck Institute for Psychiatry
D-8033 Martinsried, Federal Republic of Germany
[d]Department of Dermatology
Mount Sinai School of Medicine
One Gustave Levy Place
New York, New York 10029

INTRODUCTION

Schwann cells *in situ* ensheath axons and are themselves surrounded by a basement membrane.[1] Cultured Schwann cells have been shown to synthesize typical basement membrane components such as collagen IV[2] and laminin,[3] although in the absence of neurons production of collagen IV is reduced[2] and only irregular deposits of laminin are seen.[3,4] While the neurons themselves do not synthesize basement membrane proteins, neurons must be present in culture for the formation of organized basement membranes comprising the components synthesized by Schwann cells.[1]

A variety of cultured cells including Schwann and schwannoma cells produce molecules that form extracellular matrices which stimulate neurite outgrowth from cultured neurons.[5–7] Since laminin has recently been shown to have neurite-promoting activity,[8,9] it is likely that Schwann cell laminin is responsible for the stimulatory effects of Schwann cell conditioned medium on neurons. Excessive production of extracellular matrix material has been observed for several benign Schwann cell tumors and is particularly obvious in patients with neurofibromatosis.[10] Cell proliferation is accompanied by increased deposition of basement membrane material as shown by electron microscopy[11] and immunohistology.[12] The nature of these basement membrane components and the reasons for increased production are largely unknown.

[a]The studies were supported by grants from the Deutsche Forschungsgemeinschaft (project Ti 95/6-2). MD and MP were supported by fellowships from the European Molecular Biology Organization and the Alexander von Humboldt Foundation.

248

In the present study we have examined the biosynthetic repertoire of cultured mouse Schwann cells and a rat schwannoma cell line and found production of a laminin-like protein, nidogen, entactin, a newly described basement membrane protein, BM-40, and heparan sulfate proteoglycans. The laminin-like component, possibly in a complex with other components, is apparently responsible for neurite promotion. Similar components were detected in neurofibroma tissue by immuno-electron microscopy and were partially characterized.

SYNTHESIS OF BASEMENT MEMBRANE PROTEINS BY CULTURED SCHWANN AND SCHWANNOMA CELLS

Schwann cells from neonatal mouse sciatic nerves,[13] the rat schwannoma cell line RN22,[6] and for comparison the teratocarcinoma cell line PYS-2[14] were grown in culture and the secretion of basement membrane proteins into the medium examined by specific radioimmunoassays (TABLE 1). Schwann cells produced distinct amounts of low-density heparan sulfate proteoglycan,[15] nidogen,[16] and BM-40, a novel 40 kD basement membrane protein (Dziadek, Paulsson and Timpl, unpublished). Smaller amounts of these proteins were found in the medium of schwannoma and PYS-2 cells (except BM-40 which was higher in PYS-2 cells). Radioimmunoinhibition assays specific for laminin failed to show significant reaction in Schwann and schwannoma cell medium (not shown), but as expected[19] showed a distinct reaction with PYS-2 medium. Since such an assay may have failed to detect molecules related to but not identical with laminin, the culture media were also examined by assays detecting fragment 8 from the long arm of laminin[17] and fragment 1-4 corresponding to the short arms of laminin.[18] Both assays revealed within the limits of accuracy similar amounts of these structures in PYS-2 medium. However, when Schwann and schwannoma cell media were examined, these assays demonstrated a 5- to 50-fold higher content of short-arm structures compared to long-arm structures (TABLE 1).

The nature of the various proteins detected by radioimmunoassays was also examined by immunoblotting (FIGURE 1) and immunoprecipitation (FIGURE 2). Nidogen could be detected as a 150 kD band which corresponds to the size seen in other culture systems,[19] and BM-40 was found as a single 40 kD band (FIGURE 1). Blotting for laminin demonstrated mainly a 200 kD component from Schwann cell medium, while PYS 2 medium contained both the 200 and 400 kD chains typical for laminin (not shown).

After labeling the Schwann cells with ^{35}S-methionine, immunoprecipitation of the culture medium with antibodies to laminin revealed components having 200 kD and 150 kD molecular weights, corresponding in size to laminin B chains and nidogen, respectively (FIGURE 2). The precipitate showed only trace amounts of the 400 kD or A chain component of laminin, in contrast to the precipitates from PYS-2 cell medium. Antinidogen antibodies precipitated the same protein complex as antibodies to laminin. Since neither of the two antibody preparations showed cross-reaction with the alternate protein in radioimmunoassays or immunoblots, these data indicate the presence of a noncovalent complex between the laminin-like protein and nidogen which is similar to the complex of laminin and nidogen in mouse Reichert's membrane[19] and in the mouse EHS tumor (Dziadek *et al.*, in preparation). In addition, both antilaminin and antinidogen antibodies precipitated labeled material that was unable to enter the resolving gel. This material could possibly be heparan sulfate proteoglycan,

TABLE 1. Production of Basement Membrane Proteins by Cultured Schwann, Schwannoma, and PYS-2 Teratocarcinoma Cells[a]

Radioimmunoassay for	Amount (nM) in Culture Medium		
	Schwann Cells	Schwannoma Cells	PYS-2 Cells
Laminin, long arm	0.03	0.005	2.9
Laminin, short arm	0.16	0.26	5.3
Proteoglycan[b]	1.0	0.54	0.37
Nidogen	1.7	0.37	< 0.1
BM-40	7.5	1.1	25

[a] Schwann cells were prepared from neonatal mouse sciatic nerves by a modification of the method by Brockes et al.[13] Treatment of cultures on three alternate days with cytosine arabinoside (10^{-5} M) resulted in elimination of essentially all fibroblasts; 10^5 Schwann cells, confluent cultures of rat RN22 schwannoma cells,[6] and PYS-2 cells[14] were incubated for two days in 1.5 ml Dulbecco-modified Eagle's medium containing 10% fetal calf serum before the media were collected for radioimmunoinhibition assays.[26]
[b] Low density form of heparan sulfate proteoglycan.[15]

although antibodies to heparan sulfate proteoglycan precipitated little if any of the laminin-nidogen complex. Similarly, antibodies to BM-40 only precipitated BM-40 from conditioned medium. These data indicate that most of the heparan sulfate proteoglycan and BM-40 are not complexed with laminin-nidogen in conditioned medium.

Schwann cells were also labeled with ^{35}S-sulfate in order to analyze proteoglycans and entactin.[20] A sulfated 150 kD protein and two distinct broad bands of sulfated material could be separated from the culture medium by gel electrophoresis (FIGURE 1). After DEAE cellulose chromatography most of this sulfated material eluted late in the NaCl gradient, at a position typical for proteoglycans.[21] By molecular sieve chromatography these components were found to be of comparable size to that of heparan sulfate proteoglycans from a basement membrane mouse tumor.[21] Most of the labeled proteoglycan behaved in a CsCl gradient as material of low buoyant density ($\rho < 1.5$ g/ml), but higher density material ($\rho > 1.5$ g/ml) was also present.

Together the data demonstrate that cultured Schwann cells possess the potential to produce basement membrane proteins similar to many other cells (e.g., carcinoembryonal cells, epithelial cells). However, laminin produced by Schwann cells appears to be different, since it lacks epitopes of the long arm when analyzed by radioimmunoassay, as well as substantial amounts of an A chain detectable after gel electrophoresis. Reduced amounts of A chains have been previously reported for Schwann[3] and schwannoma[5] cell cultures. Whether this is due to artifactual proteolytic degradation or reflects the synthesis of a genetically and structurally distinct variant of laminin remains an open question. The laminin-like protein produced by Schwann cells has a distinct affinity for nidogen as found for laminin produced by other cell types.[19] A complex between laminin and an $M_r = 150,000$ protein has been observed in schwannoma cell medium but the 150 kD band was not identified.[5] The data also suggest that the binding site for nidogen is located in the laminin B chains and on the short arms of the protein.

Sulfate incorporation also demonstrated a 150 kD protein which can be tentatively identified as entactin.[20] Other studies using antisera against entactin, however, failed to demonstrate entactin in schwannoma cell cultures.[5] Studies using the EHS mouse tumor have shown the presence of a high and low density form of heparan sulfate proteoglycan[21] which may be prototypes of basement-membrane-specific proteogly-cans.[15] Schwann cells apparently produce a similar low density form of the proteoglycan detectable by radioimmunoassay (TABLE 1) and sulfate incorporation, and some pro-teoglycans of higher density which were also identified after sulfate labeling. Additional evidence shows that these cells can synthesize collagen IV[2,4] and the recently isolated protein BM-40. Thus cultured Schwann cells retain the ability to produce the other known ubiquitously occurring basement membrane proteins, and these components appear similar to those characterized from the mouse EHS tumor.

NEURITE-PROMOTING ACTIVITY OF SCHWANN CELL CONDITIONED MEDIUM

As previously reported for conditioned media from a variety of cell types,[6] both Schwann and schwannoma cell conditioned media contain components that stimulate rapid neurite outgrowth when bound to polycationic culture substrates (TABLE 2).

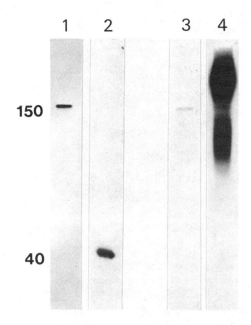

FIGURE 1. Detection of basement membrane proteins produced by Schwann cells in culture. For immunoblotting (lanes 1 and 2), conditioned medium was run on 6-15% sodium dodecyl sulfate (SDS) polyacrylamide gels and transferred to nitrocellulose.[13] Immunoperoxidase reaction with affinity-purified antinidogen antibodies (lane 1) and anti-BM-40 antibodies (lane 2) showed specific reactions with the $M_r = 150,000$ intact form of nidogen and with BM-40 respectively. ^{35}S-Sulfate-labeled Schwann cell medium was transferred to nitrocellulose after 6-15% SDS-polyacrylamide gel electrophoresis, and material on the filter (lane 3) and remaining in the gel (lane 4) was visualized after autoradiography. A distinct $M_r = 150,000$ sulfated component (lane 3) is presumably entactin. Material not transferred to the filter is resolved into two broad bands (lane 4), and was shown to be proteoglycan by other techniques (see text).

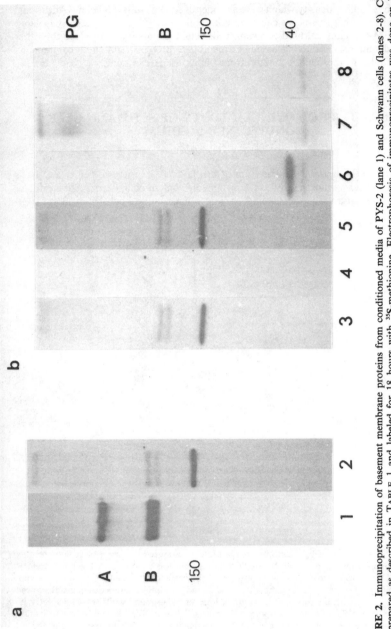

FIGURE 2. Immunoprecipitation of basement membrane proteins from conditioned media of PYS-2 (lane 1) and Schwann cells (lanes 2-8). Cultures were prepared as described in TABLE 1 and labeled for 18 hours with ^{35}S-methionine. Electrophoresis of immunoprecipitates was done on 3-10% polyacrylamide gels in the presence of SDS and mercaptoethanol, and labeled proteins were detected by fluorography. Precipitated material with affinity-purified antibodies to laminin is shown in lanes 1 and 2, with antibodies to laminin fragment 1-4 (lane 3), to laminin fragment 1-4 (lane 4), to nidogen (lane 5), to BM-40 (lane 6), to heparan sulfate proteoglycan (lane 7), and with control normal rabbit IgG (lane 8). Positions of laminin A and B chains and heparan sulfate proteoglycan are marked A, B, and PG, respectively, and the molecular weights of nidogen and BM-40 are indicated ($M_r \times 10^{-3}$).

TABLE 2. Inhibition of Neurite-Promoting Activity of Laminin and of Conditioned Culture Media by Antilaminin Antiserum[a]

Additional Substrate on Polyornithine	Percent Neurons with Neurites	
	Control	with Antilaminin[b]
None	1	1
Laminin	90 ± 5	3 ± 1
Schwann cell medium	91 ± 4	87 ± 6
Schwannoma cell medium	88 ± 7	86 ± 5

[a] Culture media were prepared as described in TABLE 1. The laminin used to coat the culture dishes (2 μg) was extracted from mouse EHS tumors, and also used to raise antisera in rabbits.
[b] Polyornithine culture dishes were coated with laminin or conditional media overnight.[9] Antilaminin antiserum was added to the cultures at a final dilution of 1:100. Neurite outgrowth was assessed after 2 hours of culture.

Laminin purified from the mouse EHS tumor has also been reported to have this ability.[8,9] The neurite-promoting activity from the conditioned media was however clearly different from laminin, since antilaminin antibodies failed to block their activity while completely inhibiting that of laminin (TABLE 2, see also References 5 and 9). However, these antibodies were able to immunoprecipitate the neurite-promoting activity (TABLE 3), indicating that this activity is, indeed, associated with the laminin-like molecules produced by the cultured Schwann cells. This conclusion was further supported by the observation that only those antibodies directed toward the laminin short arm fragment 1-4 were able to immunoprecipitate activity, whereas anti-fragment 3 antibodies directed against the long arm were inactive. In contrast, both these sets of antibodies were able to immunoprecipitate the neurite-promoting activity of laminin produced by PYS-2 cells (TABLE 3). Thus the ability of antibodies to precipitate the neurite-promoting activity of conditioned media correlates with the presence of laminin epitopes in those media (see TABLE 1). Presumably the inability of antilaminin antibodies to block the biological effect of Schwann cell laminin is due to the lack of

TABLE 3. Immunoprecipitation of Neurite-Promoting Activity from Conditioned Medium of Schwann and PYS-2 Cells[a]

Antibodies against:	Remaining Activity (units/ml)[b]	
	Schwann Cell	PYS-2 Cell
None	160	160
Laminin	< 2.5	< 2.5
Laminin fragment 3	160	< 2.5
Laminin fragment 1-4	< 2.5	< 2.5

[a] Media were prepared as described in TABLE 1 and appropriately diluted to give the same starting activity. Immunoprecipitations were performed by adding 10 μg immunoglobulin to 500 μl of conditioned medium, followed by 100 μl of a 10% Pansorbin (Calbiochem) suspension.
[b] The remaining activity was determined in the media after removal of immunoglobulin by centrifugation of the Pansorbin suspension. The media were then serially diluted and used to coat polyornithine culture substrates.[9] One unit is defined as the minimum volume of medium required to produce a detectable neurite outgrowth from neurons cultured for 2 hours.

the A chain. Consequently the molecule might lack a suitable epitope near the site that interacts with neurons. The possibility remains, however, that other molecules complexed with Schwann cell laminin in conditioned media mask epitopes that are exposed on purified mouse EHS tumor laminin.

IMMUNO-ELECTRON MICROSCOPY OF
NEUROFIBROMA TISSUE

We have recently shown by indirect immunofluorescence that skin sections from neurofibromatous lesions contain strongly stained deposits of laminin, collagen IV, and nidogen.[12] For a more precise localization of these components we have used indirect ferritin staining for laminin, collagen IV, and nidogen (FIGURE 3) by immuno-electron microscopy. Strong staining for all three proteins was found not only in the multilayered lamina densa zone surrounding Schwann cells and cytoplasmatic projections, but also in multilayered basement membranes of small blood vessels. Ferritin deposits were also observed in a few projections into the lamina rara zone, indicating close contact of these proteins with cells. Occasionally a few ferritin deposits were found in amorphous regions of the extracellular matrix that did not show the typical basement membrane morphology. Since control experiments with normal immunoglobulin G (IgG) (FIGURE 3) failed to stain basement membranes and adjacent regions, all the reactions appeared to be specific. A preferential staining for laminin and collagen IV in the lamina densa was also reported for several epithelial and renal basement membranes.[22,23] These data indicate that basement membranes in neurofibroma tissue show a normal distribution of the major components.

CHARACTERIZATION OF LAMININ AND NIDOGEN
FROM NEUROFIBROMA TISSUE

Neurofibroma tissue was extracted with 0.5 M NaCl, 0.05 M tris-HCl pH 7.4 in the presence of protease inhibitors following a standard procedure for solubilizing laminin from other tumors.[24] Passage of the extract over DEAE cellulose revealed a major peak which contained laminin and some other proteins (FIGURE 4). Final purification of laminin was achieved on a Sepharose S-400 column where it emerged in the void volume. Electrophoresis of neurofibroma laminin showed high molecular weight components which barely penetrated the gels prior to reduction, but after reduction appeared as the typical A and B chains of laminin (FIGURE 5). This

FIGURE 3. Immunoferritin localization of laminin (a), nidogen (c), and collagen IV (d) in neurofibroma tissue, compared to a control treated with normal rabbit IgG (b). The sections consist of Schwann cells (S) and cytoplasmic projections (C) surrounded by extracellular matrix. Note the strong, continuous staining of the lamina densa (arrows) and occasional staining of the lamina rara (arrowheads) and of non-basement membrane region (crosses). Lack of staining of lamina densa (arrows) is shown in the normal IgG control (b). Bars = 100 nm. This

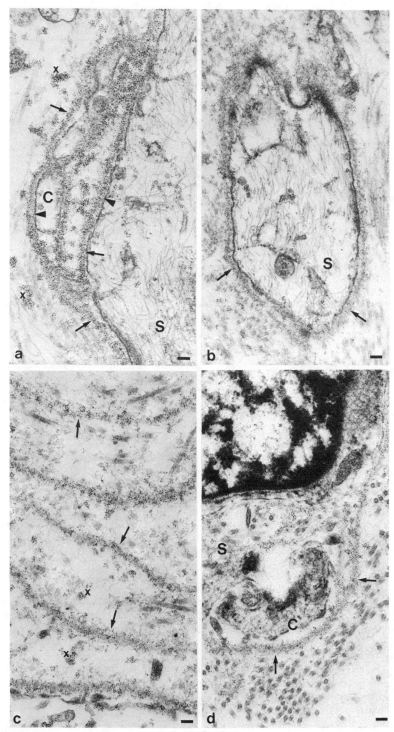

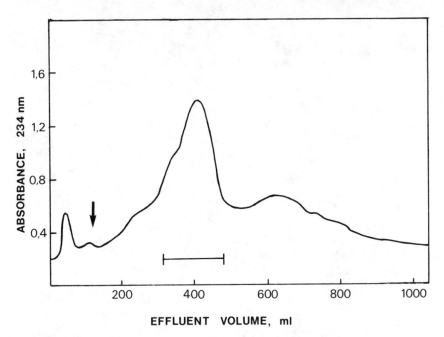

FIGURE 4. Purification of laminin from a neurofibroma extract by DEAE cellulose chroma-tography. About 10 g tissue was extracted three times with 0.5 M NaCl,[24] and the extract passed over a column (2 × 20 cm) equilibrated in 2 M urea, 0.05 M tris-HCl pH 8.6 and eluted with a linear gradient from 0-0.6 M NaCl (500/500 ml). The arrow denotes the start of the gradient, the horizontal bar the pool containing laminin.

electrophoretic pattern corresponded closely to that found for laminin from the mouse EHS tumor. Both proteins also have a similar amino acid composition.[25] About 50% of neurofibroma laminin could bind to a column of heparin-Sepharose, comparable to that observed with mouse laminin.[24]

Immunoblotting of neurofibroma laminin with antisera against human laminin demonstrated a distinct reaction with the B chains but only weak staining of A chains (FIGURE 5). The reason for the low reactivity of A chains is not clear, but may be due to lower yields of A chains from the neurofibroma, or possibly some differences in structure. Nidogen was also present in the NaCl extract but was not purified. It was identified as a 100 kD band by immunoblotting (FIGURE 5). A 100 kD form of nidogen which still has the ability to bind to laminin has been observed in other tissue extracts and is very likely generated from the genuine 150 kD form of nidogen by endogenous proteases.[19] Lower molecular weight components that reacted with an-tinidogen antibodies were observed in guanidine·HCl extracts of the neurofibroma residue after NaCl extraction (FIGURE 5), corresponding to the 80 kD and 50 kD forms of nidogen from the mouse tumor.[16]

The data suggest that laminin and nidogen extracted from neurofibroma tissue have properties corresponding to their counterparts in the mouse EHS tumor.[16,19,25] Neurofibroma laminin appears to contain an A chain, in contrast to laminin produced by cultured Schwann cells. It could indicate that laminin from culture medium is already degraded since the A chain is particularly sensitive to proteolysis.[17,18] However, it is also possible that Schwann cells in the neurofibroma tissue have switched to the production of another type of laminin or alternatively that laminin in the NaCl extract originates not from Schwann cell but rather from blood vessel basement membranes. Studies using antibodies that distinguish both types of laminin are feasible, and should help to decide between these possibilities.

SUMMARY

Mouse Schwann cells and rat RN22 schwannoma cells cultured in the absence of neurons and fibroblasts produce typical basement membrane proteins. Heparan sulfate proteoglycan (low density form), nidogen, and protein BM-40 were identified by

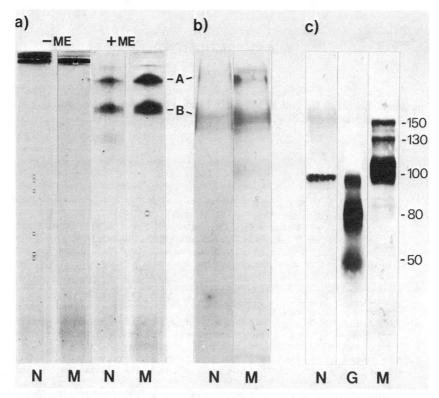

FIGURE 5. Characterization of neurofibroma laminin by electrophoresis (a), and laminin (b) and nidogen (c) by immunoblotting. In (a) electrophoresis was done using cylindrical polyacrylamide gels (3.5%) containing 2% sodium dodecyl sulfate prior to ($-$ME) and after reduction ($+$ME) with 2% 2-mercaptoethanol. N, neurofibroma laminin; M, mouse tumor laminin. In (b) equivalent samples were run on 5% polyacrylamide slab gels and transferred to nitrocellulose for immunoblotting with antibodies against human laminin.[12] Laminin A and B chains are marked. In (c), whole tissue extracts were run on 6-15% SDS-polyacrylamide gels for immunoblotting with antibodies against mouse nidogen.[16] Samples are neurofibroma extracted first with NaCl (N) followed by guanidine·HCl (G), and mouse tumor extracted with NaCl (M). Molecular weights of the nidogen forms are marked ($M_r \times 10^{-3}$).

radioimmunoassays, immunoblotting, and by immunoprecipitation after metabolic labeling. The cells also produce a laminin-like protein that differs from authentic laminin by a reduced A chain content and lack of antigenic determinants located in the long arm of laminin. Laminin possessing A and B chains is, however, produced by PYS-2 teratocarcinoma cells grown under the same conditions. Laminin from Schwann cell culture medium promotes neurite outgrowth, and this activity could be immunoprecipitated but not blocked by various antibodies against authentic laminin. In addition, Schwann cell laminin is found complexed noncovalently with nidogen. Sulfate incorporation revealed the synthesis of proteoglycans and entactin. A similar set of proteins and in addition collagen IV could be demonstrated in neurofibroma tissue by immunohistology, and were localized to the laminae densae of the multi-layered basement membranes around Schwann cells and capillaries. Laminin purified from 0.5 M NaCl neurofibroma tissue extracts possessed both A and B chains. Nidogen was identified in a partially degraded form.

ACKNOWLEDGMENTS

We thank Olivia Lovelace, Hildegard Reiter, and Vera van Delden for technical assistance. We thank Dr. S. E. Pfeiffer, University of Connecticut, for providing the rat RN22 schwannoma cells used in this study.

REFERENCES

1. BUNGE, M. B., A. K. WILLIAMS & P. M. WOOD. 1982. Neuron-Schwann cell interaction in basal lamina formation. Dev. Biol. **92:** 449-460.
2. CAREY, D. J., C. F. ELDRIDGE, C. J. CORNBROOKS, R. TIMPL & R. P. BUNGE. 1983. Biosynthesis of type IV collagen by cultured rat Schwann cells. J. Cell Biol. **97:** 473-479.
3. CORNBROOKS, C. J., D. J. CAREY, J. A. McDONALD, R. TIMPL & R. P. BUNGE. 1983. In vivo and in vitro observations on laminin production by Schwann cells. Proc. Nat. Acad. Sci. USA **80:** 3850-3854.
4. McGARVEY, M. L., A. BARON-VAN EVERCOOREN, H. K. KLEINMAN & M. DUBOIS-DALCQ. 1984. Synthesis and effects of basement membrane components in cultured rat Schwann cells. Dev. Biol. **105:** 18-28.
5. PALM, S. L. & L. T. FURCHT. 1983. Production of laminin and fibronectin by schwannoma cells: cell-protein interactions in vitro and protein localization in peripheral nerve in vivo. J. Cell Biol. **96:** 1218-1226.
6. MANTHORPE, M., S. VARON & R ADLER. 1981. Neurite promoting factor (NPF) in conditioned media from RN22 schwannoma cultures: bioassay, fractionation and other properties. J. Neurochem. **37:** 759-767.
7. LANDER, A. A., D. K. FUJI, D. GOSPODAROWICZ & L. F. REICHARDT. 1982. Characterization of a factor that promotes neurite outgrowth: evidence linking activity to a heparan sulfate proteoglycan. J. Cell Biol. **94:** 574-585.
8. BARON-VAN EVERCOOREN, A., H. K. KLEINMAN, S. OHNO, P. MARANGOS, J. P. SCHWARTZ & M. E. DUBOIS-DALCQ. 1982. Nerve growth factor, laminin and fibronectin promote neurite growth in human fetal sensory ganglia cultures. J. Neurosci. Res. **8:** 179-193.
9. EDGAR, D., R. TIMPL & H. THOENEN. 1984. The heparin-binding domain of laminin is responsible for the effects on neurite outgrowth and neuronal survival. EMBO J. **3:** 1463-1468.

10. RICCARDI, V. M. 1980. Pathophysiology of neurofibromatosis. IV. Dermatologic insights into heterogeneity and pathogenesis. J. Am. Acad. Dermatol. **3:** 157.

11. WAGGENER, J. D. 1966. Ultrastructure of benign peripheral nerve sheath tumors. Cancer **19:** 699.

12. FLEISCHMAJER, R., R. TIMPL, M. DZIADEK & M. LEBWOHL. 1985. Basement membrane proteins, interstitial collagens and fibronectin in neurofibroma. J. Invest. Dermatol. **85:** 54-59.

13. BROCKES, J. P., K. C. FIELDS & M. C. RAFF. 1979. Studies on cultured rat Schwann cells. I. Establishment of purified populations from cultures of peripheral nerve. Brain Res. **165:** 105-118.

14. OBERBÄUMER, I., H. WIEDEMANN, R. TIMPL & K. KÜHN. 1982. Shape and assembly of type IV procollagen obtained from cell culture. EMBO J. **1:** 805-810.

15. DZIADEK, M., S. FUJIWARA, M. PAULSSON & R. TIMPL. 1985. Immunological characterization of basement membrane types of heparan sulfate proteoglycan. EMBO J. **4:** 905-912.

16. TIMPL, R., M. DZIADEK, S. FUJIWARA, H. NOWACK & G. WICK. 1983. Nidogen: a new, self-aggregating basement membrane protein. Eur. J. Biochem. **137:** 455-465.

17. PAULSSON, M., R. DEUTZMANN, R. TIMPL, D. DALZOPPO, E. ODERMATT & J. ENGEL. 1985. Evidence for coiled-coil α-helical regions in the long arm of laminin. EMBO J. **4:** 309-316.

18. OTT, U., E. ODERMATT, J. ENGEL, H. FURTHMAYR & R. TIMPL. 1982. Protease resistance and conformation of laminin. Eur. J. Biochem. **123:** 63-72.

19. DZIADEK, M. & R. TIMPL. 1985. Expression of nidogen and laminin in basement membranes during mouse embryogenesis and in teratocarcinoma cells. Dev. Biol. **111:** 372-382.

20. CARLIN, B., R. JAFFE, B. BENDER & A. E. CHUNG. 1981. Entactin, a novel basal lamina associated sulfated glycoprotein. J. Biol. Chem. **256:** 5209-5214.

21. FUJIWARA, S., H. WIEDEMANN, R. TIMPL, A. LUSTIG & J. ENGEL. 1984. Structure and interactions of heparan sulfate proteoglycans from a mouse tumor basement membrane. Eur. J. Biochem. **143:** 145-157.

22. LAURIE, G. W., C. P. LEBLOND & G. R. MARTIN. 1982. Localization of type IV collagen, laminin and heparan sulfate proteoglycan to the basal lamina of basement membranes. J. Cell Biol. **95:** 340-344.

23. LAURIE, G. W., C. P. LEBLOND, S. INOUE, G. R. MARTIN & A. CHUNG. 1984. Fine-structure of the glomerular basement membrane and immunolocalization of five basement membrane components to the lamina densa (basal lamina) and its extensions in both glomeruli and tubules of the rat kidney. Am. J. Anat. **169:** 463-481.

24. TIMPL, R., H. ROHDE, L. RISTELI, U. OTT, P. GEHRON ROBEY & G. R. MARTIN. 1982. Laminin. Methods Enzymol. **82A:** 831-838.

25. TIMPL, R., H. ROHDE, P. GEHRON ROBEY, S. I. RENNARD, J.-M. FOIDART & G. R. MARTIN. 1979. Laminin—a glycoprotein from basement membranes. J. Biol. Chem. **254:** 9933-9937.

26. TIMPL, R. & L. RISTELI. 1982. Radioimmunoassays in studies of connective tissue proteins. *In* Immunochemistry of the Extracellular Matrix. H. Furthmayr, Ed. **1:** 199-235. CRC Press. Boca Raton, Fla.

Collagens in Neurofibromas and Neurofibroma Cell Cultures

JUHA PELTONEN, RISTO PENTTINEN, HANNU
LARJAVA, AND HEIKKI J. AHO[a]

Department of Medical Chemistry
University of Turku
Kiinamyllynkatu 10
SF-20520 Turku 52, Finland

INTRODUCTION

The most common connective tissue protein is collagen, comprising on average 4 kg of the adult body weight. At present 5 genetically distinct collagen types have been described fairly well, and it is expected that at least 10 more different collagen types await accurate characterization. Collagen types I, II, and III form fibrils detectable by electron microscopy, while type IV collagen is oriented to a networklike structure.[1-3] Type II collagen is restricted to hyaline cartilage, while types I and III show a more variable distribution in the body. Type IV collagen is found in no other structures than the basement membranes, and the immunohistochemical localization of type IV collagen thus reveals basement membrane zones in tissue specimens.

Neurofibromas represent a pathological proliferation of nerve supportive tissue cells and the deposition of collagen. Connective tissue-related signs often seen in neurofibromatosis (NF) are aneurysms and obstruction of arteries, and skeletal anomalies, e.g., pseudoarthrosis, kyphoscoliosis, macrocephaly, and short stature.[4] However, experimental approaches to study connective tissue components in neurofibromatosis have been rare. We have recently characterized the collagens, fibronectin, and proteoglycans in neurofibromas.[5-8] Furthermore, neurofibroma cell cultures have been studied with regard to the collagens produced by these cultures.[5,7,8]

COLLAGEN OF NEUROFIBROMAS

In light microscopy the collagen of neurofibromas is seen as thin bundles staining light red with van Gieson stain. The cell density, the amount of collagen, and mucinous material vary between different tumors and also within a single tumor.[9] Some neurofibromas contain plenty of myxomatous material which can be stained with Alcian blue, and the proportion of cells and collagen bundles is decreased, respectively. The

---

[a] Department of Pathology.

ultrastructure of neurofibromas has been studied extensively.[10-14] The diameter of collagen fibrils in neurofibromas is 30-40 nm,[11,13,14] which resembles that of human endoneurial collagen.[15] Neurofibromas also contain segmentally long spacing collagen, the so-called Luse bodies.[10]

Total Collagen of Neurofibromas

The total collagen of neurofibromas varies between 30% and 50% of the lipid-free dry weight (TABLE 1). That is about half of the corresponding value of skin, but twice that described for human endoneurial collagen.[16,17]

Types I and III Collagens

Immunohistochemical data indicate that type I collagen is found as a continuous framework throughout the neurofibroma tissue (FIGURE 1). It is absent from the endothelium of the capillaries and scant in the perineurium of the occasional nerve fascicles.[6] The distribution of type III collagen in tumors is very similar to that of type I collagen.[6]

The type III/I+III collagen ratio varies from 17.4% to 37.3% in neurofibroma samples when estimated with sodium dodecyl sulfate-polyacrylamide gel electrophoresis (SDS-PAGE) analysis of cyanogen bromide (CNBr) peptide marker peptides.[6] The corresponding values for skin samples are considerably lower (9.8-14.3%).[6] This is consistent with the fact that many developing tissues have a high type III collagen content.

Types I and III collagens have also been detected immunohistochemically in the bovine and rat endoneurium.[18,19] In this respect, too, the diffuse neurofibroma tissue collagens resemble those of the endoneurium.

The fibrous type I and type III collagens of neurofibromas may have originated from three possible sources: (1) neurofibroma fibroblasts; (2) Schwann cells; and (3) perineurial cells. The major function of fibroblasts is to synthesize connective tissue proteins, especially the mesenchymal collagens, fibronectin, and proteoglycans. They are most likely responsible for a considerable amount of the fibrous collagens deposited in neurofibroma. Bunge *et al.* demonstrated by tritiated proline incorporation, however, that Schwann cell cultures produce type I and type III collagen chains.[20] The close spatial relationship between the Schwann cells and the fibrous collagens within the endoneurium has been considered to indicate that the collagen has originated from the Schwann cells.[14,21,22] On the other hand, the collagen fibrils around Schwann cells might also be derived from endoneurial fibroblasts and the accumulation of collagen only guided by the basement membrane around Schwann cells.[23] Perineurial cells have also been postulated to be able to synthesize fibrous collagens, because collagen fibrils are seen between the lamellae of the perineurium.[15,24] However, no direct evidence of this synthetic capacity has been obtained so far.

TABLE 1. Collagen Content and the Uronic Acid/Hydroxyproline Ratio of Neurofibromas

Patient	Hydroxyproline (µg/mg dry weight)	Uronic Acid (µg/mg dry weight)	Uronic Acid: Hydroxyproline Ratio	Collagen (percent of dry weight)[a]
1.	52.9	4.1	0.078	40.7
2.	65.6	3.4	0.052	50.5
3.	49.3–55.2[b]	1.5–2.0[b]	0.027–0.040[b]	37.9–42.5[b]
4.	44.4	3.8	0.086	34.2

[a] Calculated from hydroxyproline
[b] Ranges of six samples taken from different sites of a 3 kg tumeur royale.

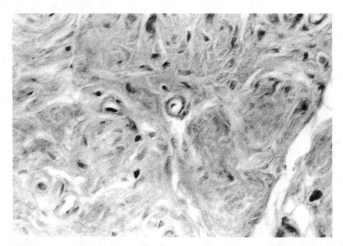

FIGURE 1. Type I collagen staining using peroxidase antiperoxidase (PAP) method.[6,7] Positive dark brown immunoreaction indicates that type I collagen forms a continuous network throughout the diffuse neurofibroma tissue. Hematoxylin counterstain. × 260.

Types IV and V Collagens

Type IV collagen was isolated from neurofibromas using pepsin treatment and fractionating salt precipitations and demonstrated electrophoretically.[7] Immunohistochemical data indicate that type IV collagen is distributed in a patchy manner in the diffuse tumor tissue (FIGURE 2). This is in line with the fact that most neurofibroma cells are surrounded by a basement membrane detectable with electron microscopy.[14]

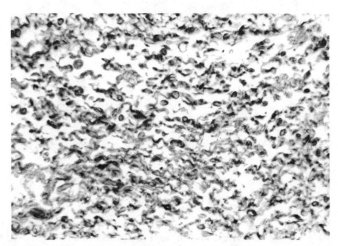

FIGURE 2. Type IV collagen staining of a neurofibroma. Note the discontinuous patchy pattern. × 260.

Some of the material stained with antibodies to type IV collagen in neurofibromas may also be intracellular.[7,25] Furthermore, type IV collagen is associated with specific structures, the dermoepidermal junction of the dermis overlying the tumors, the basement membrane of the capillary endothelium, and certain nerve structures (FIGURE 3).[7]

The visualization of type IV collagen can also be used to detect, e.g., Schwann cells and the perineurial cells which are capable of producing basement membrane components. Most of the cells in the diffuse neurofibroma tissue stain positively for type IV collagen, indicating that only a minority of the cells are fibroblasts, mast cells, macrophages, etc., that do not make type IV collagen.[7] The fact that perineurial cells do not express S-100 protein while Schwann cells do indicates that these cells are distinct entities.[26] Most of the cells in six neurofibromas produced type IV collagen and S-100 protein, indicating that the Schwann cell is the predominating cell type in neurofibromas.[7,8] Type V collagen distribution in neurofibromas resembles that of type

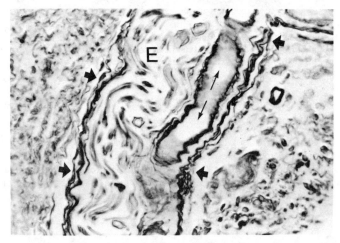

FIGURE 3. Type IV collagen staining of a neurofibroma. Perineurium (thick arrows) of a nerve fascicle in a longitudinal section is intensively stained. Endoneurium (E); small endoneurial capillary (thin arrows). × 520.

IV at the light microscopic level (FIGURE 4). Type V collagen has also been isolated from neurofibromas and demonstrated electrophoretically.[7] Type V collagen is not, however, considered as an integral component of basement membrane,[27] and it is also produced by cultured fibroblasts as estimated by SDS-PAGE of the pepsin-treated cell lysate proteins,[7] which makes it less useful as a cell type marker.

Proteoglycan / Collagen Ratio

The total uronic acid content of four neurofibromas varied from 1.5 to 4.1 μg/ mg lipid-free dry weight (TABLE 1), which is about two to five times higher than that described for human skin.[28] The uronic acid/hydroxyproline (glycosaminoglycan/

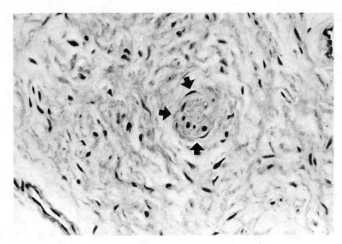

FIGURE 4. Type V collagen staining. The distribution of type V collagen resembles that of type IV at the light microscopic level. Arrow indicates the perineurium of a transected nerve. Hematoxylin counterstain. × 260.

collagen) ratio in neurofibromas was thus 4 to 10 times higher than that which can be calculated for skin.[5,28] This partly explains the typical soft consistency of the cutaneous neurofibromas. On the other hand, a high glycosaminoglycan (GAG) content may contribute to the maintenance of the extracellular milieu favoring Schwann cell proliferation. The presence of heparin in neurofibromas is explained by the presence of a large population of mast cells in the tumors.[7,28,29] Electrophoretic profiles of glycosaminoglycans, isolated from four neurofibromas, are presented in FIGURE 5.

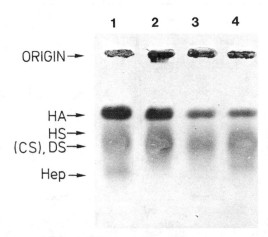

FIGURE 5. Cellulose acetate electrophoresis of glycosaminoglycans from neurofibromas of four patients.[8] The fractions were identified as described earlier.[30,31] Hyaluronic acid (HA); dermatan sulfate (DS); chonroitin sulfates (CS); heparan sulfate (HS); heparin (Hep).

Hyaluronic acid, heparan sulfate, dermatan sulfate, and heparin were demonstrated by electrophoresis after treating the samples with chondroitinase AC, ABC, or with nitrous acid.[8,30,31] Most of the nitrous acid-resistant material was also resistant to chondroitinase AC, indicating that only minor amounts of chondroitin sulfates were present.

COLLAGENS PRODUCED BY CULTURED
NEUROFIBROMA CELLS

Cultured 6th passage neurofibroma fibroblasts synthesize mostly type I collagen which can be demonstrated from the culture medium after ^{3}H-proline labeling of the cultures followed by ion exchange chromatography and SDS-PAGE analysis of the fractions (FIGURES 6 and 7). Type I collagen chains have also been demonstrated from the ^{3}H-proline-labeled tumor cell layers with SDS-PAGE/fluorography. Furthermore, two bands with relative molecular weights similar to those of type V collagen isolated from human placenta or neurofibroma have been detected in cultured neurofibroma cell layers.[7] Type III collagen of cultured neurofibroma cells has been demonstrated with indirect immunofluorescence techniques.[8]

These data indicate that the fibroblastic cell population in neurofibromas very likely has an important role in synthesizing the fibrous elements also in the tumors.[8]

Negative staining results with antibodies to type IV collagen, the determination of the 3-hydroxyproline/4-hydroxyproline ratio, and SDS-PAGE/fluorography indicate that cultured neurofibroma cells after repeated passaging do not produce type IV collagen.[5,32] This, among other cell culture data,[33] provides evidence that pure fibroblastic cell populations are obtained from neurofibromas after culturing on plastic substratum.

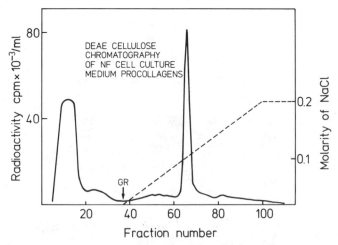

FIGURE 6. The 6th passage neurofibroma fibroblast culture medium procollagens analyzed with diethyl aminoethyl (DEAE) cellulose chromatography after ^{3}H-proline labeling of the cultures. The major peak represents type I procollagen. (See also FIGURE 7.)

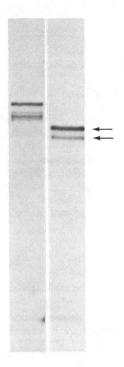

FIGURE 7. SDS-PAGE/fluorography. Lane on the left: analysis of the main peak in FIGURE 6. Lane on the right: the same sample after treatment with pepsin. The arrows indicate two bands with relative molecular weights similar to the alpha-1 and alpha-2 chains of type I collagen from human placenta.

GENERAL CONSIDERATIONS

Transection of a peripheral nerve results distally in the proliferation of Schwann cells and fibroblasts and an accumulation of collagen,[19,34,35] signs that are seen in neurofibromas, too. It would be tempting to postulate that the basic defect in neurofibromatosis in some way would result in an impaired contact between axons and the surrounding Schwann cells and thus lead to a "functional denervation," and to a massive proliferation of nerve supportive cells and an excessive synthesis of their products. Another possibility is an altered response of nerve supportive cells to the stimuli mediated by macrophages or mast cells, which are frequently seen in normal nerves and in neurofibromas and which are known to have regulatory function in connective tissue reactions.

SUMMARY

Neurofibromas contain approximately 30-50% collagen of their lipid-free dry weight, which is about half of the value of skin but approximately twice that described for peripheral nerve endoneurium.[5] Immunohistochemical stainings indicate that neurofibromas contain types I, III, IV, and V collagens and fibronectin.[6] Most of the neurofibroma cells are type IV collagen and S-100 protein positive, which provides immunohistochemical evidence that neurofibromas are mostly composed of Schwann cell-like cells.[7]

The proteoglycan/collagen ratio is 4 to 10 times higher in the neurofibromas than in the surrounding dermal tissue. This would explain the typical soft consistency of the neurofibromas and may contribute to a favorable milieu for tumor growth.[8]

Pure fibroblastic cell cultures are obtained from neurofibromas after repeated passages.[32,33] The cultured cells synthesized type I and III collagens and fibronectin, indicating that these cells are important in the production of the fibrous connective tissue proteins in neurofibromas.[5,8]

ACKNOWLEDGMENTS

Donators of the antibodies are greatly acknowledged: The anti-human type I and type III collagen antibodies were from Dr. V. Duance, Meat Research Institute, Bristol, United Kingdom; the anti-human type IV 7-S collagen antibodies were from L. and J. Risteli, University of Oulu, Oulu, Finland; the anti-human type V collagen antibodies were from Dr. J.-M. Foidart, University of Liege, Liege, Belgium.

REFERENCES

1. TIMPL, R., H. WIEDEMANN, V. VAN DELDEN, H. FURTHMAYR & K. KÜHN. 1981. A network model for the organization of type IV collagen molecules in basement membranes. Eur. J. Biochem. **120:** 203-211.
2. TIMPL, R., I. OBERBAUMER, H. FURTHMAYR & K. KÜHN. 1982. Macromolecular organization of type IV collagen. In New Trends in Basement Membrane Research. K. Kühn, H.-H. Shoene & R. Timpl, Eds.: 57-67. Raven Press. New York, N.Y.
3. SAGE, H. 1982. Collagens of basement membranes. J. Invest. Dermatol. **79:** 52s-59s.
4. RICCARDI, V. M. 1981. Von Recklinghausen's neurofibromatosis. N. Engl. J. Med. **305:** 1617-1627.
5. PELTONEN, J., T. MARTTALA, T. VIHERSAARI, S. RENVALL & R. PENTTINEN. 1981. Collagen synthesis in cells cultured from v. Recklinhausen's neurofibromatosis. Acta Neuropathol. Berlin **55:** 183-187.
6. PELTONEN, J., H. AHO, T. HALME, K. NÄNTÖ-SALONEN, M. LEHTO, J.-M. FOIDART, V. DUANCE, A. VAHERI & R. PENTTINEN. 1984. Distribution of different collagen types and fibronectin in neurofibromatosis tumours. Acta Pathol. Immunol. Microbiol. Scand. Sect. A **92:** 345-352.
7. PELTONEN, J., J.-M. FOIDART & H. J. AHO. 1984. Type IV and V collagens in von Recklinghausen's neurofibromas. An immunohistochemical and electrophoretical study. Virchows Arch. B **47:** 291-301.

8. PELTONEN, J. 1985. Connective tissue in von Recklinhausen's neurofibromatosis. An electrophoretical, immunohistochemical and cell culture study. Ph.D. Thesis. University of Turku. Turku, Finland.

9. HARKIN, J. C. & R. J. REED. 1969. Tumors of the peripheral nervous system. *In* Atlas of Tumor Pathology. 2nd ser.; fasc. 3. Armed Forces Institute of Pathology. Washington, D.C.

10. LUSE, S. A. 1960. Electron microscope studies of brain tumors. J. Neurol. Brussels **10:** 881-905.

11. LASSMANN, H., W. GEBHART & L. STOCKINGER. 1975. The reaction of connective tissue fibers in the tumor of von Recklinghausen's disease. Virchows Arch. B **19:** 167-177.

12. SMITH, T. W. & J. BHAWAN. 1980. Tactile-like structures in neurofibromas. An ultrastructural study. Acta Neuropathol. Berlin **50:** 233-236.

13. JUNQUEIRA, L. C. U., G. S. MONTES, M. D. KAUPERT, K. M. SHIGIHARA, T. M. BOLONHANI & R. M. KRISZTAN. 1981. Morphological and histochemical studies on the collagen in neurinomas, neurofibromas, and fibromas. J. Neuropathol. Exp. Neurol. **40:** 123-133.

14. WEBER, K. & O. BRAUN-FALCO. 1972. Zur ultrastruktur der Neurofibromatose. Hautarzt **23:** 116-122.

15. GAMBLE, H. J. & R. A. EAMES. 1964. An electron microscope study of the connective tissues of human peripheral nerve. J. Anat. **98:** 655-663.

16. MCFARLANE, K. R., M. POLLOCK & D. B. MYERS. 1980. Collagen and protein content of autopsied peripheral nerve. Acta Neuropathol. Berlin **50:** 167-168.

17. MCFARLANE, K. R., M. POLLOCK & D. B. MYERS. 1980. Collagen content in human ulnar nerve. Acta Neuropathol. Berlin **50:** 217-220.

18. SHELLSWELL, G. B., D. J. RESTALL, V. C. DUANCE & A. J. BAILEY. 1979. Identification and differential distribution of collagen types in the central and peripheral nervous systems. FEBS Lett. **106:** 305-308.

19. SALONEN, V., M. LEHTO, A. VAHERI, H. ARO & J. PELTONEN. 1985. Endoneurial fibrosis following nerve transection. An immunohistological study of collagen types and fibronectin in the rat. Acta Neuropathol. Berlin **67:** 315-321.

20. BUNGE, M. B., A. K. WILLIAMS, P. M. WOOD, J. UITTO & J. J. JEFFREY. 1980. Comparison of nerve cell and nerve cell plus Schwann cell cultures, with particular emphasis on basal lamina and collagen formation. J. Cell Biol. **84:** 184-202.

21. NATHANIEL, E. J. H. & D. C. PEASE. 1963. Collagen and basement membrane formation by Schwann cells during nerve regeneration. J. Ultrastruct. Res. **9:** 550-560.

22. FRIEDE, R. L. & R. BISCHHAUSEN. 1978. The organization of endoneural collagen in peripheral nerves as revealed with the scanning electron microscope. J. Neurol. Sci. **38:** 83-88.

23. THOMAS, P. K. 1964. The deposition of collagen in relation to Schwann cell basement membrane during peripheral nerve regeneration. J. Cell Biol. **23:** 375-382.

24. THOMAS, P. K. 1963. The connective tissue of peripheral nerve; an electron microscopic study. J. Anat. London **97:** 35-44.

25. GAY, R. E., S. GAY & R. E. JONES. 1983. Histological and immunohistological identification of collagens in basement membranes of Schwann cells of neurofibromas. Am. J. Dermatopathol. **5:** 317-325.

26. NAGAJIMA, T., S. WATANABE, Y. SATO, T. KAMEYA, T. HIROTA & Y. SHIMOSATO. 1982. An immunoperoxidase study of S-100 protein distribution in normal and neoplastic tissues. Am. J. Surg. Pathol. **6:** 715-727.

27. MARTINEZ-HERNANDEZ, A. & P. S. AMENTA. 1983. The basement membrane in pathology. Lab. Invest. **48:** 656-677.

28. VARMA, R. S. & R. VARMA. 1982. Glycosaminoglycans and proteoglycans of skin. *In* Glycosaminoglycans and Proteoglycans in Physiological and Pathological Processes of Body Systems. R. S. Varma & R. Varma, Eds.: 72-96. Karger. Basel, Switzerland.

29. OLSSON, Y. 1971. Mast cells in human peripheral nerve. Acta Neurol. Scand. **47:** 357-368.

30. SAITO, H., T. YAMAGATA & S. SUZUKI. 1968. Enzymatic methods for the determination of small quantities of isomeric chondroitin sulfates. J. Biol. Chem. **243:** 1536-1542.

31. LINDAHL, U., G. BÄCKSTRÖM, L. JANSON & A. HALLEN. 1973. Biosynthesis of heparin. J. Biol. Chem. **248:** 7234-7241.

32. PELTONEN, J., H. AHO, U. K. RINNE & R. PENTTINEN. 1983. Neurofibromatosis tumor and skin cells in culture. Acta Neuropathol. Berlin 61: 275-282.
33. PELTONEN, J., K. NÄNTÖ-SALONEN, H. J. AHO, T. KOURI, I. VIRTANEN & R. PENTTINEN. 1984. Neurofibromatosis tumor and skin cells in culture. II. Structural proteins with special reference to the cytoskeletal and cell surface components. Acta Neuropathol. Berlin 63: 269-275.
34. PLEASURE, D., F. W. BORA, J. LANE & D. PROCKOP. 1974. Regeneration after nerve transsection: effect of inhibition of collagen synthesis. Exp. Neurol. 45: 72-78.
35. LUGNEGÅRD, H., C.-H. BERTHOLD & M. RYDMARK. 1984. Ultrastructural morphometric studies on regeneration of the lateral sural cutaneous nerve in the white rat after transection of the sciatic nerve. II. Regeneration after nerve suture and nerve grafting. Scand. J. Plast. Reconstr. Surg. Suppl. 20: 27-64.

Connective Tissue Biochemistry of Neurofibromas[a]

JOUNI UITTO,[b,e] LOIS Y. MATSUOKA,[c] MON-LI CHU,[d]
TAINA PIHLAJANIEMI,[d] AND DARWIN J. PROCKOP[d]

[b]Department of Medicine
UCLA School of Medicine
Division of Dermatology
Harbor-UCLA Medical Center
1000 West Carson Street
Torrance, California 90509

[c]Department of Medicine
Division of Dermatology
Southern Illinois University School of Medicine
Springfield, Illinois 62708

[d]Department of Biochemistry
University of Medicine and Dentistry of New Jersey-Rutgers Medical School
Piscataway, New Jersey 08854

INTRODUCTION

Neurofibromatosis is a complex neurocutaneous syndrome inherited as an autosomal dominant trait with high penetrance of the mutated gene (for reviews, see References 1-3). Approximately half of the cases with neurofibromatosis appear to represent new mutations, and the mutation frequency of the affected gene has been estimated to be as high 4.3 $\times$ 10^{-5}.[4,5] The overall frequency of neurofibromatosis in the general population has been estimated to be 20-40 per 100,000.[4,5] Thus, neurofibromatosis is probably the most common neurocutaneous single-gene disorder.

The diagnosis of neurofibromatosis is based on clinical findings, positive family history, and associated features. The cutaneous lesions of neurofibromatosis include neurofibromas, dermal or subcutaneous tumors of varying sizes, and café-au-lait spots, pigmented cutaneous macules of varying sizes and shapes.[3,6-8] The diagnosis of neurofibromatosis can be based on the following criteria:[1,4,9]

1. The presence of at least 6 café-au-lait spots with the size of 1.5 cm or larger; or

[a]This study was supported by a grant from the National Neurofibromatosis Foundation and by Grants AM 16516, AM 28450, AM 35297, and GM 28833 from the United States Public Health Service, National Institutes of Health.

[e]Address correspondence to Dr. Uitto at the Division of Dermatology.

271

2. The presence of 20 or more neurofibromas with one biopsy being positive for neurofibroma, or at least 10 neurofibromas with one biopsy showing plexiform neurofibroma; or

3. In the absence of positive biopsy, the presence of 200 or more papular, or nodular lesions typical for neurofibroma and the presence of café-au-lait spots.

Cutaneous neurofibromas, the hallmark of neurofibromatosis, are dermal or subcutaneous lesions, which usually become manifest at puberty and which are in most cases present before the age of 20.[2] Clinically, they can have highly variable presentation varying from small, soft papules into firm, enlarged tumors producing considerable disfigurement. Histologically, neurofibromas consist of proliferation of neural structures together with the surrounding extracellular matrix.[10,11] The neural cell population has been shown to consist largely of Schwann cells together with perineurial cells.[12,13] Fibroblasts, macrophages, and mast cells have also been identified in neurofibromas.[10,14,15] The extracellular matrix is histologically composed of collagen fibers with deposition of mucinous material in the interfibrillar spaces.[10,16,17]

Neurofibromas are often cosmetically disfiguring, and their number tends to increase with advancing age. Neurofibromas frequently increase in size and number also during pregnancy, suggesting a hormonal control of the growth of the tumors. Furthermore, neurofibromas have a tendency to undergo a malignant transformation.[18,19] Thus, further understanding of the factors regulating the growth and development of the neurofibromas, as well as advanced understanding of the cell-cell[20] and cell-extracellular matrix[21] interactions, could conceivably be beneficial to patients with neurofibromatosis.

The purpose of the present study was to elucidate the connective tissue biochemistry of cutaneous neurofibromas. Toward this goal, the structural features of neurofibromas were examined by histopathology and transmission electron microscopy. The neurofibromas were further characterized by quantitative biochemical analyses for determination of the connective tissue profile of the lesions. Finally, the collagen gene expression in neurofibromas was examined by assay of the abundance of messenger RNAs (mRNA) corresponding to genetically distinct procollagen types, as detected by hybridizations with human sequence specific cDNA probes.

RESULTS

A total of nine cutaneous neurofibromas were examined by morphologic and biochemical means. The lesions were excised under local anesthesia after obtaining informed consent. The methods used are included in the accompanying references.

Structural Analyses

The neurofibromas examined in this study by biochemical means were first characterized by histopathology utilizing a variety of specific staining techniques identifying different cellular and matrix components (TABLE 1). Light microscopy revealed that all neurofibromas consisted predominantly of collagen (FIGURES 1 and 2). Cells with

TABLE 1. Special Stains Used for Histopathologic Identification of Cellular and Extracellular Components of Neurofibromas

Stain	Structures Recognized
Hematoxylin-eosin	General organization
Trichrome-Masson	Collagen
Verhoeff-van Gieson	Elastic fibers
Silver nitrate impregnation	Reticulin
Colloidal iron	Proteglycans
Toluidine blue	Proteoglycans, mast cells
Bodian luxol fast blue	Nerve fibers

spindle-shaped nuclei, mast cells, and scattered nerve fibers were enmeshed in the extracellular collagenous meshwork. Localized areas of proteoglycan (ground substance) accumulation could be detected by colloidal iron stain (FIGURE 1A). The collagen fibers appeared thinner and wavier than those present in normal skin (FIGURE 1B). Elastic and reticulin fibers were undetectable by Verhoeff-van Gieson (FIGURE 3) and silver nitrate impregnation (not shown) techniques, respectively.

Transmission electron microscopy demonstrated that the tumors contained Schwann cells with proliferating cytoplasmic processes encircling axonal-like structures (FIGURE 4A). Perineurial cells were also present. Evidence for myelinization was clearly detected, and the Schwann cells were often associated with basal lamina-like structures (FIGURE 4B). In some areas, transmission electron microscopy revealed an abundance of collagen fibers. Strikingly, the collagen fibrils demonstrated considerable variability in their diameters, and two distinct populations, one with relatively small and another one with large fibril diameter, could be recognized (FIGURE 5). Thus, on a structural basis, neurofibromas appear to contain an abundant extracellular matrix consisting predominantly of collagen.

Quantitative Biochemical Analyses of the Extracellular Components

In order to quantitate the extracellular matrix components in more precise terms, the concentrations of collagen, proteoglycans (glycosaminoglycans), and elastin were determined using hydroxyproline,[22] uronic acid,[23] and desmosine[24] as markers, respectively. The biochemical analyses indicated a connective tissue profile consisting predominantly of collagen (TABLE 2). The concentration of proteoglycans was approximately 3% of the dry weight of the tissue; this value is significantly higher than the corresponding concentration in normal human skin where approximately 0.1-0.3% of the dry weight is occupied by proteoglycans.[25,26] In contrast, elastic fibers were not detectable using an assay for desmosine, a cross-link compound present in insoluble elastic fibers.[27] Thus, the biochemical connective tissue profile of the neurofibromas indicates that collagen is indeed the predominant extracellular matrix component.

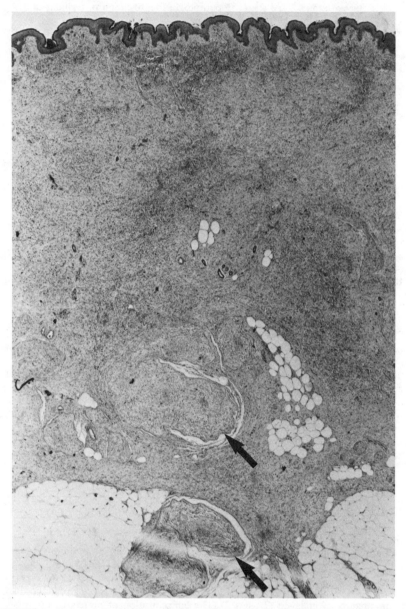

FIGURE 1. Histopathology of cutaneous neurofibromas. The tumor is predominantly composed of collagen and cells with spindle-shaped nuclei. Areas of mucoid degeneration, consisting of areas with proteoglycan (ground substance) deposition, are indicated by arrows (FIGURE 1A). Collagen fibers in some areas of the tumor are thin and wavy (FIGURE 1B). A large number of mast cells with large nuclei are also present (FIGURE 1B). FIGURE 1A (above). Colloidal iron stain; magnification 50 ×.

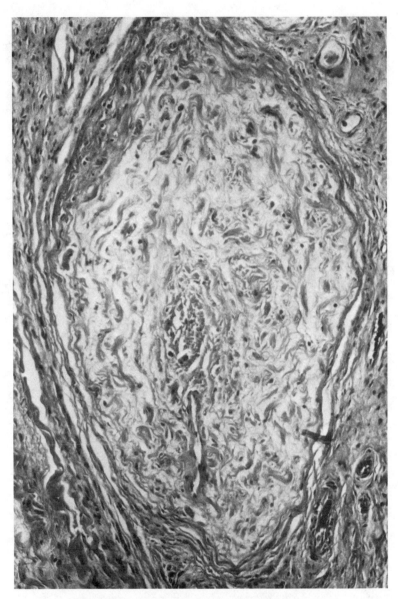

FIGURE 1B. Toluidine blue stain; magnification 200 ×.

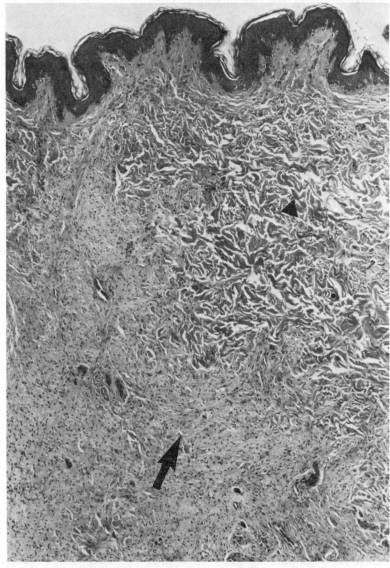

FIGURE 2. Cutaneous neurofibroma bordering normal skin. Note that the collagen fibers in the tumor are thinner and more closely packed (arrow) than the fibers in adjacent normal skin with distinct interfibrillar spaces (arrowhead). Hematoxylin-eosin stain; magnification 100 ×.

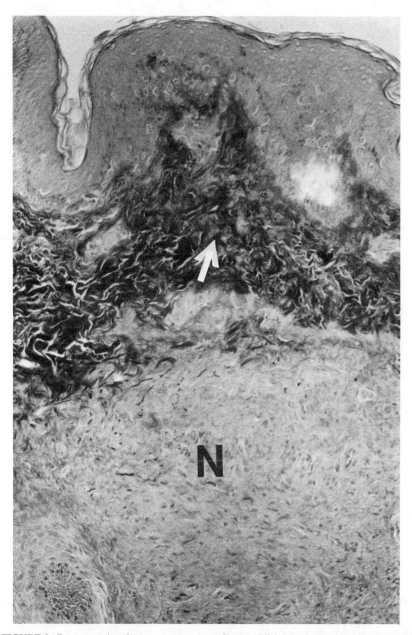

FIGURE 3. Demonstration that a cutaneous neurofibroma (N) is largely devoid of elastic fibers, while the black-staining elastic fibers are readily recognized in the bordering normal skin (arrow). Verhoeff-van Gieson stain; magnification 80 ×.

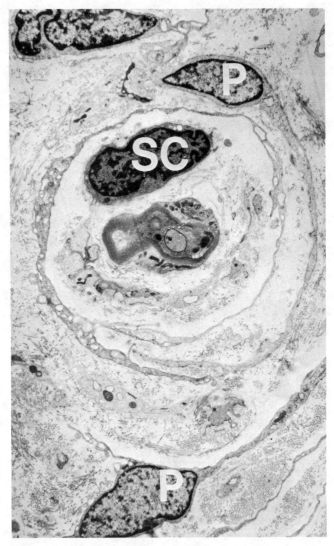

FIGURE 4. Transmission electron microscopy of cutaneous neurofibroma demonstrating the presence of Schwann cells (SC) and perineurial cells (P) (FIGURE 4A, above).

Collagen Gene Expression in Neurofibromas

A considerable amount of evidence suggests that the expression of procollagen genes in most,[28-30] but perhaps not all,[31] cases is regulated on the transcriptional level. Thus, assay of the procollagen mRNA abundance might reflect collagen production in tissues. In the present study, collagen gene expression in neurofibromas was elucidated by isolation of total RNA by CsCl density gradient centrifugation[32] and by subsequent hybridization of the messenger RNAs with human procollagen types I, III, and IV specific cDNA probes[33-35] (TABLE 3). The dot-blot hybridizations were

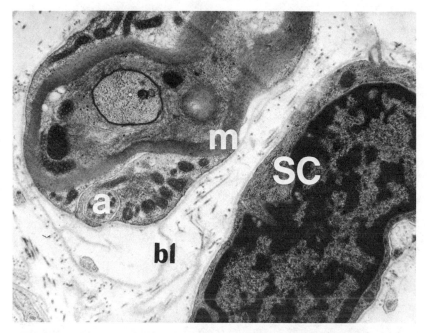

FIGURE 4B. Higher magnification reveals that the Schwann cells are associated with basal lamina (bl). Axons (a) and evidence of myelinization (m) can also be recognized. Original magnification 20,000 ×. Reduced to 83%.

performed under hybridization and washing conditions that we have previously shown to exclude cross-hybridizations between type I and type III collagen probes, as assessed by Northern blots.[40] Hybridizations with human proα1(I), proα2(I), proα1(III), and proα1(IV) cDNA probes clearly revealed the presence of types I, III, and IV collagen specific messenger RNAs, indicating transcription of the corresponding genes. Quantitation of the mRNA-[32P]cDNA hybrids by densitometric scanning of the autoradiograms[41] allowed determination of relative abundance of the corresponding mRNAs (TABLE 4). The results indicated that the abundance of type I procollagen specific mRNAs, measured by hybridization with either proα1(I) (not shown) or

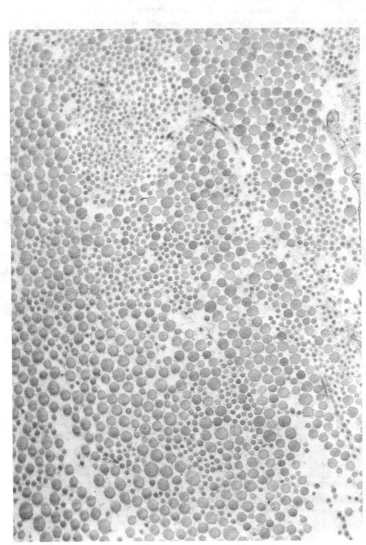

FIGURE 5. Transmission electron microscopy of collagen fibrils in a cutaneous neurofibroma. Note the presence of two distinct populations with different fibril diameters. Magnification 37,000 ×.

TABLE 2. Connective Tissue Profile of Neurofibromas[a]

Extracellular Matrix Component	Percent of Dry Weight[b]
Collagen	68.0 ± 4.7
Proteoglycans	2.9 ± 0.3
Elastin	< 1.0

[a] Neurofibromas were homogenized and assayed for hydroxyproline, uronic acid, and desmosine as markers for collagen, proteoglycans, and elastin, respectively.
[b] Mean ± standard deviation (SD) (n = 3).

TABLE 3. Characteristics of the cDNA Probes Used for Assay of Procollagen Gene Expression in Neurofibromas

Procollagen Type	Probe Designation	Size of the Probe	Corresponding Collagen Chain	Reference
I	HF 677	1.8 kb	proα1(I)	36
I	HF 1131	2.2 kb	proα2(I)	37
III	HF 934	1.2 kb	proα1(III)	38
IV	HT 21	2.6 kb	proα1(IV)	39

TABLE 4. Collagen Gene Expression in Neurofibromas[a]

Procollagen Type	mRNA Levels (U/μg RNA)[b]	Relative Abundance[c]
I	490.6 ± 84.6	11.3
III	47.4 ± 11.1	1.3
IV	58.4 ± 2.2	1.0

[a] Total RNA was isolated from three neurofibromas by CsCl density gradient centrifugation,[32] dotted on nitrocellulose filters in varying concentrations,[41] and hybridized[33-35] with ^{32}P-labeled types I, III, and IV procollagen specific cDNA probes (see TABLE 3). The mRNA-[^{32}P]cDNA hybrids were visualized by autoradiography and quantitated on the linear range of the dose-response curve by scanning densitometry at 700 nm.
[b] Arbitrary absorbance units at 700 nm (mean ± SD).
[c] Values are corrected for the length and specific activity of the probes, and for chain composition of genetically distinct procollagens.

proα2(I) (TABLE 4), was clearly predominant, being about 10 times higher than the corresponding levels of types III and IV procollagen mRNAs. Thus, the production of the extracellular matrix of neurofibromas, consisting predominantly of collagen, appears to depend on continuous expression of the collagen genes, type I collagen gene being expressed in a predominant fashion.

DISCUSSION

The results of the present study indicate that cutaneous neurofibromas contain an abundant extracellular matrix consisting predominantly of collagen. The expression of types I, III, and IV procollagen genes could be detected at the mRNA level, suggesting that the growth and development of neurofibromas are dependent on continuous expression of the collagen genes. These observations then raise the possibility that inhibition of collagen gene expression by pharmacologic means could potentially interfere with the growth and development of neurofibromas.

Previously, several pharmacologic agents have been tested for their effects on collagen metabolism, and some of these agents are currently in clinical use for treatment of fibrotic skin conditions (for reviews, see References 42 and 43). The rationale for their clinical use is largely based on their effects on collagen metabolism in isolated tissues or under cell culture conditions. Unfortunately, the effects of these pharmacologic agents are often not specific for collagen, and their clinical efficacy is frequently compromised by short-term toxicity and development of long-term side effects. In attempts to develop more specific collagen inhibitors for future clinical use, we have recently tested various agents for their effects on collagen production in vitro. The results indicate that several novel approaches are potentially applicable for further testing in in vivo models of cutaneous fibrosis.[42,43] These observations include the inhibition of collagen production by structural analogues of proline, which incorporate into the newly synthesized proteins and prevent the collagen molecules from folding into a stable triple-helical conformation.[44-46] As a consequence, the nonhelical polypeptides are degraded either intracellularly or after a slow release into the extracellular milieu.[47] As a net result of these events, the deposition of collagen in the extracellular space is arrested.

Another potentially useful approach to prevent collagen accumulation revolves around the inhibition of procollagen-to-collagen conversion by naturally occurring amino acids, polyamines, and their structural analogues.[48] Collagen is synthesized as a precursor molecule, procollagen, which contains noncollagenous extensions at both the amino- and the carboxy-terminal ends of the molecule; these precursor-specific extensions are enzymatically removed during the extracellular processing of procollagen.[49,50] Several lines of evidence suggest that if the removal of the extensions is inhibited, the formation of collagen fibers and their subsequent stabilization by intermolecular cross-links are perturbed.[49-52] Thus, a pharmacologic agent that would interfere with the enzymatic conversion of procollagen to collagen could be effective in reducing collagen accumulation in tissues. Along these lines of research, we[48,53] and others[54] have demonstrated that several amino acids, polyamines, and their structural analogues are effective in inhibiting the conversion of procollagen to collagen. Although the exact mechanism of this inhibition is currently unknown, it has been suggested that these compounds, demonstrating specific structural inhibitory features,[53] might interfere with the conversion by inhibiting the procollagen C-proteinase activity.[48]

Irrespective of the exact mechanism of the inhibition, systemic or local administration of the inhibitory compounds could lead to the accumulation of only partially converted precursor forms which are unable to form extracellular fibers of the ordinary tensile strength.

Finally, several recent studies have indicated that retinoids, synthetic vitamin A derivatives, can inhibit the deposition of extracellular matrix proteins in cell culture.[35,54-57] Specifically, some of the retinoids, including all-*trans*-retinoic acid and 13-*cis*-retinoic acid, are potent inhibitors of collagen gene expression in human skin fibroblast cultures.[35] The inhibition of collagen production by these agents occurs probably on the transcriptional level of procollagen gene expression, since the inhibition of type I collagen production is accompanied by a similar decrease in the corresponding mRNA abundance.[35] The inhibition of procollagen production in short-term cultures of human skin fibroblasts is relatively selective in that small, if any, effects were noted on the synthesis of noncollagenous proteins or on the expression of noncollagenous genes, as determined by the abundance of β-actin and fibronectin mRNA levels.[35] However, the usefulness of all-*trans*-retinoic acid and 13-*cis*-retinoic acid for treatment of fibrotic skin diseases may be limited by the fact that these two retinoids also inhibit the expression of collagenase, the enzyme initiating the extracellular degradation of collagen fibers.[54-56] Nevertheless, further development of retinoids that would favorably alter the balance between collagen production and the degradation of this protein, with appropriate tissue targeting, might potentially prove useful in the future for treatment of fibrotic conditions, such a neurofibromas.[42,43]

CONCLUSIONS

Neurofibromas, the hallmark of neurofibromatosis, are cutaneous or subcutaneous tumors consisting of proliferating neural structures and the adjacent extracellular matrix. The predominant extracellular matrix component is collagen which comprises approximately 70% of the dry weight of tissue. Significant quantities, approximately 3% of the dry weight, of proteoglycans are also present, while few, if any, elastic fibers can be demonstrated either by structural or biochemical means. The expression of procollagen genes in neurofibromas can be detected by assay of types I, III, and IV procollagen mRNAs. The levels of mRNA specific for type I procollagen are about 10 times more abundant than those of types III and IV procollagen mRNAs. It appears then that the growth and development of neurofibromas are dependent on continuous expression of collagen genes. Consequently, a pharmacologic approach that would limit collagen gene expression in cutaneous neurofibromas could be potentially beneficial for patients with neurofibromatosis.

ACKNOWLEDGMENTS

Drs. Francesco Ramirez, Karl Tryggvason, Jeane C. Myers, Markku Kurkinen, and Charles D. Boyd participated in the development of the cDNA probes used in this study. The authors thank Damon Pizzurro for technical assistance and Charlene D. Aranda for manuscript preparation.

REFERENCES

1. PELTONEN, J. 1985. Connective tissue in von Recklinghausen's neurofibromatosis. Ph.D. Thesis. University of Turku. Turku, Finland.
2. RICCARDI, V. M. 1981. Von Recklinghausen's neurofibromatosis. N. Engl. J. Med. **305:** 1617-1627.
3. ADAMS, R. D. 1979. Neurocutaneous diseases. *In* Dermatology in General Medicine. T. B. Fitzpatrick, A. Z. Eisen, K. Wolff, I. M. Freedberg & K. F. Austen, Eds. 2nd edit.: 1206-1246. McGraw Hill. New York, N.Y.
4. CROWE, F. W., W. J. SCHULL & J. V. NEEL. 1956. A Clinical Pathological and Genetic Study of Multiple Neurofibromatoses. Charles C. Thomas. Springfield, Ill.
5. SAMUELSSON, B. & R. AXELSSON. 1981. Neurofibromatosis. A clinical and genetic study of 96 cases in Gothenburg, Sweden. Acta Dermatovener Stockholm Suppl. **95:** 67-71.
6. ABELL, M. R., W. R. HART & J. R. OLSON. 1970. Tumors of the peripheral nervous system. Hum. Pathol. **1:** 503-551.
7. RICCARDI, V. M. 1981. Cutaneous manifestations of neurofibromatosis: cellular interactions, pigmentation and mast cells. Birth Defects **17:** 129-145.
8. CROWE, F. W. 1964. Axillary freckling as a diagnostic aid in neurofibromatosis. Ann. Intern. Med. **61:** 1142-1143.
9. SAMUELSSON, B. 1981. Neurofibromatosis (von Recklinghausen's disease). A clinical-psychiatric and genetic study. Ph.D. Thesis. University of Gothenburg. Gothenburg, Sweden.
10. HARKIN, J. C. & R. J. REED. 1969. Tumors of the peripheral nervous system. *In* Atlas of Tumor Pathology. 2nd ser., fasc. 3. Armed Forces Institute of Pathology. Washington, D.C.
11. LOTT, I. T. & E. P. RICHARDSON. 1981. Neuropathological findings and the biology of neurofibromatosis. Adv. Neurol. **29:** 23-32.
12. THOMAS, P. K. & Y. OLSSON. 1975. Microscopic anatomy and function of the connective tissue components of peripheral nerve. *In* Peripheral Neuropathy. V. J. Dyke, P. K. Thomas & E. H. Lambert, Eds.: 168-189. Saunders. Philadelphia, Pa.
13. LAZARUS, S. S. & L. D. TROMBETTA. 1978. Ultrastructural identification of a benign perineurial cell tumor. Cancer **41:** 1823-1829.
14. OLSSON, Y. 1971. Mast cells in human peripheral nerve. Acta Neurol. Scand. **47:** 357-368.
15. WEBER, K. & O. BRAUN-FALCO. 1972. Zur Ultrastruktur der Neurofibromatose. Hautarzt **23:** 116-122.
16. VON RECKLINGHAUSEN, F. 1882. Über die multiplen Fibrome der Haut und ihre Beziehung zu den multiplen Neuromen. Hirschwald. Berlin, Germany.
17. PELTONEN, J., H. AHO, T. HALME, K. NÄNTÖ-SALONEN, M. LEHTO, J.-M. FOIDART, V. DUANCE, A. VAHERI & R. PENTTINEN. 1984. Distribution of different collagen types and fibronectin in neurofibromatosis tumors. Acta Pathol. Microbiol. Immunol. Scand. Sect A **92:** 345-352.
18. RICCARDI, V. M. 1982. Neurofibromatosis: clinical heterogeneity. Curr. Probl. Cancer **7:** 1-34.
19. HOPE, D. G. & J. J. MULVIHILL. 1981. Malignancy in neurofibromatosis. Adv. Neurol. **29:** 33-56.
20. RICCARDI, V. M. 1979. Cell-cell interaction as an epigenetic determinant in the expression of mutant neural crest cells. Birth Defects **15:** 89-98.
21. BUNGE, R. P. & M. B. BUNGE. 1983. Interrelationship between Schwann cell function and extracellular matrix production. Trends Neurosci. **6:** 499-505.
22. KIVIRIKKO, K. I., O. LAITINEN & D. J. PROCKOP. 1967. Modification of a specific assay for hydroxyproline in urine. Anal. Biochem. **19:** 249-255.
23. BITTAR, T. & H. M. MUIR. 1962. A modified uronic acid carbazole reaction. Anal. Biochem. **4:** 330-334.
24. KING, G. S., V. S. MOHAN & B. C. STARCHER. 1980. Radioimmunoassay of desmosine. Connect. Tissue Res. **7:** 263-267.
25. PEARCE, R. H. 1965. Glycosaminoglycans and glycoproteins in skin. *In* The Amino Sugars. E. A. Balazs & R. W. Jeanloz, Eds. **11A:** 149-193. Academic Press. New York, N.Y.
26. SILBERT, J. E. 1979. Mucopolysaccharides of ground substance. *In* Dermatology in General

Medicine. T. B. Fitzpatrick, A. Z. Eisen, K. Wolff, I. M. Freedberg & K. F. Austen, Eds. 2nd edit.: 189-195. McGraw Hill. New York, N.Y.

27. UITTO, J. 1979. Biochemistry of the elastic fibers in normal connective tissues and its alterations in diseases. J. Invest. Dermatol. 72: 1-10.

28. MOEN, R. C., D. W. ROWE & R. D. PALMITER. 1979. Regulation of procollagen synthesis during the development of chick embryo calvaria. Correlation with procollagen mRNA content. J. Biol. Chem. 254: 3526-3530.

29. MERLINO, G. T., C. MCKEON, B. DECROMBRUGGHE & I. PASTAN. 1983. Regulation of the expression of genes encoding type I, II, III collagen during chick embryonic development. J. Biol. Chem. 258: 10041-10048.

30. LIAU, G., Y. YAMADA & B. DECROMBRUGGHE. 1985. Coordinate regulation of the levels of type III and type I collagen mRNA in most but not all mouse fibroblasts. J. Biol. Chem. 260: 531-536.

31. FOCHT, R. J. & S. L. ADAMS. 1984. Tissue specificity of type I collagen gene expression is determined at both transcriptional and post-transcriptional levels. Mol. Cell. Biol. 4: 1843-1852.

32. CHIRGWIN, J. M., E. PRZYBYLA, R. J. MCDONALD & W. J. RUTTER. 1983. Isolation of biologically active ribonucleic acid from sources enriched in ribonuclease. Biochemistry 18: 5294-5299.

33. THOMAS, P. S. 1980. Hybridization of denatured RNA and small DNA fragments transferred to nitrocellulose. Proc. Nat. Acad. Sci. USA 77: 5201-5205.

34. DEWET, W. J., M.-L. CHU & D. J. PROCKOP. 1983. The mRNAs for the proα1(I) and proα2(I) chains of type I procollagen are translated at the same rate in normal human fibroblasts and in fibroblasts from two variant of osteogenesis imperfecta with altered steady-state ratios of the two mRNAs. J. Biol. Chem. 258: 14385-14389.

35. OIKARINEN, H., A. I. OIKARINEN, E. M. L. TAN, R. P. ABERGEL, C. A. MEEKER, M.-L. CHU, D. J. PROCKOP & J. UITTO. 1985. Modulation of procollagen gene expression by retinoids. Inhibition of collagen production by retinoic acid accompanied by reduced type I procollagen mRNA levels in human skin fibroblast culture. J. Clin. Invest. 75: 1545-1553.

36. CHU, M.-L., J. C. MYERS, M. P. BERNARD, J.-F. DING & F. RAMIREZ. 1982. Cloning and characterization of five overlapping cDNAs specific for the human proα1(I) collagen chain. Nucl. Acids Res. 10: 5925-5934.

37. BERNARD, M. P., J. C. MYERS, M.-L. CHU, F. RAMIREZ, E. F. EIKENBERRY & D. J. PROCKOP. 1983. Structure of a cDNA for the proα2 chain of human type I procollagen. Comparison with chick cDNA for proα2(I) identified structurally conserved features of the protein and the gene. Biochemistry 22: 1139-1145.

38. CHU, M.-L., D. WEIL, W. DEWET, M. P. BERNARD, M. SIPPOLA & F. RAMIREZ. 1985. Isolation of cDNA and genomic clones encoding human proα1(III) collagen. Partial characterization of the 3'-end region of the gene. J. Biol. Chem. 260: 4357-4363.

39. PIHLAJANIEMI, T., K. TRYGGVASON, J. C. MYERS, M. KURKINEN, R. LEBO, M.-C. CHEUNG, D. J. PROCKOP & C. D. BOYD. 1985. cDNA clones coding of the proα1(IV) chain of human type IV procollagen reveal an unusual homology of amino acid sequence in two-halves of the carboxy-terminal domain. J. Biol. Chem. 260: 7681-7687.

40. UITTO, J., A. J. PEREJDA, R. P. ABERGEL, M.-L. CHU & F. RAMIREZ. 1985. Altered steady-state ratio of type I/III procollagen mRNAs correlates with selectively increased type I procollagen biosynthesis in cultured keloid fibroblasts. Proc. Nat. Acad. Sci. USA 82: 5935-5939.

41. ABERGEL, R. P., D. PIZZURRO, C. A. MEEKER, G. LASK, L. Y. MATSUOKA, R. R. MINOR, M.-L. CHU & J. UITTO. 1985. Biochemical composition of the connective tissue in keloids and analysis of collagen metabolism in keloid fibroblast cultures. J. Invest. Dermatol. 84: 384-390.

42. UITTO, J., E. M. L. TAN & L. RYHÄNEN. 1982. Inhibition of collagen accumulation in fibrotic processes: review of pharmacologic agents and new approaches with amino acids and their analogues. J. Invest. Dermatol. 79: 113s-120s.

43. UITTO, J., L. RYHÄNEN, E. M. L. TAN, A. I. OIKARINEN & E. J. ZARAGOZA. 1984. Pharmacological inhibition of excessive collagen deposition in fibrotic diseases. Fed. Proc. 43: 2815-2820.

44. UITTO, J. & D. J. PROCKOP. 1974. Incorporation of proline analogues into collagen polypeptides. Effect on the production of extracellular procollagen and on the stability of the triple helical structure of the molecule. Biochim. Biophys. Acta 336: 234-251.
45. JIMENEZ, S. A. & J. ROSENBLOOM. 1974. Decreased thermal stability of collagens containing analogs of proline or lysine. Arch. Biochem. Biophys. 163: 459-465.
46. TAN, E. M. L., L. RYHÄNEN & J. UITTO. 1983. Proline analogues inhibit human skin fibroblast growth and collagen production in culture. J. Invest. Dermatol. 80: 261-267.
47. UITTO, J. & D. J. PROCKOP. 1975. Inhibition of collagen accumulation by proline analogues: the mechanism of their action. In Collagen Metabolism in the Liver. H. Popper & K. Becker, Eds.: 139-148, Stratton Intercontinental Medical Book Corp. New York, N.Y.
48. RYHÄNEN, L., E. M. L. TAN, S. RANTALA-RYHÄNEN & J. UITTO. 1982. Conversion of type II procollagen to collagen in vitro: removal of the carboxy-terminal extension is inhibited by several naturally occurring amino acids, polyamines and structurally related compounds. Arch. Biochem. Biophys. 215: 230-236.
49. FESSLER, J. H. & L. I. FESSLER. 1978. Biosynthesis of procollagen. Annu. Rev. Biochem. 47: 129-162.
50. PROCKOP, D. J. & K. I. KIVIRIKKO. 1984. Heritable diseases of collagen. N. Engl. J. Med. 311: 376-386.
51. BAILEY, A. J. & C. M. LAPIÈRE. 1976. Effect of an additional peptide extension of the N-terminus of collagen from dermatosparactic calves on cross-linking of the collagen fiber. Eur. J. Biochem. 34: 91-96.
52. MIYAHARA, M., F. K. NJIEHA & D. J. PROCKOP. 1982. Formation of collagen fibrils in vitro by cleavage of procollagen with procollagen proteinases. J. Biol. Chem. 257: 8442-8448.
53. ZARAGOZA, E. J., L. RYHÄNEN, A. I. OIKARINEN & J. UITTO. 1986. Inhibition of type II procollagen to collagen conversion by lysine derivatives and related compounds: mapping of the inhibitory structural features. Biochem. Pharmacol. 35: 532-535.
54. ABERGEL, R. P., C. A. MEEKER, H. OIKARINEN, A. I. OIKARINEN & J. UITTO. 1985. Retinoid modulation of connective tissue metabolism in keloid fibroblast cultures. Arch. Dermatol. 121: 632-635.
55. BRINCKERHOFF, C. E., H. NAGASE, J. E. NAGEL & E. D. HARRIS. 1982. Effects of all-trans-retinoic acid (retinoic acid) and 4-hydroxyphenylretinamide on synovial cells and articular cartilage. J. Am. Acad. Dermatol. 6: 591-602.
56. BAUER, E. A., J. L. SELTZER & A. Z. EISEN. 1982. Inhibition of collagen degradative enzymes by retinoic acid in vitro. J. Am. Acad. Dermatol. 6: 603-607.
57. NELSON, D. L. & G. BALIAN. 1984. The effect of retinoic acid on collagen synthesis by human dermal fibroblasts. Collagen Rel. Res. 4: 119-128.

Genetic Linkage Analysis of Neurofibromatosis[a]

M. ANNE SPENCE,[b] DILYS M. PARRY,[c] JUDY L. BADER,[d]
MARY L. MARAZITA,[b] MAUREEN BOCIAN,[e]
STEVE J. FUNDERBURK,[b] JOHN J. MULVIHILL,[c]
AND ROBERT S. SPARKES[f]

[b]Mental Retardation Research Center
Department of Psychiatry
UCLA School of Medicine
760 Westwood Plaza
Los Angeles, California 90024

[c]Clinical Epidemiology Branch
National Cancer Institute
5a21 Landow Building
Bethesda, Maryland 20205

[d]Radiation Oncology Branch
National Cancer Institute
Landow Building
Bethesda, Maryland 20205

[e]Department of Pediatrics
University of California, Irvine
101 City Drive, South, Route 81
Orange, California 92668

[f]Department of Medicine
UCLA School of Medicine
760 Westwood Plaza
Los Angeles, California 90024

This study represents a collaborative effort primarily between the National Cancer Institute and the University of California, Los Angeles. The goal of the study has been to map the gene or genes responsible for the classical form of neurofibromatosis (NF) using the standard gene markers. Samples have been obtained from many of the families for DNA polymorphism analysis, and those results are discussed elsewhere in this volume.[1]

Key members of the families in the study have had physical examinations as well as blood drawn for the laboratory studies. The original data set consisted of 11 multigenerational families and 108 subjects.[2] We are reporting 8 additional families

[a]This research was supported in part by National Institutes of Health Grant HD-05615 and also by the generous support of the National Neurofibromatosis Foundation.

(UCLA ID numbers: NF014, NF017-023), 4 with three generations of NF. A total of 142 subjects, including 45 affected individuals, are available for analysis in this new sample. The largest pedigree (NF018) contained 27 individuals of whom 8 were affected. We had 1 black family (NF022), the other 7 were of mixed caucasian background. One pedigree (NF020) had both discordant female twins and an asymptomatic gene carrier. The asymptomatic individual had an affected father and two affected daughters. There were two additional cases of an obligate gene carrier *not* showing any clinical symptoms in the initial 11 pedigrees.[2]

For all of our families the diagnosis of neurofibromatosis was defined by standard clinical criteria as described by Crowe and his colleagues in 1956.[3] Several of the children in the new families were quite young and did not yet show any signs of NF. Since symptoms often appear, or are exaggerated, at puberty, the young children were treated as uncertain in phenotype rather than unaffected at this time.

The laboratory tests were completed at UCLA using standard published techniques.[4-6] Isoelectric focusing was done to subtype the Gc phenotypes.[7] Pedigree structures and laboratory data were coded into computer files for analysis. The lod scores, as defined by Morton,[8] were calculated using the computer program LIPED.[9] Lod scores were calculated for a matrix of recombination values where male and female recombination varied from 1% to 40%. All lod scores were calculated assuming an autosomal dominant mode of inheritance with an affected allele frequency of 0.001. Clearly documented cases of nonclinical expression in gene carriers required a reduced penetrance, and we chose 98%. For the two families with young children (NF020, NF018) we used a straight-line age-of-onset correction from 5 to 20 years.[5] The scores were summed over all informative families for each marker. The summing procedure assumes that a single locus is responsible for NF, a point we will return to later.

Four specific questions were asked with respect to the results: (1) the evidence for linkage with the markers on chromosome 1, (2) the evidence for linkage with the other 13 informative markers, (3) the evidence that classical NF is linked to the secretor locus on chromosome 19, and (4) the evidence that NF is linked to the Gc locus on chromosome 4.

The first question arises because nerve growth factor has been mapped to the short arm of chromosome 1 in the region 1pter to 1p21.[10] There is interest in the possible role of this factor in the occurrence of NF and therefore interest in whether NF would also map to chromosome 1.

TABLE 1 summarizes the results for four chromosome 1 markers: the Rh blood group, PGM1, the Duffy (Fy) blood group, and AMY2. Fy is on the long arm and Rh, PGM1, and AMY2 are on the short arm of chromosome 1. For ease of presentation, only the lod scores at equal male and female recombination frequencies are listed in the table. Recall that lod scores with values less than minus 2 are considered to give statistically significant evidence against linkage, for that value of recombination.[8] Note that for close linkage of NF with Rh, PGM1, and Fy, the scores are strikingly negative. The scores for AMY2 are positive and represent the sum over 12 informative families. AMY2 is located on the short arm of chromosome 1 in band 21 between the PGM1 and Rh loci.[10] Scores were slightly positive for PGM1 at loose linkage, and this possible location for the NF locus cannot be ruled out at this time. This location is unlikely, however, when the DNA data are considered, as discussed elsewhere in this volume.[11]

The more general issue is question 2, that of linkage with any of the other standard genetic markers. TABLE 2 lists the largest positive scores among the other markers. Here we see AMY2 again, and two other fairly small positive scores. It requires a score of at least 3.0 to have statistically significant evidence for linkage.[8] These scores are at best suggestive, and scores less than 1.0 rarely hold up to further scrutiny.

One important result, in the absence of defining a linkage with a marker, is exclusion mapping. This is the procedure whereby one excludes regions of the genome for further probing with DNA techniques on the basis of strongly negative lod scores with the readily tested standard markers. TABLE 3 gives the regions around the markers in recombination units for which the lod score was less than minus 2. Note for seven of the markers, ACP1, MNSs, GLO1, ABO, ESD, Hp, and PGP, the exclusion extends to 20% recombination. Also recall that these scores were obtained by summing over all families tested and informative for each of the markers, a procedure that requires the assumption that only one locus is responsible for NF.

Another issue raised about the location of the NF gene is that two unusual families have been reported with a disease that resembles both NF and myotonic dystrophy.[12,13] The latter disease is a member of a linkage group that has been assigned to chromosome 19. In each report the affected individuals had symptoms of both neurofibromatosis and myotonic dystrophy (MYD). Rivas and DiLiberti had eight affected individuals with one possible recombinant between the two diseases.[12] Ichikawa et al. found that the maximum lod score between the two diseases was at zero recombination,[13] subsequently confirmed by more extensive analyses of the family.[14] The NF/MYD family had positive lod scores with C3 and with secretor, both on chromosome 19.[14] We

TABLE 1. Lod Scores for Neurofibromatosis and the Gene Markers on Chromosome 1

Marker	Chromosomal Location	Recombination Frequency $\theta_m = \theta_f$					
		0.01	0.05	0.10	0.20	0.30	0.40
Rh	1p36-p34	−24.3	−13.8	− 8.4	−3.5	−1.4	−0.4
PGM1	1p22.1	−11.4	− 5.5	− 2.8	−0.7	0.1	0.2
Fy	1q12-q21	−27.9	−16.3	−10.2	−4.6	−1.9	−0.6
AMY2	1p21	0.0	0.6	0.7	0.7	0.5	0.2

have reported lod scores for NF with the secretor locus in the original 11 families.[2] Our scores were not consistent with close linkage between NF and secretor and suggest that the classical NF gene will not map to the same locus as the combined NF/MYD disorder.

The most interesting result from our original report on linkage with NF poses the final question. We had a slight suggestion of heterogeneity with the scores for the Gc locus on chromosome 4.[2] This arose because the first 5 informative families for Gc led to a combined lod score of 2.2. However, the 6th family was strikingly negative and the combined data in the original report summed over 10 informative families gave a maximum lod score of 0.89 at a male recombination frequency of 3% and a female frequency of 28%. In TABLE 4 we add 6 more informative families and see that the maximum lod score is reduced to 0.61 at a $\theta_m = 0.27$ and $\theta_f = 0.15$. It is still possible that there are some families with NF that are linked to Gc and others that are not. However, the Utah group reports results from 8 families where the diagonal lod scores ($\theta_m = \theta_f$) are negative.[15] A more detailed report of their analyses was not available at the time of this meeting, although those results should be available soon.

We tested our 16 informative families for linkage heterogeneity, that is, evidence

TABLE 2. Maximum Positive Lod Scores for Neurofibromatosis and the Standard Gene Markers

Marker[a]	Chromosome[b]	Families[c]	Maximum Lod	θ_m	θ_f
AMY2	1	12	0.74	0.1	0.5
PI	14	5	0.55	0.2	0.01
ADA	20	12	0.90	0.2	0.2

[a] For definitions of marker names, see Reference 10.
[b] Assigned chromosome, see Reference 10.
[c] Number of informative families in our sample.

that in some families NF was linked to Gc but in other families NF was not linked to Gc. The heterogeneity test uses a procedure developed by Hodge et al.[16] Our estimate of the proportion of linked families was 55% at a recombination frequency of 20%. However, the p valve was > 0.2 and did not achieve statistical significance. In the absence of data on other chromosome 4 markers, the most likely possibility is that the positive scores with Gc in some families occurred by chance.

It still remains an important issue to linkage studies whether or not there are multiple loci producing the NF phenotype. The degree of clinical variability for NF has provoked Riccardi to propose that there are four types of the disease.[17] We have not included any central NF families in our analyses. We have found some of our families to be inconsistent with respect to the proposed subtyping criteria.[17] Also, we now know that the full extreme of clinical variability for Huntington's disease is displayed in the single large Venezuelan pedigree reported by Gusella and colleagues.[18] Yet Huntington's disease in that family is due to the inheritance of a single gene identical by descent in all members of the pedigree. Further, all the Huntington's families reported to date show linkage with the same DNA polymorphism of chromosome 4.[19] Therefore, to equate clinical variability with genetic heterogeneity is

TABLE 3. Exclusion Mapping with the Informative Gene Markers; Maximum Recombination Frequency for Which the Lod Scores are Less than Minus 2

Marker[a]	Chromosome[b]	$\theta_m = \theta_f$
Jk	2	0.10
Kkp	2?	0.10
ACP1	2	0.20
MNSs	4	0.20
HLA	6	0.10
BF	6	0.10
GLO1	6	0.20
ABO	9	0.20
GPT	10?	0.10
ESD	13	0.20
Hp	16	0.20
PGP	16	0.20
ADA	20	0.01

[a] For definitions of symbols, consult Reference 10.
[b] Assigned chromosome, see Reference 10.

premature in the absence of data to support the existence of multiple loci. However, one must be alert for such a possibility and test for it statistically, since pooling heterogeneous families would obscure the linkage relations.

An intriguing point for this meeting is whether our three families with NF vs. Gc lod scores greater than 0.5 represent a different genetic entity than the four families with Gc scores less than minus 2. The families individually are too small to provide enough information for a heterogeneity test as was done by Morton for elliptocytosis and Rh.[20] Another way to address the possible heterogeneity is to query whether or not the three families with a suggestion of Gc linkage show *no* evidence of linkage with secretor and vice versa. Such a finding would be consistent with the idea that one form of the disease is linked to Gc and the other form to secretor. In fact quite the opposite is observed in our data. Of the three families with the most positive scores with Gc, two show small positive scores with secretor. And of the three families with negative scores with Gc, one also shows negative scores with secretor. The families are small, and the calculated scores subject to chance variation. Still, the picture is not suggestive of this two-locus explanation for NF. At this time no definitive statement can be made with respect to the number of NF loci because the linkage data remain inconclusive.

TABLE 4. Lod Scores for Neurofibromatosis and the Gc Locus

	Recombination Frequency $\theta_m = \theta_f$					
	0.01	0.05	0.10	0.20	0.30	0.40
First study, 10 families[2]	− 1.4	−0.1	0.4	0.7	0.6	0.3
This report, 6 families	− 10.0	−5.1	−2.8	−0.9	−0.1	0.1
Total	− 11.4	−5.2	−2.4	−0.2	0.5	0.4

In summary then, exclusion mapping has eliminated several regions of the genome for exploration with the DNA polymorphisms, as long as we accept the assumption that one locus is responsible for NF. No scores yet provide a map location for an NF gene, and there is no statistically significant evidence of heterogeneity at the genetic level to support the notion of more than one locus responsible for NF.

ACKNOWLEDGMENTS

The authors thank Maryellen Sparkes and Michol Crist for laboratory assistance; Sharon Doyle, R.N., for assistance with the families; and Alisa Goldstein for assistance with data entry.

REFERENCES

1. SEIZINGER, B. R., R. E. TANZI, T. C. GILLIAM, J. BADER, D. PARRY, A. SPENCE, M. MARIZITA, K. GIBBONS, W. HOBBS & J. F. GUSELLA. Genetic linkage analysis of neurofibromatosis with DNA markers. Ann. N.Y. Acad. Sci. (This volume.)
2. SPENCE, M. A., J. L. BADER, D. M. PARRY, L. L. FIELD, S. J. FUNDERBURK, A. E. RUBENSTEIN, P. A. GILMAN & R. S. SPARKES. Linkage analysis of neurofibromatosis (von Recklinghausen disease). 1983. J. Med. Genet. 20(5): 334-337.
3. CROWE, E. W., W. J. SCHULL & J. V. NEEL. 1956. A Clinical Pathological and Genetic Study of Multiple Neurofibromatosis. Charles C. Thomas. Springfield, Ill.
4. CRANDALL, B. F. & M. A. SPENCE. 1974. Linkage relations of the phenylcarbamide locus (PTC). Hum. Hered. 24: 247-252.
5. HODGE, S. E., M. A. SPENCE & B. F. CRANDALL. 1980. Huntington disease: linkage analysis with age of onset corrections. Am. J. Med. Genet. 5: 247-252.
6. ROBERTSON, R. D., M. A. SPENCE, R. S. SPARKES, K. NEISWANGER & L. L. FIELD. 1982. Linkage analysis with trismus-pseudocamptodactyly syndrome. Am. J. Med. Genet. 12: 115-120.
7. DYKES, D., H. POLESKY & E. COX. 1981. Isoelectric focusing of GC (vitamin D binding globulin) in parentage testing. Hum. Genet. 58: 174-175.
8. MORTON, N. E. 1955. Sequential tests for the detection of linkage. Am. J. Hum. Genet. 7: 277-318.
9. OTT, J. 1974. Estimation of the recombination fraction in human pedigrees: efficient computation of the likelihood for human linkage studies. Am. J. Hum. Genet. 26: 588-597.
10. SPARKES, R. S., K. BERG, H. J. EVANS & H. P. KLINGER, Eds. 1984. Human Gene Mapping, 7. S. Karger. Basel, Switzerland.
11. DARBY, J. K., K. GOSLIN, V. M. RICCARDI, S. HUSOM, R. FERRELL, J. KIDD, B. SEIZINGER, J. FERRIER, E. M. SHOOTER & L. L. CAVALLI-SFORZA. Linkage analysis between NGFB and other chromosome 1p markers and disseminated neurofibromatosis. Ann. N.Y. Acad. Sci. (This volume.)
12. RIVAS, M. L. & J. H. DI LIBERTI. 1984. Genetic linkage between mytonic dystrophy and neurofibromatosis. In Human Gene Mapping. R. S. Sparkes, K. Berg, H. J. Evans & H. P. Klinger, Eds. 7: 570. S. Karger. Basel, Switzerland.
13. ICHIKAWA, K., C. CROSLEY, A. CULEBRAS & L. WEITKAMP. 1981. Coincidence of neurofibromatosis and myotonic dystrophy in a kindred. J. Med. Genet. 18: 143-138.
14. PERICAK-VANCE, M. A., J. M. STAJICH, P. M. CONNEALLY, J. M. VANCE, M. H. HABSTREITH, C. J. CROSLEY & A. D. ROSES. 1984. Genetic linkage analysis of myotonic dystrophy (MYD) and neurofibromatosis (NF) with the complement component 3 (C3), secretor (Se), and Lewis (Le) loci on chromosome 19. In Human Gene Mapping. R. S. Sparkes, K. Berg, H. J. Evans & H. P. Klinger, Eds. 7: 565. S. Karger. Basel Switzerland.
15. DIETZ, J. N., T. ROBINS, C. SCHWARTZ, L. CANNON, T. MCCLELLAN, R. WILLIAMSON & M. SKOLNICK. 1985. Linkage analysis of NF to chromosome 4 and 19. Cytogenet. Cell Genet. 40: 617.
16. HODGE, S. E., C. E. ANDERSON, K. NEISWANGER, R. S. SPARKES & D. L. RIMOIN. 1983. The search for heterogeneity in insulin dependent diabetes mellitus (IDDM): linkage studies, two-locus models, and genetic heterogeneity. Am. J. Hum. Genet. 35: 1139-1155.
17. RICCARDI, V. M. 1981. Von Recklinghausen neurofibromatosis. New. Engl. J. Med. 305: 1617-1627.
18. GUSELLA, J. F., N. S. WEXLER, P. M. CONNEALLY, S. L. NAYLOR, M. A. ANDERSON, R. E. TANZI, P. C. WATKINS, K. OTINA, M. R. WALLACE, A. Y. SAKAGUCHI, A. B. YOUNG, I. SHOULSON, E. BONILLA & J. B. MARTIN. 1983. A polymorphic DNA marker genetically linked to Huntington's disease. Nature 306: 234-238.
19. FOLSTEIN, S. E., J. A. PHILLIPS, P. G. WAHER, H. H. KAZAZIAN, R. E. TANZI, W. HOBBS, K. GIBBONS, P. M. CONNEALLY & J. F. GUSELLA. 1984. Recombination between the G8 probe and the Huntington disease locus in two large kindreds. Am. J. Hum. Genet. 36(suppl.): 51S.
20. MORTON, N. E. 1956. The detection and estimation of linkage between the genes for elliptocytosis and Rh blood type. Am. J. Hum. Genet. 8: 80-96.

Parasexual Approaches to the Study of Human Genetic Disease[a]

TRACY GROSS LUGO, ROBIN J. LEACH,
AND R. E. K. FOURNIER

Department of Microbiology and
Comprehensive Cancer Center
University of Southern California
1441 Eastlake Avenue
Los Angeles, California 90033

INTRODUCTION

Parasexual genetics is an increasingly important part of the repertoire of techniques available for the study of human genetic disease. Hybrid cells containing small portions of the human genome are tools that complement pedigree analysis as a means to map disease loci. Detailed knowledge of a gene's chromosomal location and its linkage, if any, to other genetic markers makes possible more accurate diagnosis and more informative genetic counseling.

An extremely successful approach to human gene mapping, especially of autosomal loci, has been the use of somatic cell hybrids.[1] This strategy is based on the unilateral loss of human chromosomes from human × rodent hybrids, which makes it possible to establish concordance between the presence of a human gene and the presence or absence of specific human chromosomes. There have been two limitations to this technique. The first, the requirement that a human gene be expressed in the hybrids in order to be detected, has largely been eliminated by the development of recombinant DNA probes to serve as genetic markers.[2]

The second limitation is that the loss of human chromosomes from hybrids is uncontrolled and not completely random, so that large panels of independent hybrid clones are required to cover the entire chromosome complement. In addition, the karyotypic character of each hybrid line must be continuously monitored. There are a few chromosomes that can be selectively maintained in hybrids because they carry genes conferring drug resistance (e.g., thymidine kinase on human chromosome 17), but these natural selectable markers do not occur on every chromosome. They are also usually not dominant, so that cells with recessive mutations must be used as partners in the fusion. DNA-mediated transfer facilitated by calcium phosphate pre-

[a]This work was supported by grants from the National Institutes of Health and the Hereditary Disease Foundation, and by a Faculty Research Award to R.E.K.F. from the American Cancer Society. T.G.L. is a Leukemia Society of America Fellow.

cipitation has recently been used successfully to introduce dominant genes for drug resistance, some of bacterial origin, into the chromosomes of human and rodent cells.[3,4]

Several laboratories are now using microcell-mediated chromosome transfer to isolate directly hybrid cells carrying chromosomes into which selectable markers have been introduced.[3–5] Microcell-mediated chromosome transfer involves the fusion of subnuclear particles ("microcells") from donor cells with recipient cells, resulting in the transfer of single or limited numbers of intact chromosomes.[6]

Microcells can be produced efficiently from primary diploid fibroblasts, which are the donor material of choice for the construction of mapping panels because they are free of the chromosomal rearrangements characteristic of nearly all established cell lines.[7] However, the use of primary cells for these experiments has so far been constrained because of their limited proliferative potential coupled with the inefficiency of calcium phosphate-mediated gene transfer. This technique yields gene transfer at notoriously low frequencies and tends to result in the integration of multiple gene copies, few of which are expressed, at a limited number of chromosomal sites.[8] A more efficient process is required to introduce genes into the chromosomes of nonestablished cells.

Transducing retroviruses provide a very efficient way of introducing genes into primary cultured cells. Retroviral vectors carrying selectable genes have recently been constructed that can infect both human and rodent cells (amphotropic host range), and, most important, are not capable of independent replication.[9,10] The integration of these vectors into chromosomes is quasi-random, like that of the retroviruses from which they were derived; the probability of integration on a particular chromosome is a function of its size. Multiple infection of cells with such defective retroviruses permits the recovery of large numbers of independent integration events.[11] This is the approach we have used to introduce a selectable gene into the chromosomes of human diploid fibroblasts in order to construct a mapping panel.

Once a gene has been assigned to a chromosome, finer subchromosomal localization can be achieved using hybrids containing chromosome fragments.[12] Generally, cells containing either human chromosomes with terminal deletions or translocations of human fragments onto host chromosomes have been required, because fragments lacking a centromere are rapidly lost. The ability to introduce selectable genes into chromosomes provides a way to maintain fragments without centromeres in hybrid cells, by continuous application of selective pressure.

One way to produce hybrid cells containing chromosome fragments is chromosome-mediated gene transfer, in which a recipient cell is exposed to isolated metaphase chromosomes from the donor. This approach has been used successfully to produce hybrid cells containing a fragment of mouse chromosome 17 carrying a selectable gene inserted near the major histocompatibility locus.[11] However, there is no way to control the size of the piece that is transferred, and the efficiency of the process is strongly influenced by the nature of the recipient cells.

Another approach which avoids these potential difficulties is to produce chromosome fragments in intact cells by exposing them to gamma-irradiation, and then to fuse them with nonirradiated cells. Goss and Harris demonstrated that the average size of fragments transferred in this way is a function of the radiation dose,[13,14] and their technique was adapted by Cirullo et al. to produce hybrids containing fragments of a human chromosome on a hamster background.[15] This is the method we chose to construct rat cell lines containing fragments of the human X chromosome. In our experiments the selected gene was the human gene for hypoxanthine guanine phosphoribosyltransferase (HPRT), but the same strategy could be employed using an artificially introduced selectable marker.

METHODS

Human diploid fibroblasts were obtained from a sample of foreskin. They were infected with the vector pZIP-NeoSV(X)1, which is derived from the Moloney murine leukemia virus.[16] It is not capable of independent replication, because viral genes have been replaced with the bacterial neomycin-resistance gene (*neo*[R]) conferring resistance to the antibiotic G418 (Geneticin). Propagation of such a defective virus requires helper functions from an intact virus. Stocks of pZIP-NeoSV(X)1 were prepared in the packaging cell line ψ-AM2275,[9] which harbors a provirus with the envelope gene of an amphotropic retrovirus. The provirus in ψ-AM2275 cells can provide helper functions in *trans,* but it contains a mutation that prevents its own genome from being packaged into virus particles. The resulting stock of pZIP-NeoSV(X)1 is thus free of helper virus. Moreover, the pZIP-NeoSV(X)1 particles have acquired the amphotropic character of the helper virus, enabling them to infect human cells.

Microcell-mediated chromosome transfer from infected fibroblasts was carried out as described.[6,7] The cells were plated onto plastic "bullets" and subjected to prolonged (48 hours) mitotic arrest in the presence of 10 mcg/ml colcemid. Under these conditions the nuclear membrane reforms around the condensed chromosomes, partitioning them into micronuclei. The cells were eunucleated by centrifugation in the presence of 5 mcg/ml cytochalasin B. The resulting microcells (micronuclei surrounded by envelopes of plasma membrane) were fused to recipient 3T6 cells by agglutination in phytohemagglutinin P followed by application of 44% polyethylene glycol. 3T6 is an established line of mouse fibroblasts. Microcell hybrids were selected in medium containing 1 mg/ml G418.

To induce chromosome breakage, monolayers of human diploid fibroblasts were gamma-irradiated by exposure to a ^{137}Cs source. The radiation dose was controlled by varying the length of exposure. The irradiated cells were immediately transferred to flasks containing cells of the HPRT-deficient rat hepatoma line FAO-1 and fused by exposure to polyethylene glycol. Hybrids containing the human HPRT gene were selected in medium containing hypoxanthine, thymidine, and 0.25 mcg/ml aminopterin (HAT medium). Spontaneous HPRT[+] revertants of FAO-1 arise at a frequency of 10^{-8}.

RESULTS

Construction of Microcell Hybrids Containing Intact Human Chromosomes

Human diploid fibroblasts were infected at high multiplicity with pZIP-NeoSV(X)1, and infected cells from approximately 75 independent G418-resistant colonies were pooled. This population was used as the donor for microcell-mediated chromosome transfer into 3T6 cells. The presence of human chromosomes in G418-resistant microcell hybrids was confirmed by the alkaline Giemsa technique,[17] which produces differential staining of human and rodent chromosomes. (FIGURE 1).

Several of the hybrid clones examined contained three or more human chromosomes at high frequency (> 50% of the population), but two karyotypically simple

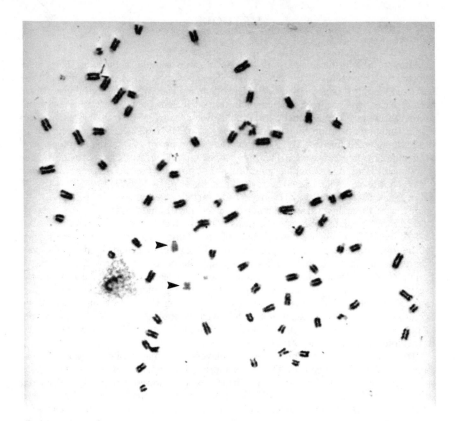

FIGURE 1. Metaphase chromosomes of microcell hybrid HDm-5 following alkaline Giemsa staining. Arrows: human chromosomes.

clones were recovered. Clone HDm-5 retained an acrocentric human chromosome (D group) in 95% of the cells, and clone HDm-9 retained a small metacentric human chromosome (F group) at high frequency (FIGURE 2). A minority of the HDm-5 population also retained a small metacentric human chromosome (evident in FIGURE 1), but the frequency of this chromosome declined rapidly with time in culture, indicating that the *neo*R gene is most likely integrated into the larger human chromosome.

Extracts of HDm-5 cells were screened electrophoretically for the presence of three human enzymes, each assigned to one of the D group human chromosomes (TABLE 1). Presence of the human form of nucleoside phosphorylase (FIGURE 3) and absence of the other two human enzymes identified the chromosome retained in HDm-5 as human chromosome 14. The F group chromosome in clone HDm-9 was determined to be human chromosome 20 in a similar manner. These chromosome identifications were confirmed by Giemsa-trypsin banding (not shown).

Construction of Hybrids Containing Fragments of the
Human X Chromosome

The effect of increasing radiation dose to the human fibroblast partner on the recovery of HPRT$^+$ hybrids is illustrated in TABLE 2. Eight hybrid cell clones from fusions in which the radiation dose was five or more krads were isolated for further analysis: five clones from experiment three, designated GHF3-1, 3-2, 3-4, 3-5, and 3-6, and three clones from experiment four, designated GHF 4-1, 4-2, and 4-3.

The hybrid cell lines were tested for the presence of human DNA by Southern blot-hybridization analysis.[18] DNA from each clone was digested with restriction endonuclease Eco RI, size fractionated by electrophoresis through agarose gels, and transferred by blotting to a nylon membrane filter. The DNA on the filters was exposed to ^{32}P-labeled genomic DNA from human fibroblasts under conditions where only

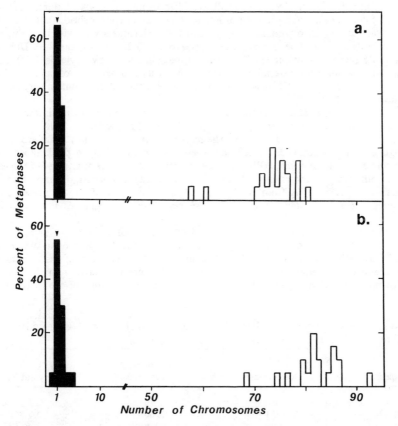

FIGURE 2. Chromosome distributions of microcell hybrids HDm-5 (a) and HDm-9 (b). Symbols: open bars, mouse chromosomes; solid bars, human chromosomes.

TABLE 1. Detection of Human Biochemical Markers in Microcell Hybrid Clones[a]

Enzyme	Corresponding Human Chromosome	HDm-5		HDm-9	
		Mouse Form	Human Form	Mouse Form	Human Form
Esterase-10	13	+	−		
Nucleoside phosphorylase	14	+	+		
Mannose phosphate isomerase	15	+	−		
Adenosine deaminase	20			+	+
Glucose phosphate isomerase	21			+	−

[a]Cell extracts were analyzed by starch gel electrophoresis followed by specific staining for enzyme activity.[1] Plus signs denote expression of enzyme from the indicated species; minus signs indicate no detectable expression.

human middle-repetitive sequences will hybridize to human DNA. Autoradiograms of the filters revealed the presence of human DNA in all eight hybrids (not shown).

Intact human chromosomes and human-rat translocations were visible in five of the hybrids after alkaline Giemsa staining (GHF 3-1, 3-2, 3-4, 3-5, and 4-3). Hybrid GHF 4-2 retained only one small human chromosome, while two hybrids, GHF 3-6 and 4-1, contained no material with the stain intensity characteristic of human chromosomes. Since human DNA is present in these cells, they clearly contain very small translocations.

A more precise estimate of the size of the X chromosome fragments in these cell lines was obtained by screening for the presence of three X-linked DNA markers, kindly provided to us by D. Drayna. The markers 52A, S21, and DX13 are arbitrary single-copy DNA sequences which have been mapped to regions of the long arm of the human X chromosome. HPRT has been mapped by pedigree analysis with respect to the other three markers on the basis of restriction fragment length polymorphism.[19] Southern blots of DNA from the hybrid cell lines were probed for the presence of sequences complementary to each of these restriction fragments as illustrated in FIGURE 4.

The results of this analysis are summarized in FIGURE 5. Only two lines, GHF 3-1 and 3-15, contained all four markers; these lines contained large amounts of human DNA as indicated by alkaline Giemsa staining and the presence of many human middle-repetitive sequences. Both of these hybrids were recovered from the fusion with fibroblasts that received the 5 krad dose of radiation. None of the three lines

TABLE 2. Recovery of HPRT[+] Hybrids following Fusion of Gamma-Irradiated Human Fibroblasts with FAO-1 Rat Cells

Experiment	Dose (krads)	Number of Hybrids Recovered	Hybrid Yield
1	0	70	2.3×10^{-5}
2	0.1	80	2.6×10^{-5}
3	5	6	2×10^{-6}
4	10	3	1×10^{-6}
5	20	0	$<3 \times 10^{-6}$

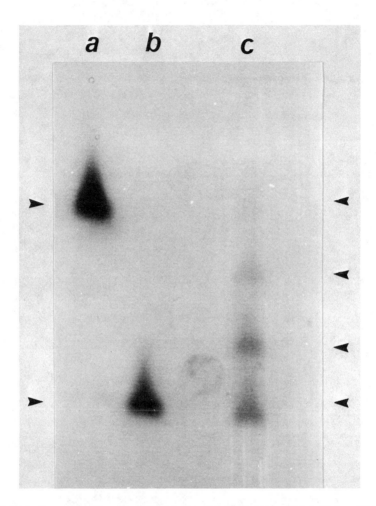

FIGURE 3. Expression of human nucleoside phosphorylase in microcell hybrid clone HDm-5. Starch gel electrophoresis of cell extracts was used to separate human and mouse forms of the enzyme, which was visualized by specific staining.[1] Lane a, HT1080 (human fibrosarcoma); lane b, 3T6 (mouse fibroblasts); lane c, HDm-5 (microcell hybrid). Interspecific heteropolymers are evident in the extract of HDm-5. The gene encoding nucleoside phosphorylase has been assigned to human chromosome 14.[1]

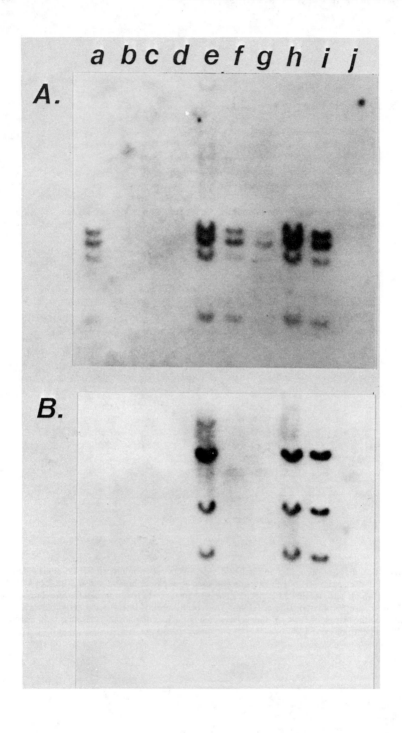

from the fusion with fibroblasts that received the higher dose contained marker S21, the most proximal marker. In general, hybrids with fibroblasts receiving the 10 krad dose of radiation were recovered at lower frequency and retained less human DNA.

DISCUSSION

The work described in this report demonstrates the feasibility of rapidly constructing panels of hybrid cells that will permit the mapping of genes on all the human chromosomes and will in many cases provide subchromosomal localizations as well. Such panels will facilitate the development of DNA markers that reveal restriction fragment length polymorphisms in human populations, thereby accelerating human gene mapping by means of pedigree analysis.[20]

Hybrids containing very small pieces of human chromosomes are also useful starting materials for the isolation of particular human genes. One well-established strategy involves the preparation of a library of cloned sequences from such a hybrid, from which clones of human origin can be identified by virtue of species-specific repetitive DNA sequences.[2] Depending on the amount of human DNA present in the hybrid, a considerable enrichment for the gene of interest can be achieved without the use of specific probes.

Some genetic diseases are the result of known biochemical defects (e.g., phenylketonuria, the hemoglobinopathies). In these instances, isolation of the defective gene provides the means for definitive diagnosis. However, other diseases are probably the result of disruptions in patterns of gene expression, and the deleterious effects of many mutations are likely due to changes in gene action in certain tissues but not in others.

The parasexual genetic strategies we have described afford the possibility of establishing models for features of such diseases in tissue culture. It is clear that the expression of genes in microcell hybrids can be modulated in a tissue-specific manner.[21] The insertion of selectable markers into human chromosomes means that these chromosomes can now be transferred into cultured cells of virtually any kind, so that the effects of genes residing on them can be studied against a variety of histiotypic backgrounds. The development of *in vitro* model systems for tissue-specific gene expression may well be the most important future application of these techniques.

SUMMARY

We have used two different strategies to construct hybrid cells in which specific, individual human chromosomes or fragments thereof are maintained by direct selective

---

FIGURE 4. Southern blot analysis of hybrid cell lines. The photographs depict autoradiograms of filters that were hybridized with ^{32}P-labeled DNA restriction fragments DX13 (panel A) and S21 (panel B). DNA from cell lines was digested with restriction endonuclease Taq I. Lane a, hybrid GHF 4-3; lane b, hybrid GHF 4-2; lane c, hybrid GHF 4-1; lane d, hybrid GHF 3-6; lane e, hybrid GHF 3-5; lane f, hybrid GHF 3-4; lane g, hybrid GHF 3-2; lane h, hybrid GHF 3-1; lane i, human diploid fibroblast; lane j, FAO-1 (rat parent). DX13 and S21 do not cross-hybridize with any rat sequences under the hybridization conditions used.

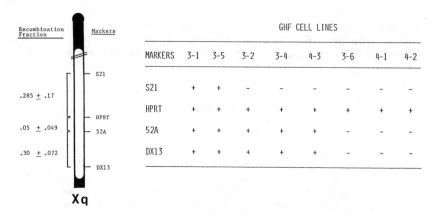

FIGURE 5. Detection of human X chromosome-specific sequences in gamma hybrids. A linkage map of the long arm of the human X chromosome adapted from Reference 19 showing the relative positions of the four markers is provided at left. Plus signs denote detection of a marker sequence in the indicated hybrid cells. The hybrids are presented in decreasing order based on the amount of X chromosome-specific DNA they contained. All lines were scored as positive for HPRT because of their ability to grow in HAT medium.

pressure. Our first approach was to introduce a drug-resistance gene into human chromosomes using a retroviral vector, and to transfer the marked chromosomes via microcells into mouse cells. The second method was to fuse gamma-irradiated human cells with rodent cells to produce hybrids containing fragments of the human X chromosome. Such hybrid cell lines should greatly facilitate both human gene mapping and the isolation of human genes by molecular cloning. The gene-transfer technologies described here can also be used to construct cell lines in which the expression of genes involved in human diseases can be studied *in vitro*.

ACKNOWLEDGMENTS

We would like to thank D. Housman for the vector pZIPNeoSV(X)1 and D. Drayna for the X chromosome-specific DNA markers 52A, S21, and DX13. We also wish to acknowledge the expert technical assistance of M. J. Przyborski, F. Parker, and M. Smith.

REFERENCES

1. RUDDLE, F. H. & R. P. CREAGAN. 1975. Annu. Rev. Genet. **9**: 407-486.
2. GUSELLA, J. F., C. KEYS, A. VARSANYI-BREINER, F.-T. KAO, C. JONES, T. T. PUCK & D. HOUSMAN. 1980. Proc. Nat. Acad. Sci. USA **77**: 2829-2833.

3. ATHWAL, R. S., M. SMARSH, B. M. SEARLE & S. S. DEO. 1985. Somatic Cell Mol. Genet. **11:** 177-187.
4. SAXON, P. J., E. S. SRIVATSAN, G. V. LEIPZIG, J. H. SAMESHIMA & E. J. STANBRIDGE. 1985. Mol. Cell. Biol. **5:** 140-146.
5. DHAR, V., B. M. SEARLE & R. S. ATHWAL. 1984. Somatic Cell Mol. Biol. **6:** 547-559.
6. FOURNIER, R. E. K. 1981. Proc. Nat. Acad. Sci. USA **78:** 6349-6353.
7. MCNEILL, C. A. & R. L. BROWN. 1980. Proc. Nat. Acad. Sci. USA **77:** 5394-5398.
8. ROBINS, D. M., S. RIPLEY, A. S. HENDERSON & R. AXEL. 1981. Cell **23:** 29-39.
9. CONE, R. D. & R. C. MULLIGAN. 1984. Proc. Nat. Acad. Sci. USA **81:** 6349-6353.
10. MILLER, A. D., M.-F. LAW & I. VERMA. 1985. Mol. Cell. Biol. **5:** 431-437.
11. WEIS, J. H., D. L. NELSON, M. J. PRZYBORSKI, D. D. CHAPLIN, R. C. MULLIGAN, D. E. HOUSMAN & J. G. SEIDMAN. 1984. Proc. Nat. Acad. Sci. USA **81:** 4879-4883.
12. GUSELLA, J. G., A. VARSANYI-BREINER, F.-T. KAO, C. JONES, T. T. PUCK, S. ORKIN & D. HOUSMAN. 1979. Proc. Nat. Acad. Sci. USA **76:** 5239-5243.
13. GOSS, S. J. & H. HARRIS. 1977. J. Cell Sci. **25:** 17-37.
14. GOSS, S. J. & H. HARRIS. 1977. J. Cell Sci. **25:** 39-57.
15. CIRULLO, R. E., S. DANA & J. J. WASMUTH. 1983. Mol. Cell. Biol. **3:** 892-902.
16. CEPKO, C. L., B. E. ROBERTS & R. C. MULLIGAN. 1984. Cell **37:** 1053-1062.
17. FRIEND, K. K., S. CHEN & F. H. RUDDLE. 1976. Somatic Cell Genet. **2:** 183-188.
18. SOUTHERN, E. M. 1975. J. Mol. Biol. **98:** 503-517.
19. DRAYNA, D., K. DAVIES, D. HARTLEY, J.-L. MANDEL, G. CAMERINO, R. WILLIAMSON & R. WHITE. 1984. Proc. Nat. Acad. Sci. USA **81:** 2836-2839.
20. WHITE, R., M. LEPPERT, D. T. BISHOP, D. BARKER, J. BERKOWITZ, C. BROWN, P. CALLAHAN, T. HOLM & L. JEROMINSKI. 1985. Nature **313:** 101-105.
21. KILLARY, A. M. & R. E. K. FOURNIER. 1984. Cell **38:** 523-534.

Genetic Linkage Analysis of Neurofibromatosis with DNA Markers[a]

B. R. SEIZINGER,[b] R. E. TANZI,[b] T. C. GILLIAM,[b]
J. L. BADER,[c] D. M. PARRY,[d] M. A. SPENCE,[e]
M. L. MARAZITA,[e] K. GIBBONS,[b] W. HOBBS,[b]
AND J. F. GUSELLA[b]

[b]Neurogenetics Laboratory
Massachusetts General Hospital
Department of Genetics
Harvard Medical School
Boston, Massachusetts 02114

[c]Radiation Oncology Branch
National Cancer Institute
NCI-Navy Radiation Oncology Section
Bethesda, Maryland 20205

[d]Clinical Epidemiology Branch
National Cancer Institute
Bethesda, Maryland 20205

[e]Departments of Psychiatry and Biomathematics
UCLA School of Medicine
Los Angeles, California 90024

INTRODUCTION

Peripheral neurofibromatosis (PNF), as described by von Recklinghausen, is one of the most common single-gene disorders affecting the nervous system. It is transmitted in an autosomal dominant fashion, with high penetrance but remarkably variable phenotype expression (for review see References 1 and 2). While multiple cell types can be affected, the most common abnormalities are in cells of neural crest origin, causing neoplasia or dysplasia. Typical clinical features include neurofibromas (disordered growth of Schwann cells) and café-au-lait spots (dysregulated growth of melanocytes).

[a]This work was supported by NINCDS grants NS22224 and NS20012. B.R.S. was supported by a research fellowship by the Max-Planck-Society for the Advancement of Sciences, West Germany. T.C.G. was supported by the Anna Mitchell Fellowship from the Hereditary Disease Foundation.

The primary defect causing PNF has not yet been identified. Although it might be possible to determine the primary defect by searching for a defective protein, there is so far no strong evidence to implicate any particular candidate. Moreover, it is possible that the primary defect of PNF is in a DNA region that does not encode a protein, but is rather a regulatory site. If so, one might search for quantitative rather than qualitative alterations in expression of particular proteins. Differences in level of expression, however, might easily represent secondary effects of the disease state.

In view of these uncertainties, we have chosen a strategy that is independent of any assumptions concerning the exact nature of the primary defect. The approach is that of genetic linkage analysis in families displaying PNF with the goal of identifying polymorphic DNA markers that are coinherited with the disease gene. The rapid development of recombinant DNA technology in recent years has provided a vast new supply of DNA markers, which detect heritable sequence variations (polymorphisms) in the patterns of restriction endonuclease digests of human genomic DNA. They have therefore been termed "restriction fragment length polymorphisms" (RFLPs).[3,4] DNA markers can be used in family studies to investigate putative coinheritance of RFLPs with the defective gene of a disease and may therefore lead to the chromosomal localization of the genetic defect. More than 200 DNA markers useful for genetic linkage analysis have already been described, and the rate of discovery of new polymorphic DNA loci is accelerating.[5] As a single gene disorder with autosomal dominant inheritance, PNF is an ideal candidate for the application of genetic linkage analysis with DNA markers. The feasibility of this approach has recently been demonstrated by our laboratory for another neurological disease with autosomal dominant inheritance, Huntington's disease, which was found to be linked to a polymorphic DNA marker on chromosome 4.[6]

STRATEGIES FOR LINKAGE ANALYSIS

The basis for any successful linkage analysis is the quality of family material available for study. Pedigrees are chosen for study because they contain a large number of individuals of defined genotype at the disease locus. These "informative" individuals represent the offspring of parents who definitely carry the defect, but may be either affected or unaffected so long as the diagnosis is clear-cut. In a disease such as neurofibromatosis, the diagnosis is usually more definitive in the case of affected family members. Each informative individual represents one potential test for coinheritance of a genetic marker with the disease. Consequently, families with large numbers of informative individuals (> 10) are favored since they can each yield a significant score for correlation between the marker locus and the disease gene.

If the pedigrees being used are too small, scores from separate kindreds can be summed. In the latter case, the investigator makes the assumption that the disease locus is the same in all families, and risks missing a positive linkage if the disease displays nonallelic heterogeneity (i.e., if mutations at more than one locus can cause symptoms of the disease). FIGURE 1 displays the four families used thus far in our studies. Members of each family were examined, and affected individuals diagnosed by previously described criteria.[7] In each case, permanent lymphoblastoid cell lines were initiated from all informative individuals as well as unaffected parents.[8] These lines act as a permanent source of DNA from members of the family in the event that several hundred markers must be tested to identify the map location of the disease gene. We continue to collect additional families of this type, but are also searching for larger pedigrees to eliminate the difficulties engendered by possible heterogeneity.

Given DNA from PNF families, there are two possible strategies that can be pursued in an attempt to identify the chromosomal position of the disease locus—the candidate gene approach and the random DNA marker approach.

THE CANDIDATE GENE APPROACH

In the candidate gene approach, the investigator can choose a gene for which a DNA probe exists that might be a candidate for being the PNF gene itself. Once an

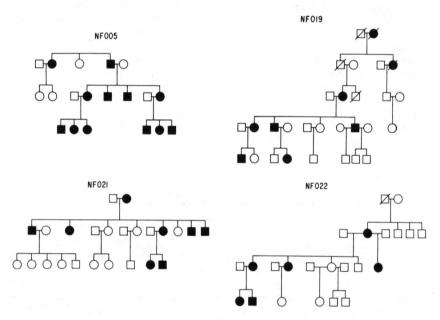

FIGURE 1. Peripheral neurofibromatosis families. Affected individuals are shown as solid symbols. Circles, females; squares, males. A slashed symbol indicates that an individual is deceased. EBV-transformed lymphoblastoid cell lines were established for the individuals.[8]

RFLP has been identified using this probe, it is then straightforward to test the possibility that the gene under investigation might represent the primary defect in the disease. The RFLP is traced in the PNF families using Southern transfer and hybridization.[3,4] An affected child is chosen at random to determine which allele at the marker locus would have to represent the defective gene if the hypothesis were correct. Each additional informative child then represents a test of the hypothesis. The detection of even a single affected sibling possessing the alternate allele from the affected parent indicates that a recombination event has taken place between the disease gene and the DNA marker locus. Since on average, two loci will display only 1% recombination if they are approximately 10^6 base pairs apart, the chances of observing such a recombination event if the candidate gene truly represents the PNF gene are negligible. PNF involves hyperplasia of Schwann cells, a phenomenon that could involve the activation of a cellular oncogene. As an example of the above strategy, we chose to investigate the possibility that PNF is caused by a mutation at or near the locus encoding platelet-derived growth factor on chromosome 22. This gene, the SIS locus, is homologous to the v-sis oncogene (for review see Reference 9). A probe for the v-sis sequence has previously been shown to detect a frequent HindIII polymorphism in the cellular gene.[10,11] We have traced the inheritance of this RFLP in our PNF families. An example of the results of these experiments is shown in FIGURE 2. In this nuclear family, the mother was affected with neurofibromatosis and passed the gene on to three of her children, one female and two males. The mother was also heterozygous for the HindIII polymorphism while her husband was homozygous for the most frequent 1 allele. The female child received both the PNF gene and the 2 allele from her mother. Both of her brothers however received the 1 allele from the mother but also inherited PNF, thereby eliminating the locus as a candidate for causing the disease in this family. It is still possible that the platelet-derived growth factor plays a primary role in other PNF families, or plays a secondary role in PNF in general since these possibilities are not addressed by this experiment. Furthermore, the detection of a single recombination event does not eliminate the possibility that the PNF gene is located on chromosome 22 several hundred thousand or more base pairs from the SIS locus.

THE RANDOM MARKER APPROACH

If no candidate gene yields positive results, the investigator is then left with the possibility of applying any DNA probes that are known to detect polymorphisms in a standard linkage analysis. Whether these problems detect known genes or are anonymous is of no import in this approach which is aimed only at detecting significant correlation in the pattern of inheritance of the disease gene and the DNA marker. In practice, positive linkage scores are most easily obtained when the two loci coinherit greater than 90% of the time. Since this will occur if the two are within 10^7 base pairs of each other, it would theoretically take only 150-200 equally spaced genetic markers to test all regions of the genome. Since not all markers will be informative in any given set of pedigrees, and equally spaced markers are not yet available for most chromosomal regions, the investigator should be prepared to type several hundred DNA markers. The redeeming feature of committing to this effort is that with adequate family material, the endeavor is virtually assured of eventual success.

In the above example using the v-sis probe, it was very easy to exclude the cellular gene as the primary cause of PNF by detecting a single recombination event. The v-sis probe is still useful to test additional families, however, since it is possible to statistically exclude the presence of the PNF gene over a large stretch of chromosome 22 by detecting additional recombination events. Once the v-sis polymorphism was traced through our families, we tested the data for evidence of genetic linkage to PNF by calculating lod scores. The lod score is the ratio (expressed as the logarithm) of the likelihood of observing the pattern of inheritance of the marker assuming linkage to the disease gene at a distance θ versus observing the same data assuming 50% recombination (no linkage). A lod score > 3 constitutes evidence for linkage of the

Sis Oncogene Hind Ⅲ RFLP

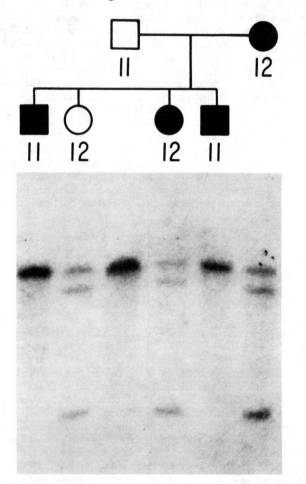

FIGURE 2. Hybridization of the v-sis oncogene probe to HindIII-digested DNA from a PNF family. DNA was prepared from lymphoblastoid cell lines as described.[6] Five micrograms of each DNA was digested to completion with the restriction enzyme HindIII. DNA fragments were fractionated on a 0.8% horizontal agarose gel, subsequently transferred to positively charged nylon filters by the Southern blot procedure, and finally hybridized against nick-translated v-sis probe DNA. (v-sis-DNA was obtained by Oncor, Gaithersburg, Md.) These procedures have been described in detail elsewhere.[6] The v-sis probe detects a restriction fragment length polymorphism (RFLP) in HindIII-digested human genomic DNA. A 21.8 kb fragment represents the 1 allele, the 15.5 and 6.8 fragments the 2 allele.

marker and the gene, while a score < -2 indicates odds of greater than 200:1 against linkage. In our analysis with v-sis, the lod score remained less than -2 as θ was varied from 0 to 0.5 indicating that the PNF gene does not map within 5% recombination of the locus encoding platelet-derived growth factor, a region of approximately 5×10^6 base pairs (see TABLE 1).

The same analysis could be carried out using any DNA probe that detects a polymorphism and eventually all regions of the genome can be tested until the location of the PNF gene is found. The size of the area that can be tested using each marker will depend on the total number of cases in which cosegregation of the marker and the disease gene can be followed. The most efficient use is made of the PNF pedigrees, therefore, when the marker is heterozygous in all affected parents. In order to approximate this ideal, we are currently concentrating on DNA markers that detect multiple RFLPs usually with different restriction enzymes. These polymorphic sites are so close together in the genome that they can be combined to generate many haplotypes at a single marker locus in much the same way that haplotypes are generated to make the HLA complex the most useful classical marker.

There are currently two clues to the potential location of the PNF gene that can be addressed using the DNA marker approach. In a study of PNF using the limited

TABLE 1. Lod Score Analysis for SIS Locus versus PNF[a]

		θ (Recombination Fraction)			
0.01	0.05	0.10	0.20	0.30	0.40
-4.99	-2.67	-1.57	-0.59	-0.22	$+0.08$

[a] Scores were calculated using LIPED with data for all four PNF pedigrees shown in FIGURE 1.

number of protein polymorphisms available as genetic markers, Spence et al. eliminated some areas of the genome from the possibility of containing the PNF gene.[7] These investigators also obtained some evidence of possible linkage of the PNF gene to the GC locus in a subset of their families. GC represents a protein polymorphism mapping to the region below the centromere on chromosome 4. A second possible location of the PNF gene has been introduced by the observation of two families in which myotonic muscular dystrophy and PNF appear to be cosegregating.[12] Myotonic muscular dystrophy has previously been mapped to chromosome 19.[13] Both chromosomes 4 and 19 are currently the subjects of intensive investigation since they contain the Huntington's disease gene[6] and the myotonic muscular dystrophy gene[13] respectively. Large numbers of new DNA markers are being generated, and complete linkage maps are being constructed at a rapid pace. These should soon allow the definitive test of whether PNF maps to either of these two chromosomes. If the defect is not localized in these studies, it will then be straightforward to sequentially test every other human chromosome by the same technique. The location of the PNF gene is therefore likely to be found within the next few years. This event will likely lead to prenatal diagnosis in this disorder, as well as opening many new avenues of research into the primary defect, including the possibility of isolating the disease gene itself based on its map location.

ACKNOWLEDGMENT

We wish to thank Karen Griffin for typing the manuscript.

REFERENCES

1. RICCARDI, V. M. 1981. N. Engl. J. Med. **305:** 1617-1627.
2. KANTER, J. R., R. ELDRIGE, R. FABRICANT, J. C. ALLEN & T. KOERBER. 1980. Neurology **30:** 851-859.
3. BOTSTEIN, D., R. L. WHITE, M. SKOLNICK & R. DAVIS. Am. J. Hum. Genet. **32:** 314-331.
4. HOUSEMAN, D. & J. F. GUSELLA. 1981. *In* Genetic Strategies for Psychobiology and Psychiatry. E. S. Gershon, S. Matthysse, X. O. Breakfield & R. D. Ciaranello, Eds.: 125-140. Boxwood.
5. SPARKES, R. S., K. BERG, H. J. EVANS & H. P. KLINGER, Eds. 1984. Human Gene Mapping 7. Karger. Basel, Switzerland.
6. GUSELLA, J. F., N. WEXLER & P. M. CONNEALLY, *et al.* 1983. Nature **306:** 234-238.
7. SPENCE, M. A., J. BADER, D. M. PARRY, *et al.* 1983. J. Med. Genet. **20:** 334-337.
8. ANDERSON, M. A. & J. F. GUSELLA. 1984. In Vitro **11:** 856-858.
9. BISHOP, J. M. 1983. Annu. Rev. Biochem. **52:** 301-354.
10. BARKER, D. & R. WHITE. 1984. Cytogenet. Cell Genet. **37:** 250.
11. JULIER, C., *et al.* 1985. Cytogenet. Cell Genet. **40:** 664.
12. ICHIKAWA, K., C. J. CROSLEY, A. CULEBRAS & L. WEITKAMP. 1981. J. Med. Genet. **18:** 134-138.
13. DAVIES, K. E., J. JACKSON, R. WILLIAMSON, P. HARPER, S. BALL, M. SAFARAZI, L. MEREDITH & G. FEY. 1983. J. Med. Genet. **20:** 259-263.

Linkage Analysis between the β-Nerve Growth Factor Gene and Other Chromosome 1p Markers and Disseminated Neurofibromatosis[a]

JOHN K. DARBY, KIM GOSLIN, VINCENT M. RICCARDI,[b]
SUSAN M. HUSON,[c] ROBERT FERRELL,[d]
JUDY KIDD,[e] BARND R. SEIZINGER,[f] JAMEY FERRIER,
ERIC M. SHOOTER, AND LUIGI L. CAVALLI-SFORZA

Department of Genetics
Stanford University School of Medicine
Stanford, California 94305

INTRODUCTION

β-Nerve growth factor (β-NGF) plays a critical role in the development and metabolism of sympathetic and some sensory neurons.[1] It is also a key factor in the growth or regeneration of neurites, and these processes are controlled by the uptake of β-NGF at growth cones or nerve endings.[2] This uptake is mediated by high- and low-affinity receptors[3] (also M. Hosang and E. M. Shooter, unpublished data).

In 1967 the β-NGF protein was isolated from the mouse submandibular gland,[4] where it is present in a multisubunit complex, 7SNGF, which contains the active β-NGF dimer, two copies of a trypsin-like subunit (γ-NGF), two copies of an acidic protease subunit (α-NGF), and two zinc ions.[5] The β-NGF protein is processed from a prepro-NGF of 33 kilodaltons (kD) through a series of cleavages to a 13.5 kD monomeric form.

[a]This work was supported by Grants GM-28428 from the National Institutes of Health and a grant from the National Neurofibromatosis Foundation.

[b]Neurofibromatosis Program, Baylor College of Medicine, 1 Baylor Plaza, Houston, Texas 77030.

[c]Department of Medical Genetics, University of Wales College of Medicine, Heath Park, Cardiff, Wales CF4 4XN. Present address: Research Registrar/Medical Genetics, Clinical Research Center, Northwick Park Hospital, Harrow, Middlesex, United Kingdom.

[d]Center for Demographic and Population Genetics, University of Texas at Houston, Houston, Texas 77225.

[e]Department of Human Genetics, Yale University School of Medicine, New Haven, Connecticut 06510.

[f]Neurogenetics Laboratory, Massachusetts General Hospital, Boston, Massachusetts 02114.

The β-NGF protein appears to be produced by sympathetic effector tissues,[6,7] but it is also found in the central nervous system[7] where its function is unaccounted for.

β-NGF has been implicated in several disorders of altered peripheral nerve growth or development: (1) impaired sympathetic and sensory nerve development in familial dysautonomia;[8-11] (2) dysplastic and hyperplastic neurofibromas in disseminated neurofibromatosis (NF)[12-14] and intestinal ganglioneuromatosis;[15] and (3) neoplasia in neuroblastoma.[16]

The identification and cloning of the β-NGF gene (NGFB)[17,18] have made possible new approaches to testing for NGFB gene alteration in these disorders. For example, Breakefield et al. reported exclusion of the NGFB locus (with BglII and HincII polymorphisms) in familial dysautonomia by discordant sibship and linkage analysis.[19] The NGFB gene has been mapped to chromosome 1p22.1[16,20] in proximity to N-ras[16,21,22] and PGM$_1$.

This paper reviews the NGFB gene TaqI and BglII restriction fragment length polymorphisms (RFLP)[23] and presents linkage analyses between five chromosome 1p markers and disseminated neurofibromatosis. Restriction analysis of the NGFB gene in neurofibroma tumor tissue is also presented.

METHODS

Cellular DNA was extracted from 30 ml blood samples[24] per standard protocols. Restriction enzymes were used to digest 2.5 to 8 μg of DNA, and restriction fragments were separated in 0.8% agarose gels. Transfer to nitrocellulose (S&S) or Zetabind (AMF) was by the method of Southern.[25] Probes were nick-translated with 32-P-dATP and 32-P-dCTP (3000 Ci/mmol; Amersham) to a specific activity of 1-5 $\times$ 10^8 cpm/μg.[26] Hybridization was done using 6-20 $\times$ 10^6 cpm of labeled probe (10-30 ng/ml) in 50% formamide, 5 $\times$ SSPE, 1 $\times$ Denhardt's at 40°C for 48 hours, followed by high stringency washes (twice for 30 minutes in 0.1 $\times$ SSPE, 0.1% sodium dodecyl sulfate at 65°C). Filters were autoradiographed on Kodak XAR-5 film with DuPont lightning plus intensifying screens at -70°C for 5-12 days. All results were duplicated for verification.

NGFB POLYMORPHISMS

The human NGFB gene was obtained by library screen, subcloned at the Eco R1 sites, and the BglII and TaqI polymorphism sites were mapped.[23] As can be seen in FIGURE 1 the two polymorphic sites are approximately 6 kilobases (kb) apart.

The loss of the TaqI restriction site between the 5' 4.3-kb fragment and the 1.7-kb fragment produces the 6-kb polymorphic fragment. The appearance of this RFLP in homozygote and heterozygote forms on wide comb gels (8 μg DNA) can be seen in FIGURE 2.

Parents from 35 families were screened, and the two alleles (4.3 kb and 6 kb) were found to be in Hardy-Weinberg equilibrium with allelic frequencies of 83% and 17%, respectively (see TABLE 1). This test indicates that the TaqI RFLP is not associated with any lethal condition.

The parents were also screened with *Bgl*II and the allelic fragments (1.4 kb and 5.6 kb) were in Hardy-Weinberg equilibrium with frequencies of 78% and 22%, respectively. The *Bgl*II and *Taq*I alleles (5.6 and 6.0 kb) show significant linkage disequilibrium, and no *Taq*I 6-kb and *Bgl*II 5.6-kb haplotypes were found (TABLE 2).

The simultaneous appearance of the *Bgl*II and *Taq*I hybridizing fragments can be seen in the autoradiograph (FIGURE 3) where small gel combs (4 μg DNA) were used.

CLINICAL PATIENT SAMPLES

Blood samples (30 ml) were obtained from 17 families with NF. These families were comprised of 188 persons of whom 85 individuals were affected with NF. One-half of the subject population was collected in Cardiff, Wales and one-half was from Texas. Informed consent was obtained from all participants.

TABLE 1. χ^2 Test of Hardy-Weinberg Law on Parents of Families for *Taq* I Polymorphism[a]

Genotype (kb)	Observed	Expected	$(O-E)^2/E$
4.3/4.3	49	47.9	0.026
4.3/6.0	17	19.1	0.248
6.0/6.0	3	1.9	0.593
Total	69	69	$\chi^2 = 0.867$
			$df = 1$
			$p = 0.34$

[a] Allele frequencies: 4.3 kb; 0.833; 6 kb; 0.167.

Each member of the disseminated NF pedigrees was extensively evaluated and affected members exhibited multiple café-au-lait spots and diffuse neurofibromas (in adults), and penetrance in these pedigrees was assumed to be virtually complete.[27] Standard protein markers and several RFLPs have been tested for linkage to NF in these families, and no evidence of inheritance incompatibilities was detected.

NGFB and NF

Three methods were employed to analyze the NGFB gene in NF:

1. Restriction fragment analysis. This test was used to screen for any gross NGFB gene alteration in NF patients. Restriction analysis of six patients with NF

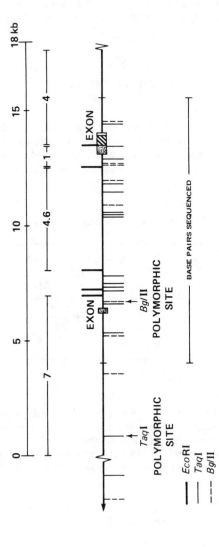

FIGURE 1. Restriction endonuclease cleavage sites in the 17 kb human NGFB DNA insert in phage charon 4A-H16. (1) Above the figure is the 0-18 kb scale. (2) Eco R1 subcloned fragments are bracketed as 7, 4.6, 1, and 4 kb fragments between the upright Eco R1 restriction sites. (3) Exons marked as: stippled box = preproNGF; hatched box = mature NGF; blank box = 3' sequence - function unknown. (4) 12 kb bracketed section of NGF gene sequenced by Ullrich et al. (5) BglII and TaqI restriction sites and polymorphic sites marked with downward verticals.

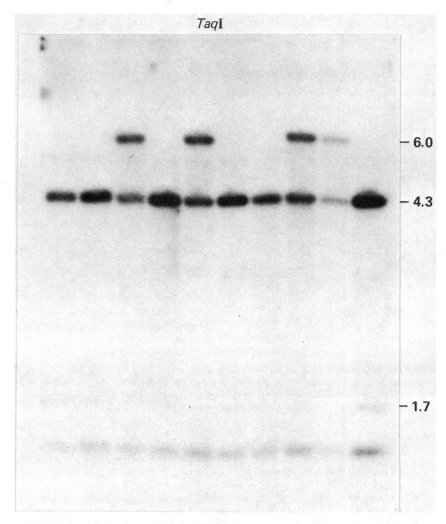

FIGURE 2. Autoradiogram of a nitrocellulose filter after hybridization of ^{32}p-7 kb NGFB subclone to large comb *Taq*I digestions of normal subjects DNA. Molecular lengths of the hybridizing fragments are given in kb as judged by log scale graphs.

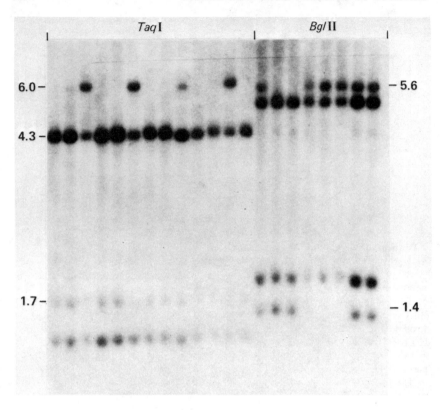

FIGURE 3. Autoradiogram of a nitrocellulose filter after hybridization of [32]p-7 kb NGFB subclone to small comb BglII and TaqI digestions of NF family DNA. Molecular lengths of the hybridizing fragments are given in kb as judged by log scale graphs.

(from separate families) was carried out with six enzymes (EcoRI, MspI, SstI, TaqI, BglII, HindIII) and probed with the EcoRI 7-kb and 4-kb subclones. Fragment sizes were identical with normals and in agreement with the restriction map (FIGURE 1).

2. Discordant sibship analysis. This technique of linkage analysis is useful in excluding a locus when few informative families are available. If genetic heterogeneity is present, however, the strength of the technique is compromised. Five families informative for this method were identified, and two are illustrated in FIGURE 4. In family 125, the affected father has passed the same NGFB allele to all three offspring, one of whom does not have NF. The father's unaffected sister is also concordant for the BglII 1.4-kb NGFB allele. In family 135, the affected mother has transmitted separate NGFB alleles to each of two affected offspring. In addition, the mother is discordant for T2 NGFB alleles seen in two of her affected sibs. These two informative families each have at least one parent heterozygous for both the DNA polymorphism and NF. They show that NF segregates independently from the NGFB gene polymorphism

and therefore preclude direct linkage involvement of the gene in these families. If genetic heterogeneity were present, however, the NGFB gene would theoretically be involved in other families. This possibility of genetic heterogeneity in NF was raised in a prior linkage study with the GC marker.[28]

3. Lod score analysis. Positive or negative linkage to a disease is more reliably tested by making a statistical analysis of the frequency with which two markers segregate together in many families. This is done by a mathematical computation of the odds for and against linkage[29] that was initially programmed in 1974.[30] The assignment of haplotypes for *Bgl*II and *Taq*I RFLPs further strengthens the linkage analysis by providing more NGFB gene markers in the pedigrees. TABLE 3 lists the lod scores for various recombination fractions between NGFB haplotypes and NF. These results exclude linkage to 15 map units on each side of the NGFB locus for the 12 families currently completed.

DISI AND NF

Harper and Saunders originally mapped the random phage probe DISI by *in situ* hybridization to chromosome 1p.[31] DISI RFLPs can be seen with both *Stu*1 and *Hin* DIII restriction endonucleases.[32] Goode, Ledbetter, and Daiger and Carritt, Welch, and Parry-Jones have recently described homologous DISI DNA fragments on both chromosomes 1 and 3.[33,34] Carritt, Welch, and Parry-Jones have mapped the *Stu*1 RFLPs to chromosome 1p.[34] The *Hin* DIII RFLP has been mapped to chromosome 3p by somatic cell hybridization by both Carritt and associates[34] and M. Goode (personal communication).

The lod scores between the DISI RFLPs and NF are indicated in TABLE 4. It can be seen that NF can be excluded from linkage to the *Stu*1 RFLP for 4-5 map units. The *Hin* DIII RFLP (on chromosome 3p) can apparently also be excluded from linkage to NF for 5 map units; however, some degree of individual family lod score variation is observed.

The average lod score for 11 informative families with the *Hin* DIII DISI RFLP is illustrated in FIGURE 5 where the vertical axis shows the lod score and the horizontal axis indicates the recombination fraction.

However, FIGURE 6 illustrates the plots for each of the 11 families individually. It can be seen here that 6 families show positive scores while 5 show negative scores.

TABLE 2. χ^2 Test of Linkage Equilibrium for *Taq* I and *Bgl* II Alleles

Taq I Allele	*Bgl* II Allele	Haplotypes		
		Ob	Ex	$(O-E)^2/E$
4.3	1.4	89	93.26	0.195
6.0	1.4	21	16.74	1.084
4.3	5.6	28	23.74	0.764
6.0	5.6	0	4.26	4.260
	Totals	138	138	$\chi^2 = 6.303$
				$df = 1$
				$p < 0.05$

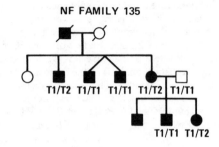

NF FAMILY 135

T1/T2 T1/T1 T1/T1 T1/T2 T1/T1

T1/T1 T1/T2

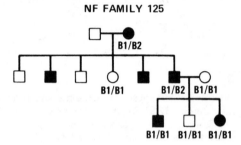

NF FAMILY 125

B1/B2

B1/B1   B1/B2 B1/B1

B1/B1 B1/B1 B1/B1

FIGURE 4. Pedigrees of two informative disseminated NF families. Key to NGFB alleles: B1 = *Bgl*II 1.4 kb; B2 = *Bgl*II 5.6 kb; T1 = *Taq*I 4.3 kb; T2 = *Taq*I 6 kb.

This is most likely due to statistical variance as the Morton test[35] for genetic heterogeneity fails to reach statistical significance. More families need to be tested to definitely exclude the DISI *Hin* *D*III RFLP.

NF AND GENE PRODUCT MARKERS

By combining our own gene product marker linkage analysis with NF[38] with previously published information,[28] we can strengthen the chromosome 1p negative linkage findings to date. TABLE 5 summates these findings.

It can be seen that NF is excluded from linkage with Rh to 18 map units, PGM$_1$ to 9 map units; and with Duffy to 27 map units.

TABLE 3. Lod Scores for Recombination Fractions between NGFB-Linked Restriction Fragment Length Polymorphism Haplotypes and Disseminated Neurofibromatosis

Marker	Families	Recombination Fraction							
		0.01	0.05	0.10	0.15	0.20	0.25	0.30	0.40
NF	12	−17.2	−8.4	−4.8	−2.0	−1.7	−1.0	−0.5	0

INTERMARKER DISTANCE

The intermarker distances between Rh and PGM_1 and Duffy have been compiled and estimated by McKusick.[36] By linkage analysis of NGFB and DISI *Stu*1 RFLPs with these existing gene product markers, we are able to provide further chromosome

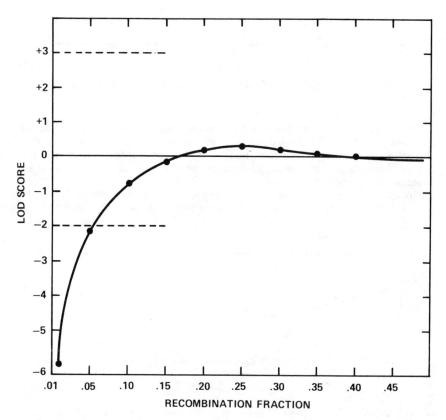

FIGURE 5. Graphic representation of total lod score for 11 informative NF-DISI *Hin* DIII families. (1) Lod score on vertical axis. (2) Recombination fraction on horizontal axis. (3) Significant positive lod score at +3.0 and negative score at −2.0.

lp mapping data. The *Stu*1 DISI RFLP was found to be greater than 3 map units distant from Rh, and other cytological and somatic cell hybridization[34] and related linkage data suggest it is more than 14-20 map units distal to Rh (Carritt, personal communication). NGFB was found to be proximal to PGM_1 by more than 16 map units and linked to Duffy at 17 map units.[37] FIGURE 7 illustrates the placement and approximate linkage relationships found for these five markers by using our RFLP linkage data.

TABLE 4. Lod Scores for Recombination Fractions between DISI-Linked Restriction Fragment Length Polymorphisms and Neurofibromatosis

Marker	Families	Recombination Fraction						
		0.01	0.05	0.10	0.15	0.20	0.30	0.40
NF and *Hin D*III	11	−6.1	−2.1	−0.73	−0.14	0.11	0.14	0.0
NF and *Stu*1	8	−3.8	−1.8	−1.1	−0.7	−0.5	−0.2	−0.1

NF AND CHROMOSOME 1p LINKAGE SUMMATION

By utilizing our intermarker distances and compiling this information with our own and published NF linkage data,[28] we can then compile a chromosome 1p map that suggests exclusion of NF from most of this region. FIGURE 8 illustrates our information to date. Gene product intermarker distances and centromere position are based on McKusick.[36]

In summary, approximately 123 centimorgans (cm) of chromosome 1p can be excluded from linkage to NF. While this preliminary evidence suggests there is no

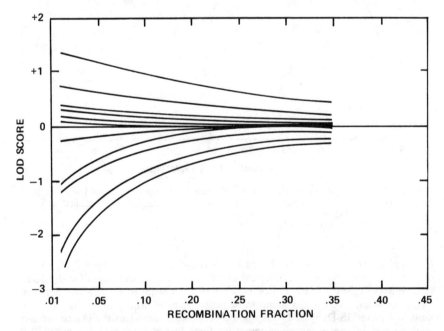

FIGURE 6. Graphic representation of 11 individual family lod scores informative for *Hin D*III DISI-NF linkage. (1) Lod score on vertical axis. (2) Recombination fraction on horizontal axis.

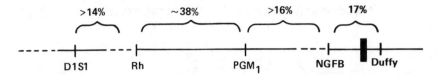

FIGURE 7. Approximate placement and known linkage relationships for five chromosome 1p markers: (1) > indicates greater than; (2) ~ indicates established approximate number (from Reference 36); (3) broken line scale indicates no linkage determined; (4) vertical box indicates centromere position (from Reference 36).

NF-chromosome 1p linkage, several caveats are evident: (1) potential linkage sites with NF still exist distal to DISI, between DISI and Rh, between Rh and PGM₁, and between PGM₁ and NGFB; (2) the *Hin* DIII DISI RFLP on chromosome 3p heterogeneity issue has not been definitively excluded. Further testing in more families is necessary to definitively clarify these two issues.

NEUROFIBROMA TUMOR DNA

The evidence presented excludes a primary role for the inheritance of the NGFB and DISI loci in NF. We are also interested in the somatic cell NGFB and DISI DNA gene structure in neurofibromas and related tumors to search for any secondary events that might occur. Three principal lines of evidence point to a need to evaluate the somatic cell DNA in these tumors:

1. Cytogenetic studies have indicated marked chromosomal aberrations in many malignant tumors and some of these tumors are associated with NF (V. Riccardi, personal communication).

TABLE 5. Lod Scores for Recombination Fractions between Three Chromosome 1p Gene Product Markers and Disseminated Neurofibromatosis

Linkage Markers	Data Source (reference no.)	Families	Recombination Fraction					
			0.01	0.05	0.10	0.20	0.30	0.40
NF-Rh	28	10	−9.7	−4.6	−2.4	−0.7	−0.1	0.0
	38	10		−3.5	−2.0	−0.7	−0.2	0.0
	Total	20		−8.1	−4.4	−1.4	−0.3	0.0
NF-PGM₁	28	11	−6.9	−3.3	−1.6	−0.3	0.2	0.2
	38	7		−0.7	−0.1	0.1	0.2	0.1
	Total	18		−4.0	−1.7	−0.2	0.4	0.3
NF-Duffy	28	10	−17.4	−10.5	−6.8	−3.2	−1.4	−0.4
	38	6		−1.6	−0.8	−0.2	−0.1	0.0
	Total	16		−12.1	−7.6	−3.4	−1.5	−0.4

INTERMARKER DISTANCES   NF LINKAGE EXCLUSIONS

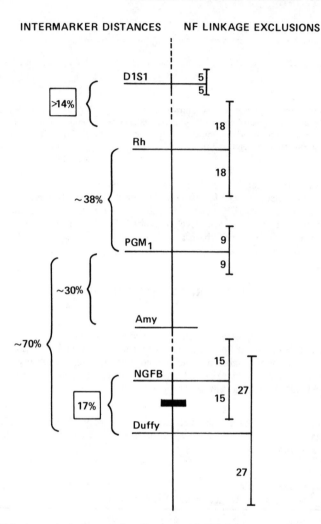

FIGURE 8. Approximate intermarker distances with NF linkage exclusions for five markers on chromosome 1p: (1) > indicates greater than; (2) ~ indicates approximated linkage (from Reference 36); (3) horizontal crossbar indicates centromere (Reference 36); (4) vertical brackets indicate NF exclusion by lod score of −2.0.

2. Somatic cell deletions and/or translocations have been described for retino-blastoma,[39] Wilm's tumor,[40] and chronic myelogenous leukemia.[41] In 1983, Francke *et al.* postulated that chromosome 1p breakage at the N-ras locus might alter β-NGF synthesis and its differentiation effect upon target cells thereby leading to a proliferative response via dedifferentiation.[16]

3. Tumors may exhibit an autocrine response[42] with alterations in growth factor production.

We have performed restriction analysis of NGFB and DISI in NF associated tumors to commence a general assessment of their gene structure.

In TABLE 6 are shown the results of probing of neurofibroma tissue DNA with the 7-kb and 4-kb NGFB subclones and the DISI phage clone.

These data indicate grossly normal DNA gene structure in NF neurofibromas. Further testing of more neurofibromas and associated tumors is indicated to discover if any gross gene structural alterations occur in associated malignant tumors.

FIGURE 9 illustrates two sample radiographs of the 7-kb NGFB subclone probed onto seven neurofibromas cut with MSPI, four neurofibromas cut with *Bgl*II, and two neurofibromas cut with *Taq*I. All signals appear equal to controls and compatible with restriction fragment maps in normals and sequencing data.

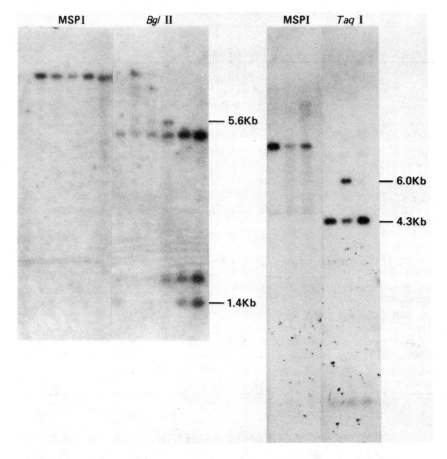

FIGURE 9. Two autoradiograms of nitrocellulose fibers after hybridization of the [32]p NGFB 7 kb subclone to MSP I, *Bgl*II and *Taq*I digestions of neurofibroma tumor DNA. (1) MSP I—lane 5 is control. (2) *Bgl*II—lanes 5 and 6 are controls. (3) *Taq*I—lane 2 is control. (4) Molecular lengths of hybridizing fragments are given in kb as judged both by log scale graphs and sequencing data.

CONCLUSION

We have illustrated a basic methodology for studying linkage between a chromosomal arm (1p) and a disease (NF). While we can exclude approximately 123 centimorgans of chromosome 1p from linkage to NF, the entire arm cannot be excluded. Further, the length of the arm is not known and cytological distances may not show direct relationship to recombination fractions.[37] Further testing to exclude any probability for NF heterogeneity and the DISI *Hin* DIII RFLP on chromosome 3p is required.

The Southern analysis of neurofibroma DNA with gene probes is another important approach. While we have preliminary evidence showing no gross NGFB locus alteration, this does not exclude an aberration of β-NGF synthesis. Northern blot analysis will be required to address this further question.

TABLE 6. DNA Probes of Neurofibroma Tumor DNA

Enzyme	Number of Solid Tumor Neurofibromas	Number of Neurofibroma Explant Cell Cultures	Number of NF Patients Normal Skin Culture	Assessment Fragment Sizes
NGFB—7 kb subclone				
Bgl II	6	3	2	Normal
Taq I	1	—	2	Normal
Eco RI	6	3	1	Normal
MSP I	4	3	2	Normal
Hinc II	5	2	—	Normal
Hin DIII	1	—	1	Normal
Hpa I	1	—	—	Normal
Sst I	2	—	—	Normal
Bam HI	2	2	—	Normal
Pst I	1	1	—	Normal
Kpn I	3	—	—	Normal
NGFB—4 kb subclone				
Eco RI	1	—	—	Normal
Hin DIII	2	—	1	Normal
Taq I	4	—	—	Normal
Bgl II	4	—	—	Normal
DISI probe				
Hin DIII	3	—	—	Normal
Bam HI	2	—	—	Normal

ACKNOWLEDGMENTS

We thank Ken Kidd, M.D., for filters and intermarker data analyses. We thank Mark Selby, Ph.D., and William Rutter, Ph.D., for the β-NGF mouse clone and Mary Harper, Ph.D., for the use of DISI. Finally, we gratefully acknowledge the families and the National Neurofibromatosis Foundation for their participation in this study.

REFERENCES

1. LEVI-MONTALCINI, R. & P. U. ANGELETTI. 1968. Nerve growth factor. Physiol. Rev. **48:** 534-569.
2. THOENEN, H. & Y. A. BARDE. 1980. Physiology of nerve growth factor. Physiol. Rev. **60:** 1284-1335
3. SUTTER, A., R. J. RIOPELLE, R. M. HARRIS-WARRICK & E. M. SHOOTER. 1979. Nerve growth factor receptors: characterization of two distinct classes of binding sites on chick embryo sensory ganglia cells. J. Biol. Chem. **254:** 1516-1523.
4. VARON, S., J. NOMURA & E. M. SHOOTER. 1967. The isolation of the mouse nerve growth factor protein in a high molecular weight form. Biochemistry **6:** 2202-2209.
5. SERVER, A. C. & E. M. SHOOTER. 1977. Nerve growth factor. Adv. Prot. Chem. **31:** 339-409.
6. HEUMANN, R., S. KORSCHING, J. SCOTT & H. THOENEN. 1984. Relationship between levels of nerve growth factor (NGF) and its messenger RNA in sympathetic ganglia and peripheral target tissues. EMBO J. **3**(13): 3183-3189.
7. SHELTON, D. L. & L. F. REICHARDT. 1984. Expression of the β-nerve growth factor gene correlates with the density of sympathetic innervation in effector organs. Proc. Nat. Acad. Sci. USA **81:** 7951-7955.
8. PEARSON, J., F. B. ALEXROD & J. DANCIS. 1974. Current concepts of dysautonomia: neuropathological defects. Ann. N.Y. Acad. Sci. **228:** 288-300.
9. SIGGERS, D. C., J. G. ROGERS, S. H. BOYER, *et al.* 1976. Increased nerve growth factor chain cross reacting material in familial dysautonomia. N. Engl. J. Med. **295:** 629-634.
10. GORIN, P. D. & E. M. JOHNSON, JR. 1980. Effects of exposure to nerve growth factor antibodies on the developing nervous system of the rat: an experimental autoimmune approach. Dev. Biol. **80:** 313-323.
11. SCHWARTZ, J. P. & X. O. BREAKEFIELD. 1980. Altered nerve growth factor in fibroblasts from patients with familial dysautonomia. Proc. Nat. Acad. Sci. USA **77:** 1154-1158.
12. SCHENKEIN, I., E. D. BUEKER, L. HELSON, F. AXELROD & J. DANCIS. 1974. Increased nerve growth factor stimulating activity in disseminated neurofibromatosis. N. Engl. J. Med. **290:** 613-614.
13. SIGGERS, D. C., S. M. BOYER & R. ELDRIDGE. 1975. Nerve growth factor in disseminated neurofibromatosis. N. Engl. J. Med. **292:** 1134.
14. FABRICANT, R. N. & G. J. TODARO. 1981. Increased serum levels of nerve growth factor in von Recklinghausen's disease. Arch. Neurol. **38:** 401-405.
15. DESCHRYVER-KECSKEMETI, D., R. E. CLOUSE, M. N. GOLDSTEIN, D. GARSELL & L. O'NEAL. 1983. Intestinal ganglioneuromatosis. A manifestation of overproduction of nerve growth factor? N. Eng. J. Med. **308:** 635-639.
16. FRANCKE, U., L. COUSSENS & A. ULLRICH. 1983. The human gene for the β subunit of nerve growth factor is located on the proximal short arm of chromosome 1. Science **222:** 1248-1250.
17. SCOTT, J., M. SELBY, M. URDEA, M. QUIROGA, G. BELL & W. J. RUTTER. 1983. Isolation and nucleotide sequence of a cDNA encoding the precursor of mouse nerve growth factor. Nature **302:** 538-540.
18. ULLRICH, A., A. GRAY, C. BERMAN & T. J. DULL. 1983. Human β nerve growth factor gene sequence highly homologous to that of mouse. Nature **303:** 821-825.
19. BREAKEFIELD, X. O., G. ORLOFF, C. M. CASTIGLIONE, F. B. AXELROD, L. COUSSENS & A. ULLRICH. 1983. Genetic linkage analysis in familial dysautonomia using a DNA probe for the β nerve growth factor gene. *In* Biochemical and Clinical Aspects of Neuropeptides: Synthesis, Processing, and Gene Structure. G. Koch & D. Richter, Eds. Academic Press. New York, N.Y.

20. ZABEL, B. U., R. L. EDDY, J. SCOTT & T. B. SHOWS. 1983. The human nerve growth factor gene (β-NGF) is located on the short arm of chromosome 1. Abstract Gene Mapping Workshop. University of California. Los Angeles, Calif.

21. MARTINVILLE, B., M. J. CUNNINGHAM, M. J. MURRAY & U. FRANCKE. 1983. The N-ras oncogene assigned to chromosome 1 (p31 - cen) by somatic cell hybrid analysis. Abstract. Human Gene Mapping Conference. University of California. Los Angeles, Calif.

22. DAVIS, M., S. MALCOLM & A. HALL. 1983. The N-ras oncogene is located on the short arm of chromosome 1. Abstract. Gene Mapping Workshop. University of California. Los Angeles, Calif.

23. DARBY, J. K., J. FEDER, M. SELBY, V. RICCARDI, R. FERRELL, D. SIAO, K. GOSLIN, W. RUTTER, E. M. SHOOTER & L. L. CAVALLI-SFORZA. 1985. A discordant sibship analysis between β-NGF and neurofibromatosis. Am. J. Hum. Genet. 37: 52-59.

24. STEFFEN, D. & R. A. WEINBERG. 1978. The integrated genome of murine leukemia virus. Cell 15: 1003-1010.

25. SOUTHERN, E. M. 1975. Detection of specific sequences among DNA fragments separated by gel electrophoresis. J. Mol. Biol. 98: 503-517.

26. RIGBY, P. W. J., M. DIECKMANN, C. RHODES & P. BERG. 1977. Labeling deoxyribonucleic acid to high specific activity in vitro by nick translation with DNA polymerase 1. J. Mol. Biol. 113: 237-251.

27. RICCARDI, V. M. 1981. von Recklinghausen neurofibromatosis. N. Engl. J. Med. 305(27): 1617-1626.

28. SPENCE, M. A., J. L. BADER, D. M. PARRY, et al. 1983. Linkage analysis of neurofibromatosis. J. Med. Genet. 20: 334-337.

29. MORTON, N. E. 1955. Sequential tests for the detection of linkage. Am. J. Hum. Genet. 7: 277-318.

30. OTT, J. 1974. Estimation of the recombination fraction in human pedigrees; efficient computation of the likelihood for human linkage studies. Am. J. Hum. Genet. 26: 588-597.

31. HARPER, M. E. & G. F. SAUNDERS. 1981. Localization of single copy DNA sequences on G banded chromosomes by in situ hybridization. Chromosoma Berlin 83: 431-439.

32. GOODE, M. E. & S. P. DAIGER. 1983. Restriction fragment length polymorphisms detected by λH3. Genetics 104: 530.

33. GOODE, M. E., D. H. LEDBETTER & S. P. DAIGER. 1984. Failure of in situ hybridization to detect the primary copy of λH3. (Abstr. 406) Am. J. Hum. Genet. 36: 138S.

34. CARRITT, B., H. M. WELCH & N. J. PARRY-JONES. 1986. Sequences homologous to the human DISI locus present on chromosome 3. Am. J. Hum. Genet. 38: 428-436.

35. MORTON, N. E. 1956. The detection and estimation of linkage between the genes for elliptocytosis and the Rh blood group. Am. J. Hum. Genet. 8: 80-96.

36. McKUSICK, V. A. 1983. Mendelian Inheritance in Man. Johns Hopkins University Press. Baltimore, Md.

37. DARBY, J. K., J. R. KIDD, A. J. PAKSTIS, R. S. SPARKES, H. M. CANN, R. E. FERRELL, D. G. GERHARD, V. RICCARDI, J. A. EGELAND, E. M. SHOOTER, L. L. CAVALLI-SFORZA & K. K. KIDD. 1985. Linkage relationships of the gene for the β subunit of nerve growth factor (NGFB) with other chromosome 1 marker loci. J. Cytogenet. Cell Genet. 39: 158-160.

38. DUNN, B. G., R. FERRELL & V. RICCARDI. 1985. A genetic linkage study in 15 families with von Recklinghausens neurofibromatosis. Am. J. Med. Genet. 22: 403-407.

39. CAVENEE, W. K., T. P. DRYJA, R. A. PHILLIPS, W. F. BENEDICT, R. GODBOUT, B. L. GALIE, A. L. MURPHREE, L. C. STRONG & R. L. WHITE. 1983. Expression of recessive alleles by chromosomal mechanisms in retinoblastoma. Nature 305: 779-784.

40. KOUFOS, A., M. F. HANSEN, B. C. LAMPKIN, M. L. WORKMAN, N. G. COPELAND, N. A. JENKINS & W. K. CAVENEE. 1984. Loss of alleles at loci on human chromosome 11 during genesis of Wilm's tumor. Nature 309: 170-172.

41. LEDER, P., J. BATTERY, G. LENOIR, G. MOULDING, W. MURPHY, H. POTTER, T. STEWART & R. TAUB. 1983. Translocations among antibody genes in human cancer. Science 222: 765-771.

42. SPORN, M. B. & A. B. ROBERTS. 1985. Autocrine growth factors and cancer. Nature 313: 745-747.

Oncogene Expression in Neurofibromatosis[a]

PETER T. ROWLEY,[b,c] BARBARA KOSCIOLEK,[b]
AND JUDITH L. BADER[d]

[b]Division of Genetics
[c]Department of Medicine
University of Rochester School of Medicine
601 Elmwood Avenue
Rochester, New York 14642

[d]Radiation Oncology Branch
National Cancer Institute
Building 10, Room B3B69
Bethesda, Maryland 20892

INTRODUCTION

Oncogenes are a class of structural genes hypothesized to have a causal role in neoplasia.[1] The more than 20 oncogenes now known have been recognized in one of two ways. The first is their recognition in the genome of RNA tumor viruses (retroviruses) where they have been shown to account for transforming activity by analysis of mutants. The second is their recognition in tumor cell DNA; DNA of certain tumors transforms test cells by transfection.

Viral oncogenes are thought to have arisen from cellular oncogenes. Cellular oncogenes exist in normal cells as protooncogenes. Their physiological role is poorly understood, but regulation of cellular differentiation, possibly in a tissue-specific manner, has been proposed. In many tumor cell lines, the malignant phenotype is associated with either a mutation in a protooncogene or its hyperexpression secondary to some other genetic change. In fresh tumor tissue, the same types of changes can be found, but data are more limited.

Carcinogenesis is commonly said to involve multiple steps.[2] Dominantly inherited syndromes predisposing to neoplasia constitute an important resource for study because individuals at high risk for malignancies of specific types are identifiable years in advance. Furthermore, the sequence of mutations leading to malignancy may be identifiable by a comparison of malignant tissue, unaffected tissue from the same individual, and tissue from control individuals. Of inherited syndromes predisposing to neoplasia, neurofibromatosis is the most suitable for analysis because it is dominant, common, and involves multiple tumors of multiple types at accessible sites.[3]

[a]This research was supported by the National Neurofibromatosis Foundation.

327

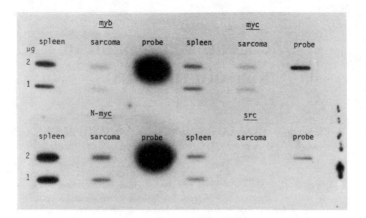

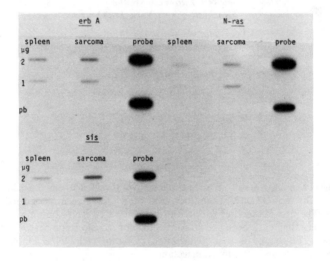

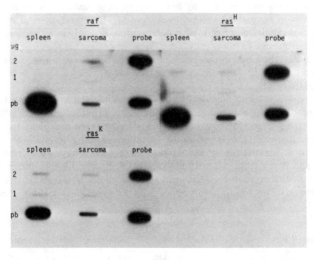

METHODS

Tissues were frozen immediately upon removal from the subject. After tissue disruption by a Polytron homogenizer (Kinematica, Luzern, Switzerland), total RNA was purified by precipitation from guanidine isothiocyanate and from guanidine hydrochloride.[4] Residual protein was removed by proteinase K digestion followed by phenol extraction and ethanol precipitation. Poly A$^+$ RNA was purified by oligo(dT)-cellulose chromatography.[5] Plasmids containing a specific oncogene were grown up in bacteria and radioactively labeled by nick translation using ^{32}P-deoxycytidine triphosphate (dCTP) to a specific activity of 1-8 $\times$ 10^8 cpm/μg.[6] Oncogene transcripts were analyzed by slot blots using a GeneScreen membrane (New England Nuclear, Boston, Mass.) and a manifold II (Schleicher and Schuell, Keene, N.H.). Autoradiograms were quantitated using a Kipp and Zonen BD40 densitometer.

We wish to thank the following individuals for specific oncogene probes: S. Aaronson (v-*abl*, v-*mos*, and v-*sis*), J. Bishop (v-*erb*A, v-*erb*B, v-*myb*, v-*myc*, v-*src*), G. Cooper (c-B*lym*), P. Balduzzi (v-*ros*), N. Kohl (N-*myc*), K. Robbins (v-*fgr*), C. Sherr (v-*fes*/*fps*), U. Rapp (v-*raf*), I. Verma (v-*fos*), R. Weinberg (N-*ras*, v-*ras*^{Harvey}, v-*ras*^{Kirsten}), and M. Yoshida (v-*yes*).

RESULTS

Oncogene transcripts from a neurofibrosarcoma and from control (spleen) tissue from a patient with hereditary neurofibromatosis (NF) were quantitated by slot blot analysis. The radiograms of some of these are shown in FIGURE 1. Relative intensities were quantitated by densitometry and the results are shown in TABLE 1. In the malignant compared to the control tissue, *sis* and N-*ras* were moderately hyperexpressed (over 3$\times$). *Raf*, *Blym*, and *erb*A were slightly hyperexpressed (1.5-2$\times$). *Abl*, *erb*B, *fes*/*fps*, *fgr*, *fos*, *mos*, *myb*, *myc*, N-*myc*, *ras*^{Harvey}, *ras*^{Kirsten}, *ros*, *src*, and *yes* were not hyperexpressed.

DISCUSSION

Since a survey has been completed on only one patient, no conclusion is warranted about neurofibrosarcoma in neurofibromatosis in general. However, the oncogenes found most expressed in this tumor are of special interest in relation to this hereditary predisposition to neural tumors.

FIGURE 1. Slot blots of poly A$^+$ RNA from neurofibrosarcoma and from spleen from a patient with hereditary neurofibromatosis. Poly A$^+$ RNA (2 and 1 μg) was applied to GeneScreen. Hybridization was done with 1 $\times$ 10^7 cpm of each oncogene probe labeled with ^{32}P-dCTP to a specific activity of 1-8 $\times$ 10^8 cpm/μg by nick translation in 5 ml 10% dextran sulfate-50% formamide-5$\times$SSC (SSC = 0.15 M NaCl-0.015 M Na citrate, pH 7.0) at 42° for 36 hours. Washing was done in 0.1$\times$ SSC at 50°C. Autoradiography was performed using Kodak SL1 film and intensifying screens for 27 hours.

Sis is the transforming gene of simian sarcoma virus,[7] the only known acute transforming virus of primate origin. *Sis* is expressed as a 4.2 kb transcript in highest amounts in the human glioblastoma cell line A172 and slightly less in different cell lines derived from fibrosarcomas and osteosarcomas.[8,9] The product of the *sis* oncogene is the protein p28^{sis}.[7] This protein is closely related in its predicted amino acid sequence and structural properties to a polypeptide of platelet-derived growth factor (PDGF) or its precursor.[10–16] PDGF is thought to be synthesized by megakaryocytes, stored and transported by platelets, released at the site of endothelial injury, and to have a role in repair. PDGF is the most potent mitogen in the serum for cells of mesenchymal origin[17,18] and has been shown to have a growth-promoting effect on human glial cells in culture.[19] Normally located on chromosome 22, the gene is translocated in chronic

TABLE 1. Expression of Oncogenes in NF Neurofibrosarcoma[a]

	Oncogene	Hybridizable poly A$^+$ RNA (neurofibrosarcoma/control)
Moderately hyperexpressed:	*sis*	3.22 ± 0.42[b]
	N-*ras*	3.01 ± 0.57
Slightly hyperexpressed:	*raf*	2.03 ± 0.78
	Blym	1.76 ± 0.15
	*erb*A	1.46 ± 0.06
Not hyperexpressed:	Ha-*ras*	0.83 ± 0.01
	Ki-*ras*	0.53 ± 0.01
	fos	0.42 ± 0.01
	fes/fps	0.34 ± 0.01
	myc	0.31 ± 0.04
	yes	0.27 ± 0.03
	ros	0.26 ± 0.02
	mos	0.23 ± 0.03
	N-*myc*	0.22 ± 0.02
	myb	0.14 ± 0.01
	*erb*B	0.10 ± 0.04
	fgr	0.07 ± 0.01
	src	0.06 ± 0.01

[a] Autoradiograms were quantitated by an integrating densitometer. For other experimental details, see FIGURE 1 legend.
[b] Mean ± standard error.

myelogenous leukemia. Thus, it is of some interest that a gene we have found hyperexpressed in an NF neurofibrosarcoma is already known to be characteristically expressed in gliomas, sarcomas, and to be translocated in chronic myelogenous leukemia, all conditions occurring with increased frequency in neurofibromatosis.

N-*ras* is the transforming gene of several human malignant cell lines, including neuroblastoma,[20] sarcoma,[21,22] fibrosarcoma,[21] rhabdomyosarcoma,[23] teratocarcinoma,[24] acute promyelocytic leukemia,[22] and of some primary hematopoietic tumors.[25] The gene is homologous to *ras*^{Harvey} and *ras*^{Kirsten}, but no corresponding retrovirus has been discovered. The gene is located on chromosome 1.[21,26,27] In tumors, the gene contains nucleotide substitutions,[23,24] but is not amplified or rearranged.[21] Its 2.2 kb transcript is present in increased amount in some cases.[21] Since N-*ras* appears to cause malignancy by structural changes, rather than simply by hyperexpression, the significance of hyperexpression in the present NF tumor is not obvious.

To pursue the significance of these initial findings, we are analyzing the DNA from this patient and examining neoplasms from additional neurofibromatosis patients.

SUMMARY

To investigate the role of oncogenes in malignancies characteristic of neurofibromatosis, oncogene transcripts were quantitated in a neurofibrosarcoma and in control tissue from a patient with hereditary neurofibromatosis. *Sis* and N-*ras* were moderately hyperexpressed, *raf*, B*lym*, and *erb*A were slightly hyperexpressed, and *abl*, *erb*B, *fes/fps*, *fgr*, *fos*, *mos*, *myb*, *myc*, N-*myc*, *ras*[Harvey], *ras*[Kirsten], *ros*, *src*, and *yes* were not hyperexpressed in the tumor compared to the control tissue. Although additional tumors will be assayed before conclusions are possible, it may be significant that the two oncogenes most hyperexpressed are prior suspects for a pathogenetic role in tumors of the nervous system.

ACKNOWLEDGMENTS

We express our gratitude to Dr. Arjang Miremadi of the National Naval Medical Center for assisting with tissue procurement from a patient with neurofibromatosis and neurofibrosarcoma. We thank Dr. Allan Rubenstein for tissue solicitation.

REFERENCES

1. BISHOP, J. M. 1983. Annu. Rev. Biochem. **52:** 301-354.
2. BODMER, W. F. 1982. Cancer Surveys **1:** 1-15.
3. RICCARDI, V. M. & J. J. MULVIHILL, Eds. 1981. Neurofibromatosis (von Recklinghausen Disease). Raven Press. New York, N.Y. (Adv. Neurol. **29.**)
4. CHIRGWIN, J. M., A. E. PRZYBYLA, R. J. MACDONALD & W. J. RUTTER. 1979. Biochem. **18:** 5294-5299.
5. AVIV, H. & P. LEDER. 1972. Proc. Nat. Acad. Sci. USA **69:** 1408-1412.
6. RIGBY, P. W. J., M. DIECKMANN, C. RHODES & P. BERG. 1977. J. Mol. Biol. **113:** 237-251.
7. ROBBINS, K. C., S. G. DEVARE, E. P. REDDY & S. A. AARONSON. 1982. Science **218:** 1131-1133.
8. WOLFE, L. G., F. DEINHARDT, G. H. THEILEN, H. RABIN, T. KAWAKAMI & L. K. BUSTAD. 1971. J. Nat. Cancer Inst. **47:** 1115-1120.
9. EVA, A., K. C. ROBBINS, P. R. ANDERSEN, S. ALAGARSAMY, S. R. TRONICK, E. P. REDDY, N. W. ELLMORE, A. T. GALEN, J. A. LAUTENBERGER, T. S. PAPAS, E. H. WESTIN, F. WONG-STAAL, R. C. GALLO & S. A. AARONSON. 1982. Nature **295:** 116-119.
10. DEVARE, S. G., E. P. REDDY, J. D. LAW, K. C. ROBBINS & S. A. AARONSON. 1983. Proc. Nat. Acad. Sci. USA **80:** 731-735.
11. ANTONIADES, H. N. & L. T. WILLIAMS. 1983. Fed. Proc. **42:** 2630-2634.

12. DOOLITTLE, R. F., M. W. HUNKAPILLER, L. E. HOOD, S. G. DEVARE, K. C. ROBBINS & S. A. AARONSON. 1983. Science 221: 275-276.
13. WATERFIELD, M. D., G. T. SCRACE, N. WHITTLE, P. STROOBANT, A. JOHNSSON, A. WASTESON, B. WESTERMARK, C.-H. HELDIN, J. S. HUANG & T. F. DEUEL. 1983. Nature 304: 35-39.
14. JOHNSSON, A., C. H. HELDIN, A. WASTESON, B. WESTERMARK, T. F. DEUEL, J. S. HUANG, P. H. SEEBURG, A. GRAY, A. ULLRICH, G. SCRACE, P. STROOBANT & M. D. WATERFIELD. 1984. EMBO J. 3: 921-928.
15. JOSEPHS, S. F., L. RATNER, M. F. CLARKE, E. H. WESTIN, M. S. REITZ & F. WONG-STAAL. 1984. Science 225: 636-639.
16. DEUEL, T. F. & J. J. HUANG. 1984. Blood 65: 951-958.
17. ROSS, R. & A. VOGEL. 1978. Cell 14: 203-210.
18. SCHERR, C. D., R. C. SHEPARD, H. N. ANTONIADES & C. D. STILES. 1979. Biochim. Biophys. Acta 560: 217-241.
19. WESTERMARK, B. & A. WASTESON. 1975. Adv. Metab. Disorders 8: 85-100.
20. SHIMIZU, K., M. GOLDFARB, Y. SUARD, M. PERUCHO, Y. LI, T. KAMATA & J. FERAMISCO. 1983. Proc. Nat. Acad. Sci. USA 80: 2112-2116.
21. HALL, A., C. J. MARSHALL, N. K. SPURR & R. A. WEISS. 1983. Nature 303: 396-400.
22. MURRAY, M. J., J. M. CUNNINGHAM, L. F. PARADA, F. DAUTRY, P. LEBOWITZ & R. A. WEINBERG. 1983. Cell 33: 749-757.
23. BOS, J. L., M. VERLAAN-DE VRIES, A. M. JANSEN, G. H. VEENEMAN, J. H. VAN BOOM & A. J. VAN DER EB. 1984. Nucleic Acids Res. 12: 9155-9163.
24. TAINSKY, M. A., C. S. COOPER, B. C. GIOVANELLA, E. STAVNEZER, J. FOGH, M. H. WIGLER & G. F. VANDE WOUDE. 1984. Science 225: 643-645.
25. EVA, A., S. R. TRONICK, R. A. GOL, J. H. PIERCE & S. A. AARONSON. 1983. Proc. Nat. Acad. Sci. USA 80: 4926-4930.
26. RYAN, J., C. P. HART & F. H. RUDDLE. 1984. Nucleic Acids Res. 12: 6063-6072.
27. RABIN, M., M. WATSON, P. E. BARKER, J. RYAN, W. R. BREG & F. H. RUDDLE. 1984. Cytogenet. Cell Genet. 38: 70-72.

DNA Transfection Analysis of the Tumors of Neurofibromatosis

LEE B. JACOBY AND ROBERT L. MARTUZA

Department of Surgery
Harvard Medical School
and Neurosurgical Service
Massachusetts General Hospital
Boston, Massachusetts 02114

Neurofibromatosis (NF) is a relatively common autosomal dominant disorder affecting the nervous system by causing dysplasia of various cells of neural crest origin. Although recognized for more than two centuries, the biochemical or genetic basis of this disease has not been defined nor has any major advance in treatment been developed. From the geneticist's point of view, the most pressing problems in NF research are to find the gene or genes responsible for NF, to learn how these genes cause the tumors of NF, and ultimately to learn how these genes can be controlled. Although the NF gene(s) is present within all cells of a patient's body, it is primarily expressed in two cells of neural crest origin: Schwann cells and melanocytes. While fibroblasts form a component of neurofibromas, fibroblasts are only involved when associated with other involved neural crest cells and are otherwise unaffected in skin or connective tissue. Thus it would be worthwhile to study the gene(s) of NF within a cell that normally expresses this gene, and for these studies, we have chosen the Schwann cell because Schwann cell tumors constitute the most serious neurologic problem in NF and because Schwann cell culture conditions have been studied in detail.

Our overall objective is to use DNA transfection analysis to try to detect the genes responsible for NF and for the tumors associated with NF including neurofibromas, neurofibrosarcomas, and acoustic neuromas. DNA will be extracted from tumor cells and introduced into normal Schwann cells and fibroblasts growing in culture. Foci of morphologically transformed cells will be identified and grown, and their DNA sequences will be isolated and characterized because these sequences are likely to be important in the tumors of NF.

Our first goal has been to optimize the conditions for efficient DNA absorption, integration, and expression in human and rodent Schwann cells and fibroblasts. For these experiments we have used pSV2gpt and pSV2neo, two hybrid plasmids constructed by Berg and his colleagues that contain the bacterial xanthine-guanine phosphoribosyltransferase gene (*gpt*) or neomycin resistance gene (*neo*) adjacent to SV40 promoter and termination signals.[1,2] When these plasmid DNAs were introduced into mouse NIH 3T3 fibroblasts using the calcium phosphate precipitation technique described by Wigler *et al.*,[2] transformants arose at frequencies of about 1-2×10^{-4} (TABLE 1).

Introducing the same pSV2gpt or pSV2neo DNAs into rat Schwann cells has proven more difficult. Schwann cells were cultured from rat sciatic nerve according to techniques modified from Brockes *et al.*[4] Neonatal rat sciatic nerves were removed and digested with 0.25% trypsin and 0.03% collagenase. The cells were plated in

333

TABLE 1. DNA Transfer into Mouse NIH 3T3 Fibroblasts[a]

Plasmid DNA	Total Colonies	Colonies per 10^6 Cells per μg DNA
0	0	< 0.25
pSV2gpt	692	173
0	0	< 0.25
pSV2neo	476	119

[a] Two micrograms plasmid DNA and 18 μg salmon sperm carrier DNA were precipitated with calcium phosphate and added to 10^6 3T3 cells in replicate 100 mm petri dishes. After six hours, cells were exposed to 15% glycerol for three minutes and then refed with complete medium. Two days later, gpt^+ transfectants were selected in HATMAX medium containing 15 μg/ml hypoxanthine, 4 μg/ml amethopterin, 10 μg/ml thymidine, 25 μg/ml mycophenolic acid, 25 μg/ml adenine, and 250 μg/ml xanthine and neo^+ transfectants were selected in medium containing 800 μg/ml of G418 (GIBCO). Colonies were counted after Giemsa staining about 12 days later. The frequency of transfection was corrected for one population doubling which occurred between DNA treatment and time of selection.

Dulbecco's medium and treated with 10^{-5} M cytosine arabinoside to kill the dividing fibroblasts. A few days later they were treated in suspension with monoclonal anti-mouse Thy1.1 plus rabbit complement and this treatment was repeated as necessary to remove any residual fibroblasts. The remaining cells were plated in Dulbecco's medium supplemented with partially purified glial growth factor, shown by Brockes and co-workers to be an effective mitogen for Schwann cells.[5,6] Plasmid DNAs were introduced into rat Schwann cells on several occasions by the calcium phosphate technique. No stable transfectants were observed for either the gpt or neo genes among 2-6 $\times$ 10^7 cells treated (TABLE 2). This result was disappointing but not altogether unexpected since primary or early passage cultures are generally difficult to transfect and the optimal conditions for Schwann cell transfection have not yet been defined.

To confirm that foreign DNA enters rat Schwann cells we introduced by transfection pBAG, a plasmid DNA that contains the bacterial beta-galactosidase and neomycin resistance genes under the control of mammalian promoters (Cepko, personal communication). Three days later we measured the transient expression of beta-galactosidase and selected for stable transfectants resistant to the neomycin analogue G418. Beta-galactosidase activity was detected in treated Schwann cells at levels comparable to those measured in NIH 3T3 cells (TABLE 3). No stable G418-resistant transfectants, however, were isolated from replicate Schwann cell cultures (data not

TABLE 2. DNA Transfer into Rat Schwann Cells[a]

DNA	Number of Colonies	Number of Cells Screened
pSV2gpt	0	2.6 $\times$ 10^7
pSV2neo	0	5.7 $\times$ 10^7

[a] Transfections were performed as described in TABLE 1 except that 2-5 $\times$ 10^6 Schwann cells were treated with 2-4 μg plasmid DNA and 20-40 μg carrier DNA in 75 cm^2 flasks. Cells were replated in selective medium 2-3 days later and refed twice weekly for 4-6 weeks, at which time they were stained with Giemsa.

TABLE 3. Transient Expression of Beta-Galactosidase following DNA Transfer[a]

Cells	DNA	Beta-galactosidase (units/mg protein)
NIH 3T3	pBAG	1.5
Rat Schwann	pBAG	3.1

[a] Transfections were performed as described in TABLES 1 and 2. Beta-galactosidase activity was measured 72 hours later in duplicate cultures as described by Norton and Coffin.[7] One unit equals 1 nmol substrate hydrolyzed per minute at 37°C.

shown). Thus it appears that foreign DNA enters Schwann cells but either is not integrated into the Schwann cell DNA or is not efficiently expressed, possibly because the Schwann cells are dividing slowly under our culture conditions.

Ultimately the gene transfer frequency into Schwann cells must be high enough to allow us to screen genomic DNAs. We plan to continue to optimize conditions for transfer of DNA into primary Schwann cells. For certain experiments, we shall use primed Schwann cells, that is, cells that have been made more receptive to the uptake and expression of foreign DNA, for example, cells that have lost some normal growth control due to the introduction of an oncogene or SV40 genome. Should it prove impossible or inefficient to transfect primary Schwann cells it may be necessary to use fibroblasts as recipients when screening genomic DNAs and to use Schwann cells exclusively as recipients for cloned genes. We hope that such techniques will not only allow isolation of the NF gene(s) but also provide a cell culture system in which to study the expression of the NF gene. Additionally, studies defining the optimal conditions necessary for Schwann cell transfection will also allow research into the control mechanisms of the Schwann cells in the normal state and in other disease states.

REFERENCES

1. MULLIGAN, R. C. & P. BERG. 1980. Science **209:** 1422-1427.
2. SOUTHERN, P. J. & P. BERG. 1982. J. Mol. Appl. Genet. **1:** 327-341.
3. WIGLER, M., S. SILVERSTEIN, L.-S. LEE, A. PELLICER, Y. CHENG & R. AXEL. 1977. Cell **11:** 223-232.
4. BROCKES, J. P., K. L. FIELDS & M. C. RAFF. 1979. Brain Res. **165:** 105-118.
5. BROCKES, J. P., G. E. LEMKE & D. R. BALZER, JR. 1980. J. Biol. Chem. **255:** 8374-8377.
6. LEMKE, G. E. & J. P. BROCKES. 1984. J. Neurosci. **4:** 75-83.
7. NORTON, P. A. & J. M. COFFIN. Mol. Cell. Biol. **5:** 281-290.

Sensitivity of Cultured Skin Fibroblasts from Patients with Neurofibromatosis to DNA-Damaging Agents[a]

WILLIAM G. WOODS, BRUCE McKENZIE,
MARY A. LETOURNEAU, AND
TIMOTHY D. BYRNE

Department of Pediatrics
Box 454 Mayo Building
University of Minnesota
420 Delaware Street S.E.
Minneapolis, Minnesota 55455

INTRODUCTION

Neurofibromatosis (NF) is an autosomal dominant disease associated with constitutional abnormalities in organs of neuroectodermal origin as well as with a striking predisposition for malignancy.[1,2] Although classically defined as "neurocristopathy,"[3] NF may not be limited to cells of neural crest origin, based on the patterns of cancer in this disease. For example, there appears to be an increased incidence of leukemia,[4] rhabdomyosarcoma,[5] and Wilms' tumor[6] in children with neurofibromatosis.

Little is known about the *in vitro* characteristics of cultured cells from individuals with neurofibromatosis. Several investigators have examined the growth and morphology of NF skin fibroblasts in tissue culture. Krone and colleagues showed that the doubling time of NF cells in early passage (less than 10) is faster than that of normal fibroblasts.[7] However, Zelkowitz and Stambouly found that NF fibroblasts grew slower and incorporated ^{3}H-thymidine at a lower rate than normal skin cells did when grown in Dulbecco's modified Eagle's medium.[8] NF cells were larger, more pleomorphic, and appeared to be more contact inhibitable in that they stopped growing at a lower population density than normal cells.[8] NF cells also appeared to bind epidermal growth factor less than normal cells did, possibly explaining why fibroblasts from these individuals were not normally stimulated after exposure to epidermal growth factor.[9] These studies suggest that there may be an underlying abnormality of growth regulation in NF cells not originating in the neural crest. Whether NF fibroblasts actually exhibit *in vitro* premature senescence as hinted in studies by Zelkowitz and Stambouly[8] is unknown.

[a] Supported in part by Grant EY04612 from the U.S. National Eye Institute (WGW) and by a grant from the National Neurofibromatosis Foundation, Inc. (WGW).

Individuals with NF appear to have an increased incidence of radiation-induced neoplasia, especially neurofibrosarcoma.[6,10] Other genetic disorders have been described in man that are associated with a predisposition to cancer and *in vivo* sensitivity to known DNA-damaging agents.[11] *In vitro* cultured cells from individuals with these disorders exhibit a chromosomal and/or cellular sensitivity to the DNA-damaging agent which is suspected to lead to *in vivo* malignant transformation, and may exhibit biochemical evidence of defective DNA repair.[11] Among the best examples of these diseases is xeroderma pigmentosum, which is associated with skin cancer, increased *in vitro* cytotoxicity after ultraviolet light exposure, and a cellular inability to repair ultraviolet light-induced DNA pyrimidine dimers.[12]

We have hypothesized that neurofibromatosis involves a global defect rather than one limited to the neural crest. Furthermore, this defect may manifest itself as a cellular sensitivity, as measured by cytotoxicity, to DNA-damaging agents, thus predisposing NF individuals to primary and secondary neoplasia. Studies were performed on cultured skin fibroblast cell strains from three individuals with NF to examine the sensitivity of these cells to different types of DNA damage at various *in vitro* ages, or passage numbers. The results suggest that cultured NF fibroblast cell strains exhibit early *in vitro* senescence which sometimes is associated with an inability to handle certain DNA-damaging agents.

METHODS

Fibroblast Cell Strains and Cell Maintenance in Tissue Culture

Nontransformed human fibroblasts from patients with neurofibromatosis were obtained as follows. Strain GM0622, originally derived from an 8-year-old male, was obtained in passage 6 from the NIGMS Human Genetic Mutant Cell Repository, Camden, New Jersey. GM1639, originally derived from a 19-year-old female, was also obtained from the Human Genetic Mutant Cell Repository in passage 6. SB23, derived from an 8-year-old male who developed a neurofibrosarcoma, was initiated in primary tissue culture by this laboratory using techniques previously described.[13] In addition, nine normal nontransformed human fibroblast cell strains initiated in this laboratory were used as controls. All fibroblasts were maintained in Dulbecco's modified Eagle's medium (MEM) with 10% fetal calf serum, L-glutamine, sodium pyruvate, 100 IU/ml penicillin, 100 mg/ml streptomycin, 10 mcg/ml gentamicin, and 2.5 mcg/ml amphotericin. Both normal and NF cell strains were split 1:3 every 7-14 days, with each split considered a passage and all studies performed between passages 3-18. As growth rates declined with increasing passage number in NF strains, plates were eventually split every 20-40 days. Studies were performed at various passages as described below.

Fibroblast cell strains were tested periodically for presence of *Mycoplasma* using a fluorescent microscopic technique with Hoescht stain 33258.[14]

Cytotoxicity Assay to Detect Sensitivity of Cultured Fibroblasts to DNA-Damaging Agents

Fibroblasts from NF patients in both early (7-9) and middle (11-13) passage and from normal individuals were tested for survival after exposure to various DNA-damaging agents, including gamma radiation, which leads to DNA scission and causes free radical mediated base changes; actinomycin D, a DNA intercalating agent; and mitomycin C, a bifunctional alkylating agent which causes DNA-DNA and DNA-protein cross-links. For gamma radiation survival experiments, fibroblasts in log phase growth were trypsinized (0.25%) at 37°C for five minutes, scraped off plates, spun down, resuspended in Dulbecco's MEM and replated in known amounts of 10^2 to 2×10^4 cells/75 cm^2 tissue culture plate as above. Eighteen hours later individual plates were irradiated at various doses at room temperature by exposure to a ^{137}Cs radiation source (JL Sheperd, Mark I) at a rate of 150 cGy (rad) per minute and then reincubated at 37°C in a 5% CO_2 water-jacketed incubator for 15-40 days, with media changes weekly. At the end of the incubation time, during which surviving cells would have divided sufficiently to form colonies of greater than 30-50 cells, plates were stained with 1% methylene blue and colonies counted. The surviving fraction, after "correcting" for low density plating efficiency (the percent of 100-500 surviving cells per plate after no radiation exposure), was then plotted semilogarithmically versus gamma radiation dose.

Five to six radiation dose points with a minimum of six plates per dose were used between 0 and 800 rad for each experiment. Furthermore, all cell strains were studied between two and five times at a particular passage number, with the vast majority of strains tested three or more times. Survival curves for NF cells at various passage numbers were compared to results from controls using D_0, the inverse of the slope of the straight line portion of the survival curve, and theoretically the dose in rad that leads to one lethal hit per cell, or 37% cell survival; and D_{10}, the dose of radiation necessary for 90% cell kill.

Although low density plating efficiency can vary from cell to cell and experiment to experiment,[15,16] no relationship was found between this variable and passage number or survival ability in the nine normal cell strains used as controls. For both NF and control cells, however, the effect of increasing numbers of cells on improving the plating efficiency was minimized in the cytotoxicity experiments by keeping the number of cells plated below 4×10^4 per 75 cm^2 surface area in all experiments.[15] Satellite colony formation was not observed under these conditions.

Studies of the sensitivity of NF and control fibroblast cell strains to both actinomycin D and mitomycin C were carried out in a similar fashion. Fibroblasts were prepared and plated at a known cell number as in the radiation experiments above and then exposed to one of several doses of actinomycin D (0-0.1 mcg/ml) or mitomycin C (0-2.0 mcg/ml) for one hour in Dulbecco's MEM. The drug-containing medium was then removed and the cells washed extensively several times in phosphate-buffered saline (0.15 M NaCl, 0.7 mM KH_2PO_4, 4.3 mM K_2HOP_4) before being reincubated in normal medium for 15-40 days. Plates were then treated with 1% methylene blue and the number of colonies scored as in the radiation sensitivity experiments above. D_0's and D_{10}'s were again determined and compared at various passage numbers to control strains using at least five drug doses and six plates per drug dose point.

Growth Studies

Simultaneously with the survival experiments performed above, NF fibroblast cell strains at various passage numbers were examined for their growth rate, expressed as the fractional increase in cell number per day. Cells were plated in triplicate at 3 ×

10^5 per 75 cm^2 tissue culture plate, with plating efficiencies at this concentration noted between 75 and 90%, even for NF strains at presenescent cell passage. Cells were then incubated in Dulbecco's MEM as above and examined every one to three days until the plates reached visual confluency, as determined by a single observer. Plates were then scraped and washed extensively in medium, with the cells spun down, resuspended, and counted in a hemocytometer using all quadrants to increase accuracy. Growth rates per day, *r*, were calculated by the following formula:

$$r = \frac{\left[\ln \dfrac{N_1}{N_0}\right]}{t}$$

where N_1 was the number of cells at time *t*, N_0 the number of cells originally plated (3×10^5), and *t* the number of days cells were incubated. The nine normal fibroblast cell strains exhibited growth rates of approximately 15-30% per day at passages used for performing the cytotoxicity studies below (3-18).

Statistical Considerations

Results of cytotoxicity assays of NF cell strains at specific passage numbers were compared to the same strains at different passage numbers as well as to results from the nine normal cell strains for each DNA-damaging agent studied. Results from NF experiments were compared to controls using a t-test for results of D_0 and D_{10}, with the straight line portion of the survival curves determined using linear regression analysis.

Plating efficiencies and growth rates in NF cell strains were compared to passage number and to each other using linear regression analysis.

RESULTS

Sensitivity of NF Cell Strains to DNA-Damaging Agents

Neurofibromatosis fibroblast cell strains GM0622, GM1639, and SB23 were studied for sensitivity to gamma radiation, actinomycin D, and mitomycin C. For gamma radiation survival experiments, all three cell strains studied in early passage (7-9) exhibited normal D_0's (143-178 rad) compared to pooled data of nine normal cell strains [D_0 155 ± 4 standard error of the mean (SEM) rad; TABLE 1]. Because of early senescence, as described below, NF strain GM1639 was unable to be passaged further in tissue culture and thus was only studied in passages 7 and 8. NF strain GM0622, on the other hand, was studied between passages 11 and 13, with a mean D_0 of 106 ± 10 rad (p < 0.001) and a mean D_{10} of 303 ± 32 rad compared with normal D_{10}'s of 379 ± 12 rad (p = 0.04). FIGURE 1 demonstrates the marked increase

TABLE 1. Sensitivity of 3 Neurofibromatosis Cell Strains to Gamma Radiation

Strain	Passage	D_0 (rad)	p Value	D_{10} (rad)	p Value
9 Normals	3-18	155 ± 4 (SEM)	—	379 ± 12	—
GM0622	7-9	178	NS[a]	380	NS
	11-13	106	0.001	303	0.04
GM1639	7-8	176	NS	330	NS
SB-23	7-8	143	NS	330	NS
	12-13	145	NS	382	NS

[a] NS means not significant.

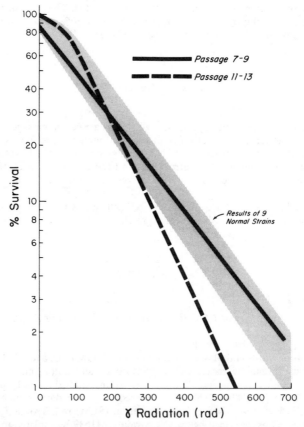

FIGURE 1. Sensitivity of neurofibromatosis (NF) fibroblasts at various *in vitro* passages to gamma radiation. NF strain GM0622 was exposed to varying doses of gamma radiation and studied for survival ability in early (7-9) and middle (11-13) passage as described in Methods. The shaded area represents the accumulative results of studies performed on nine normal cell strains.

TABLE 2. Sensitivity of 3 Neurofibromatosis Cell Strains to Actinomycin D

Strain	Passage	D_0 (μg/ml)	p Value	D_{10} (μg/ml)	p Value
9 Normals	3-17	0.039 ± 0.003 (SEM)	—	0.099 ± 0.007 (SEM)	—
GM0622	7-8	0.044	NS	0.107	NS
	9-10	0.026	0.04	0.074	0.07
	11-12	0.024		0.068	
GM1639	8-9	0.017	0.04	0.050	0.05
SB-23	7-8	0.045	NS	0.117	NS
	12-13	0.061	NS	0.148	NS

in sensitivity of GM0622 cells when studied in middle passage compared both to nine normal cell strains and to GM0622 studied in passages 7-9. NF strain SB23 continued to exhibit normal survival after gamma radiation exposure at passages 12-13. Neither strain GM0622 nor SB23 was studied at passages greater than 13 because of prohibitively low growth rates and low density plating efficiencies.

As with gamma radiation, strains GM0622 and SB23 exhibited normal sensitivity after actinomycin D exposure in early (7-8) cell passage, compared to the results of nine normal cell strains studied (mean D_0 0.039 ± 0.003 mcg/ml and D_{10} 0.099 ± 0.007 mcg/ml; TABLE 2). In contrast, strain GM1639 exhibited a marked increase in sensitivity after actinomycin D exposure at passages 8 and 9 (D_0 0.017 mcg/ml, p=0.04, and D_{10} 0.050 mcg/ml, p=0.05; FIGURE 2). At later passage, NF strain GM0622 demonstrated increased sensitivity as manifested by a decreased D_0 (0.025 mcg/ml for all experiments done in passages 9-12) and D_{10} (0.071 mcg/ml). NF strain SB23 continued to exhibit normal survival after actinomycin D exposure as it had after gamma radiation.

In 23 experiments performed in seven normal fibroblast cell strains, mean D_0's after mitomycin C exposure were 0.32 ± 0.04 mcg/ml, with mean D_{10}'s of 0.83 ± 0.09 mcg/ml. All three NF strains studied in early cell passage and the two studied in middle cell passage exhibited normal survival after exposure to this bifunctional alkylating agent (TABLE 3).

Growth Rates of NF Cell Strains

Growth rates of the three NF cell strains were examined at various *in vitro* passages. Normal cell strains consistently exhibited a fractional increase of approximately

TABLE 3. Sensitivity of 3 Neurofibromatosis Cell Strains to Mitomycin C

Strain	Passage	D_0 (μg/ml)	p Value	D_{10} (μg/ml)	p Value
7 Normals	4-18	0.32 ± 0.04 (SEM)	—	0.83 ± 0.09 (SEM)	—
GM0622	7-8	0.32	NS	0.77	NS
	13	0.27	NS	0.88	NS
GM1639	7-8	0.27	NS	0.71	NS
SB-23	7-8	0.34	NS	0.88	NS
	12-13	0.29	NS	0.78	NS

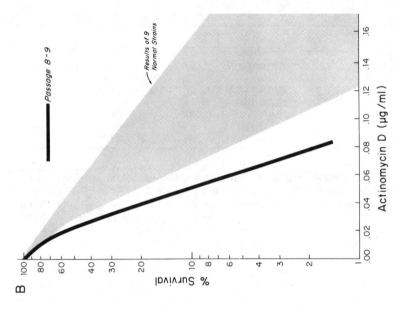

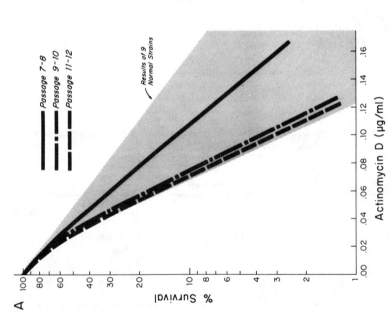

FIGURE 2. Sensitivity of NF fibroblasts at various *in vitro* passages to actinomycin D. NF strains GM0622 (A) and GM1639 (B) were exposed to varying doses of actinomycin D and studied for survival ability at different passages as described in Methods. The shaded area represents the accumulative results of studies performed on nine normal cell strains.

15-30% per day through all passages studied (less than 18). NF strain GM0622 was studied only in passages 12, 13, and 14; the fractional increase per day varied from 3.6% to 7.5%. NF strain GM1639 was studied six times at passage 8 with increases of only 0-2.4% per day found; doubling times were calculated at greater than 28 days, or about tenfold longer than those of normal cell strains.

The effect of passage number between 8 and 15 on the growth rate of NF strain SB23 was able to be examined (FIGURE 3). SB-23 cells increased in number by 17-22% per day in passages 8 and 9. Subsequently, a dramatic decrease in growth rate was

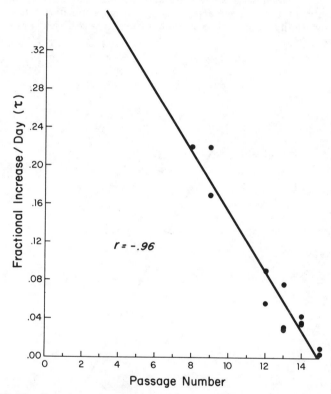

FIGURE 3. The effect of passage number on the growth rate of NF fibroblast strain SB23. The fractional increase in cell number per day was determined as described in Methods at various passage numbers and is plotted versus passage number.

noted such that by passage 15 SB-23 cells were exhibiting less than 0.7% increase per day, representing a doubling time of greater than 125 days. A strong negative correlation between passage number and fractional increase per day was found ($r = -0.96$, $p < 0.01$; FIGURE 3).

Plating efficiencies for the NF growth rate studies, in which 3×10^5 cells were grown on 75 cm^2 tissue culture plates, showed no decrease at high passage, with values noted between 75 and 90%. However, the low density plating efficiency of 100-500 cells per 75 cm^2 surface area dramatically decreased with passage number. For example, plating efficiency in strain SB23 went from an average of 25% at passage 7 to 2-3% at passage 13 ($r = -0.90$, $p < 0.01$; FIGURE 4). Similar values were obtained for NF strain GM0622 (20 points compared between passages 7 and 13 with a correlation coefficient $r = -0.62$, $p < 0.01$; data not shown). In NF strain GM1639, correlations of plating efficiency and passage number were not feasible, as cells were unable to be studied past passage 9. However, plating efficiencies were consistently between 1 and 8% in the eight experiments performed.

Because both growth rates and low density plating efficiencies decreased with passage number, the relationship between growth rate and plating efficiency was examined in NF strain SB23 where there were sufficient data for such analysis. As can be seen in FIGURE 5, there appears to be a strong correlation between growth rate and low density plating efficiency, with a correlation coefficient r of 0.96 ($p < 0.01$).

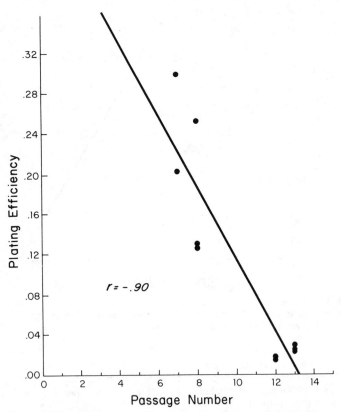

FIGURE 4. The effect of passage number on the low density plating efficiency of NF fibroblast strain SB23. The plating efficiency of 100-500 cells per 75 cm² surface area, determined as part of the cytotoxicity assays described in Methods, is plotted versus passage number.

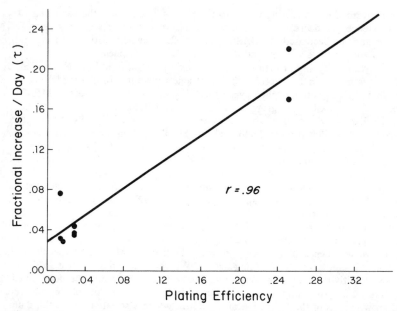

FIGURE 5. The correlation of growth rate and low density plating efficiency in NF fibroblast strain SB23. The fractional increase in cell number per day determined at a particular passage is plotted versus the plating efficiency of 100-500 cells per 75 cm² surface area at the same passage.

DISCUSSION

We have demonstrated that sensitivity of cultured cells from neurofibromatosis patients to certain DNA-damaging agents, specifically gamma radiation and actinomycin D, may be increased at *in vitro* passage levels that represent presenescence. Although increased sensitivity to gamma radiation and actinomycin D was not a consistent finding, it could be argued that were studies possible in slightly later passages in the cell lines exhibiting normal sensitivity (for example, SB23), decreased survival would have been documented.

A striking and consistent finding in all three neurofibromatosis cell strains studied was the fact that growth rates markedly decreased at *in vitro* passages at which normal cell strains exhibit normal growth rates. Associated with this finding was the observation that low density plating efficiency of NF cells (100-500 per 75 cm² surface area) also dramatically decreased with increased passage number. Although a correlation was seen between low density plating efficiency and growth rates (FIGURE 5), the two phenomena appear to be independent, as plating efficiencies observed in the growth rate studies using 300,000 cells/75 cm² surface area were consistently high, even at passage numbers indicating cell presenescence. Furthermore, the increased sensitivity of NF strains seen after exposure to gamma radiation and actinomycin D was not related to low density plating efficiency, as all survival studies were performed by correcting values to the plating efficiency of the particular experiment. Hence, the decreased survival seen in NF cell strains after exposure to DNA damage and the decreased low density plating efficiency seen with increasing *in vitro* age also appear to be separate, although possibly related, phenomena.

All cytotoxicity and growth rate studies performed above utilized NF and control cell strains grown in Dulbecco's modified Eagle's medium. In one study, decreased growth and changes in morphology seen in NF cells grown in Dulbecco's MEM were reversible when cells were grown in Ham's F12 medium.[8] It is not known whether or not cell sensitivity studies would also revert to normal if NF cells at presenescent passage were switched from Dulbecco's to Ham's F12 medium. Such studies are currently in progress in this laboratory.

It has been hypothesized that cellular decline in the ability to handle DNA-damaging agents may be associated with, or the primary cause of, aging.[17,18] For example, certain types of DNA repair appear to decrease in late passage fibroblasts *in vitro*.[19,20] Furthermore, there appears to be reduced DNA repair in cells from older individuals;[21] and organisms that have a short life span appear to have less ability to excise ultraviolet light-induced DNA damage than do organisms with longer life spans.[22] The results obtained above suggest that there is a correlation between the premature senescence of NF cells grown in Dulbecco's MEM and the diminished capacity to handle DNA-damaging agents. Whether the aging process leads to increased sensitivity to DNA-damaging agents or vice versa cannot be determined. It is of interest that there appeared to be a steady decline in low density plating efficiencies and growth rates in the NF cell strains studied, whereas sensitivity to DNA damage appeared normal or appeared to decline only at the most senescent cell passages. Regardless, the data suggest that there are altered growth properties in cultured skin fibroblasts from patients with neurofibromatosis, supporting the hypothesis that this disease represents a biochemically global defect, rather than one limited to cells of neural crest origin. As a corollary, the use of cultured skin cells from NF patients may be an excellent human model to study *in vitro* aging processes.

In summary, the results of these studies suggest that cultured fibroblast cell strains from patients with neurofibromatosis exhibit early *in vitro* senescence which can be associated with an inability to handle certain DNA-damaging agents. Future studies will pursue these observations by continuing to examine the hypothesis that the increased incidence of neoplasms seen in individuals with NF may be associated with an altered ability to handle DNA damage.

SUMMARY

Neurofibromatosis (NF) is an autosomal dominant disorder associated with various constitutional abnormalities as well as a striking predisposition for malignant and nonmalignant neoplasms, both in cells originating in and not originating in the neural crest. We have examined the sensitivity of cultured skin fibroblasts from patients with neurofibromatosis to several types of DNA damage. Fibroblasts in Dulbecco's modified Eagle's medium were plated at 10^2 to 2×10^4 cells per 75 cm^2 tissue culture plates, and exposed to various doses of gamma radiation (leads to DNA scission), actinomycin D (a DNA intercalating agent), or mitomycin C (a bifunctional alkylating agent leading to DNA cross-links). Cells were reincubated for 15 to 40 days until surviving colonies exhibited greater than 30-50 cells. Plates were then stained with 1% methylene blue and the colonies counted, with surviving fraction determined relative to plating efficiency. Nine skin fibroblast cell strains from normal individuals were studied as controls. One neurofibromatosis (NF) cell strain, SB23, exhibited normal sensitivity to all three DNA-damaging agents studied in early (7-8) and middle (12-13) *in vitro* passage. Strain GM0622, on the other hand, exhibited normal sensitivity to the three DNA-damaging agents studied at early passage, but showed a significant decrease in survival after exposure to both gamma radiation (D_0 = 106 rad) and actinomycin D (D_0 = 0.024 mcg/ml) with increasing passage. Strain GM1639 exhibited decreased survival after actinomycin D exposure at early passage (D_0 = 0.017 mcg/ml), with normal survival after exposure to gamma radiation and mitomycin C at the same passage. Cell strains exhibited decreasing low density plating efficiencies and growth rates with increasing passage such that study of cytotoxicity was not feasible after middle passage in strains SB23 and GM0622, and after early passage in strain GM1639. The results suggest that cultured fibroblast cell strains from patients with NF exhibit early *in vitro* senescence which sometimes is associated with an inability to handle certain DNA-damaging agents.

REFERENCES

1. RICCARDI, V. M. 1981. Von Recklinghausen neurofibromatosis. N. Engl. J. Med. **305:** 1617-1627.
2. MULVIHILL, J. J. & D. G. HOPE. 1981. Malignancy in neurofibromatosis. Adv. Neurol. **29:** 32-56.
3. BOLANDE, R. P. 1981. Neurofibromatosis—the quintessential neurocristopathy: pathogenic concepts and relationships. Adv. Neurol. **29:** 67-75.
4. BADER, J. L. & R. W. MILLER. 1978. Neurofibromatosis and childhood leukemia. J. Pediatr. **92:** 925-929.
5. McKEEN, E. A., J. BODURTHA, A. T. MEADOWS, E. C. DOUGLASS & J. J. MULVIHILL. 1978. Rhabdomyosarcoma complicating multiple neurofibromatosis. J. Pediatr. **93:** 992-993.
6. STAY, E. J. & G. VAWTER. 1977. The relationship between nephroblastoma and neurofibromatosis (von Recklinghausen's disease). Cancer **39:** 2550-2555.
7. KRONE, W., S. ZORLEIN & R. MAO. 1981. Cell culture studies on neurofibromatosis (von Recklinghausen). I. Comparative growth experiments with fibroblasts at high and low concentrations of fetal calf serum. Hum. Genet. **58:** 188-193.
8. ZELKOWITZ, M. & J. STAMBOULY. 1981. Neurofibromatosis fibroblasts: slow growth and abnormal morphology. Pediatr. Res. **15:** 290-293.
9. ZELKOWITZ, M. & J. STAMBOULY. 1980. Diminished epidermal growth factor binding by neurofibromatosis fibroblasts. Ann. Neurol. **8:** 296-299.
10. DUCATMAN, B. S. & B. W. SCHEITHAUER. 1983. Post-irradiation neurofibrosarcoma. Cancer **51:** 1028-1033.
11. SETLOW, R. B. 1978. Repair deficient human disorders and cancer. Nature **271:** 713-717.
12. CLEAVER, J. E. 1968. Defective repair replication of DNA in xeroderma pigmentosum. Nature **218:** 652-656.
13. WOODS, W. G. 1981. Quantitation of the repair of gamma radiation-induced double strand DNA breaks in human fibroblasts. Biochim. Biophys. Acta **655:** 342-348.
14. CHEN, T. R. 1977. *In situ* detection of *Mycoplasma* contamination in cell cultures by fluorescent Hoechst 33258 stain. Exp. Cell Res. **14:** 255-262.
15. WEICHSELBAUM, R. R., J. NOVE & J. B. LITTLE. 1980. X-Ray sensitivity of 53 human diploid fibroblast cell strains from patients with characterized genetic disorders. Cancer Res. **40:** 920-925.

16. ARLETT, C. F. & S. A. HARCOURT. 1980. Survey of radiosensitivity in a variety of human cell strains. Cancer Res. **40:** 926-932.
17. LITTLE, J. B. 1976. Relationship between DNA repair capacity and cellular aging. Gerontology **22:** 28-55.
18. HART, R. W., S. M. D'AMBROSIO, K. J. NG & S. P. MODAK. 1979. Longevity, stability and DNA repair. Mech. Ageing Dev. **9:** 203-223.
19. MATTERN, M. R. & P. A. CERUTTI. 1975. Age-dependent excision repair of damaged thymine from gamma irradiated DNA by isolated nuclei from human fibroblasts. Nature **254:** 450-452.
20. LAMPIDIS, T. J. & G. E. SCHAIBERGER. 1975. Age-related loss of DNA repair synthesis in isolated rat myocardial cells. Exp. Cell Res. **96:** 412-416.
21. LAMBERT, G., U. RINGBORG & L. SKOOG. 1979. Age-related decrease in ultraviolet light-induced DNA repair synthesis in human peripheral leukocytes. Cancer Res. **39:** 2792-2795.
22. FRANCIS, A. A., W. H. LEE & J. D. REGAN. 1981. The relationship of DNA excision repair of ultraviolet light-induced lesions to the maximum life span of mammals. Mech. Ageing Dev. **16:** 181-189.

Evidence against Linkage of von Recklinghausen Neurofibromatosis and Chromosome 19 Markers

S. M. HUSON,[a,c] A. L. MEREDITH,[a] M. SARFARAZI,[a]
D. J. SHAW,[a] D. BROOK,[a] D. A. S. COMPSTON,[b]
AND P. S. HARPER[a]

[a]Section of Medical Genetics
[b]Department of Neurology
University of Wales College of Medicine
Heath Park, Cardiff, Wales

INTRODUCTION

There have been two three-generation families reported in which myotonic dystrophy (DM) and von Recklinghausen neurofibromatosis (NF) appear to segregate together, suggesting that the two diseases may be closely linked. The first family was reported by Ichikawa et al. in 1981.[1] In this family the origin of NF in generation I is clear but that of DM is uncertain. In generations II and III however there are seven double heterozygotes. If one assumes that the mother in generation I who had NF also had DM, then this family gives a lod score of 2.4 between NF and DM with no recombination. If, however, her husband had DM then the evidence from this family would be strongly against linkage between NF and DM.

The second family was reported by Rivas at the seventh workshop in human gene mapping.[2] In this family there are seven double heterozygotes in four generations, and only one possible recombinant—a 23-year-old female with NF only. If one assumes that this girl will develop DM then this family gives a lod score of 3.01 with no recombination between NF and DM. If she does not develop DM then the lod score is only 0.7 with a recombination fraction of 0.20.

If the clinical assumptions in these families are correct then the combined lod score from the two families for NF-DM would be 5.41 with no recombination. This would strongly suggest that the NF gene lies close to the myotonic dystrophy gene, which is part of a well-studied linkage group on chromosome 19. DM was in fact the first serious autosomal genetic disease for which linkage was established.

In 1954 Mohr reported a suggestion of linkage between DM, the Lutheran blood group (Lu), and the secretion of ABH blood group substances (Se).[3] This linkage was confirmed by the studies of Renwick et al. in 1971[4] and Harper et al. in 1973.[5] Further linkage studies added the Lewis blood group (Le) and the third component of human

[c]Present address: Research Registrar/Medical Genetics, Clinical Research Center, Northwick Park Hospital, Harrow, Middlesex, United Kingdom.

349

complement (C3)[6] to this group, and the whole linkage group was assigned to chromosome 19 with the assignment of C3 to that chromosome by Whitehead *et al.* in 1982.[7]

Since that time several additional loci have been assigned to this linkage group including peptidase D (PEPD)[8] and the apolipoproteins E (APOE)[9] and CII (APOC2).[10] The orientation of this linkage group on chromosome 19 has also been established.[11] To investigate the possible linkage between NF and DM further we studied the segregation of five markers in this linkage group in families with NF.

MATERIALS AND METHODS

The families were ascertained through two sources, the records of the Department of Medical Genetics, University Hospital of Wales, and the British Neurofibromatosis Patients Association, LINK. The families were contacted by letter and if they agreed to take part were visited at home by one of us (S.M.H.). All the family members were examined personally, and specimens of blood and saliva taken.

The criteria used for the diagnosis of NF were as follows:

1. *In adults*—six or more café-au-lait spots > 1.5 cm diameter and multiple peripheral neurofibromas.
2. *In children*—an affected parent and six or more café-au-lait spots > 1.5 cm diameter.

Family members were typed for the following markers: Se, Lu, PEPD and the restriction fragment length polymorphisms identified by the gene probes for C3 and APOC2 when total human DNA is digested using the restriction enzymes Sst1 and Taq1 respectively. Both these polymorphisms have previously been reported in detail.[12,10]

Fifty-seven affected individuals and 41 normal relatives were studied from six three-generation and three two-generation families. Three children were excluded from the study because of equivocal clinical findings. They were age 7, 6, and 5 years and had one, two, and one café-au-lait spots greater than 1.5 cm in diameter respectively. They had no smaller café-au-lait spots and no other stigmata of NF. We feel that these children probably do not have NF but because of the slight uncertainty excluded them from the linkage analysis.

Linkage analysis was done using the program LIPED.[13] No evidence of nonpenetrance of the NF gene was found in the families studied, and penetrance was assumed to be complete for the linkage analysis. In the case of unaffected relatives only those over the age of 5 were included because of the uncertainty as to the age by which affected individuals will have manifested café-au-lait spots.

RESULTS

The lod scores for various values of recombination fraction from 0.01 to 0.40 for Se, the C3 and APOC2 polymorphisms are shown in TABLE 1. Results are given assuming equal male and female recombination frequencies. None of the families were informative for Lu and PEPD.

TABLE 1. Lod Scores, Assuming $\theta_m = \theta_f$, between NF and APOC2, C3 and Se

	Number of Families	Lod Scores at Various Values of θ					
		0.01	0.05	0.10	0.20	0.30	0.40
NF-APOC2	6	−22.63	−11.85	−7.42	−3.48	−1.65	−0.70
NF-C3	3	− 3.79	− 1.82	−1.08	−0.50	−0.26	−0.11
NF-Se	4	− 4.12	− 2.08	−1.25	−0.52	−0.19	−0.05

The three informative markers all show significant evidence against linkage (lod ≤ −2.0) for at least some values of θ. There was also no significant evidence of linkage when male and female recombinations were analyzed separately. No family gave a positive lod score for any of the markers that might have suggested the possibility of genetic heterogeneity.

DISCUSSION

The probable linkage relationships of the markers studied and their orientation on chromosome 19 are shown in FIGURE 1. PEPD and APOC2 are the closest markers

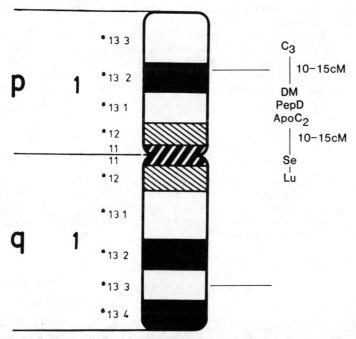

FIGURE 1. Relationship between genetic and physical maps of chromosome 19. The markers C3, PEPD, and APOC2 have been analyzed by genetic linkage and by use of hybrid cells, thus allowing the orientation to be established.

for the DM locus available at the present time. PEPD gives a maximum lod score of 3.5 at $\theta = 0^8$ and APOC2 a maximum lod score of 7.87 at $\theta = 0.04$.[14] Both these markers have been localized to the region 19p13-19q13 using somatic cell hybrids.[11,14] Recent results show that APOC2 is at 19p13-19cen (unpublished data). C3 has been localized to the region 19p13.2-Pter,[11] and linkage analysis shows C3 to be between 5 and 15 cm from DM. The C3 and Se loci probably flank the DM gene as shown in FIGURE 1.[6]

Our study shows evidence against linkage of APOC2 to NF to a distance of 30 cm, of C3 to NF to a distance of 10 cm, and of Se to NF to a distance of 10 cm. This excludes the NF gene from a considerable region of chromosome 19 around the DM locus. In terms of the physical map of chromosome 19 these results probably exclude the NF gene from the short arm of this chromosome.

This study was prompted by previous suggestions of linkage between DM and NF from two families in which the diseases appeared to segregate together. We must now find an explanation for this other than linkage between NF and DM. One explanation would be that there is more than one genetic locus for von Recklinghausen neurofibromatosis; another that the affected individuals in these families actually have a disease in which the features of NF and DM are combined. We feel that both these possibilities are unlikely and that the explanation is that the clinical assumptions that have to be made to show linkage between NF and DM in these families are incorrect.

The family reported by Ichikawa et al. is the only one for which full clinical details have been published.[1] In this family the origin of NF in generation I is clearly from the mother but that of DM is uncertain. If her husband had DM then there is no evidence of linkage in this family. This would be supported by the fact that in generation IV (not included in the linkage analysis) there is an individual who has congenital DM and no stigmata of NF at the age of two. This would be very unusual if he has inherited the NF gene.

From a clinical viewpoint our results are important but disappointing. Not only would a closely linked marker for von Recklinghausen neurofibromatosis be useful clinically to identify the status of at-risk individuals, but the mapping of the gene would be a major step toward our understanding of the disease and its relationship to other forms of neurofibromatosis.

SUMMARY

In this paper we report the study of the segregation of three chromosome 19 markers known to be linked to myotonic dystrophy in nine families with von Recklinghausen neurofibromatosis. Clear evidence against linkage was found for all three markers excluding the von Recklinghausen neurofibromatosis gene from the myotonic dystrophy region of chromosome 19.

ACKNOWLEDGMENTS

We would like to thank Dr. G. Fey for the C3 probe, Dr. O. Myklebost for the APO2 probe, Dr. P. Tippett for Lutheran typing, and Professor E. B. Robson for peptidase D typing. We are grateful to all the family members and to the association LINK for their cooperation.

REFERENCES

1. ICHIKAWA, K., C. J. CROSLEY, A. CULEBRAS & L. WEITKAMP. 1981. Coincidence of neurofibromatosis and myotonic dystrophy in a kindred. J. Med. Genet. **18:** 134-138.
2. RIVAS, M. L. & J. H. DI LIBERTI. 1984. Genetic linkage between myotonic dystrophy and neurofibromatosis. Birth Defects **20:** 570.
3. MOHR, J. 1954. A Study of Linkage in Man. Munksgaard. Copenhagen, Denmark.
4. RENWICK, J. H., S. E. BUNDEY, M. A. FERGUSON-SMITH & M. M. IZATT. 1971. Confirmation of the linkage of the loci for myotonic dystrophy and ABH secretion. J. Med. Genet. **8:** 407-416.
5. HARPER, P. S., M. L. RIVAS, W. B. BIAS, J. R. HUTCHINSON, P. R. DYKEN & V. A. McKUSICK. 1972. Genetic linkage confirmed between the locus for myotonic dystrophy and the ABH—secretion and Lutheran blood group loci. Am. J. Hum. Genet. **24:** 310-316.
6. EIBERG, H., J. MOHR, L. S. NIELSEN & N. SIMONSON. 1983. Genetics and linkage relationships of the C3 polymorphisms. Discovery of C3-Se linkage and assignment of LES-C3-DM-Se-PEPD-Lu synteny. Clin. Genet. **24:** 159-170.
7. WHITEHEAD, A. S., E. SOLOMAN, S. CHAMBERS, W. F. BODMER, S. POVEY & G. FEY. 1982. Assignment of the structural gene for the third component of human complement to chromosome 19. Proc. Nat. Acad. Sci. USA. **79:** 5021-5025.
8. O'BRIEN, T., S. BALL, M. SARFARAZI, P. S. HARPER & E. B. ROBSON. 1983. Genetic linkage between the loci for myotonic dystrophy and peptidase D. Ann. Hum. Genet. **47:** 117-121.
9. GEDDE-DAHL, T., B. OLAISEN, P. TELSBERG, M. C. WILHEMY, B. MEVAG & R. HELLAND. 1984. The locus for apolipoprotein E (APOE) is close to the Lutheran (Lu) blood group locus on chromosome 19. Hum. Genet. **67:** 178-182.
10. MYKLEBOST, O., S. ROGNE, B. OLAISEN, T. GEDDE-DAHL & H. PRYDZ. 1984. The locus for apolipoprotein CII is closely linked to the apolipoprotein E locus on chromosome 19 in man. Hum. Genet. **67:** 309-312.
11. BROOK, J. D., D. J. SHAW, A. L. MEREDITH, G. A. P. BRUNS & P. S. HARPER. 1984. Localization of genetic markers and orientation of the linkage group on chromosome 19. Hum. Genet. **68:** 282-285.
12. DAVIES, K. E., J. JACKSON, R. WILLIAMSON, P. S. HARPER, S. BALL, M. SARFARAZI, A. L. MEREDITH & G. FEY. 1983. Linkage analysis of myotonic dystrophy and sequences on chromosome 19 using a cloned complement 3 gene probe. J. Med. Genet. **20:** 259-263.
13. OTT, J. 1974. Estimation of the recombination fraction in human pedigrees: efficient computation of the likelihood for human linkage studies. Am. J. Hum. Genet. **26:** 588-589.
14. SHAW, D. J., A. L. MEREDITH, M. SARFARAZI, S. M. HUSON, J. D. BROOK & P. S. HARPER. 1985. The apolipoprotein CII gene: subchromosomal localisation and linkage to myotonic dystrophy. Hum. Genet. **70:** 271-273.

Cell Culture Studies on Neurofibromatosis (von Recklinghausen)

Characterization of Cells Growing from Neurofibromas

W. KRONE, R. MAO, O. S. MÜHLECK, H. KLING,
AND T. FINK

Department of Human Genetics
University of Ulm
Post Office Box 4066
D-7900 Ulm, Federal Republic of Germany

Investigations of neurofibromatosis (NF) cells in culture have so far yielded a rather modest amount of information. The research on this subject is guided by the very justified assumption that these cells, so readily available, conceal at least part of the secret, and that it only depends on the skill of the investigator to unravel it. All kinds of approaches, however, using fibroblast-like cells (FLC) run into the well-known difficulties that arise from the wide range of interindividual variability influencing many qualitative and all quantitative parameters of this system. The results reported here also reflect to some extent this kind of problem. We have tried to investigate a series of parameters related to cell biology and biochemistry, and the various approaches will be discussed briefly below.

THE DESCRIPTIVE LEVEL

What can be seen in primary cultures derived from neurofibromas? First of all, the small fragments of tumor tissue used to establish conventional stem cultures commence growth with FLC much more frequently than do explants of unaffected skin from NF patients or from skin of healthy donors. Of 104 explants derived from peripheral neurofibromas of 11 NF patients, 84 (81%) started with FLC and most of them never developed epitheloid outgrowth later on. In contrast, the large majority (more than 90%) of the explants of unaffected skin began outgrowth with epitheloid cells generally surrounding the explants before any FLC became visible. Explants from the skin overlying neurofibromas showed an intermediate distribution. Since we

354

also observed analogous behavior in primary cultures from other types of fibromas, it may be in some way related to the contribution of FLC to this kind of tumor.

Secondly, among the FLC growing from explants of neurofibromas there is a conspicuously high number of binuclear and oligonuclear cells. We have seen this in all of our primary cultures from 30 NF patients, and it was photographically documented in 18 of these; examples are shown in FIGURE 1. The presence of similar bi- and oligonuclear cells in stem cultures made with collagenase/trypsin-dissociated tumor tissue can thus not be attributed to the proteolytic digestion procedure. The most important mechanisms by which binuclear cells can arise are cell fusion and inhibition of cytokinesis ensuing karyokinesis. Tetraploid cells will emerge from synchronous mitosis of the two nuclei, and tetraploidy has been suspected as one of the initial steps in the development of aneuploidy which can become the cause of neoplasia.[1,2] Hence the elucidation of the origin of these bi- and oligonuclear cells may contribute to our understanding of tumor growth also in NF. Similar binuclear cells were observed in cultures from acoustic neuromas by Cravioto and Lockwood.[3]

Cell morphology and growth pattern are different from those of normal FLC in many but not all FLC strains derived from neurofibromas, as noted by others.[4,5] This deviant, somewhat bizarre morphology is not, however, necessarily related to poor growth. There are NF strains with the typical morphology that achieve very high cell population densities and normal numbers of cell population doublings *in vitro*. The growth pattern suggests a higher affinity of the cells to each other than to the substratum; it is a fascicular pattern consisting of a system of dense ridges or arrays leaving relatively scarcely populated spaces in between. There is a larger variety of cells emerging from explants of neurofibromas than from explants of normal skin. Also the samples from neurofibromas dissociated by collagenase/trypsin digestion yield four or five types of cells which can be distinguished by morphology. Besides the two types of FLC—the normal fusiform, regularly arranged type and the bizarre, irregularly growing type, respectively—there are (1) epitheloid cells growing as a close sheet, (2) spindle-shaped immature Schwann cells, (3) macrophages, (4) a small type of cell presumably arising from the endothelium of small blood vessels, and (5) a highly refractile, rare type of cell, which we call "hyaline" cell just to give them a name alluding to their glassy appearance. While this latter type of cell as well as the putative endothelial cells await identification by more sophisticated methods, the macrophages and the Schwann cells were identified by some of their respective specific properties. Offering an insoluble dye like neutral red to cultures containing the cells in question leads to rapid engulfing of the dye particles by these cells, which also express large amounts of the so-called unspecific esterase, as detected cytochemically (FIGURE 2). An explant shedding macrophages will invariably round up within a few days, probably due to proteolysis which also becomes recognizable by the spontaneous detachment and contraction of the cell lawn in the vicinity of the explant.

The spindle-shaped Schwann cells have occurred in the primary cultures of neurofibromas from all of our 30 patients. The yield of spindle cells is generally better in the collagenase/trypsin-dissociated material than in conventional stem cultures. We have never seen larger groups of spindle cells in cultures established from normal skin, although isolated sporadic cells with a comparable morphology occur occasionally.

The morphological features of these cells and their behavior in culture have been described in detail earlier.[6] Their identification as immature Schwann cells is based upon the expression of S-100 protein and of galactocerebroside, as detected by immunocytochemistry. In contrast to fibroblasts they show a mitogenic response to dibutyryl cyclic AMP (dbcAMP) and methylisobutylxanthine (an inhibitor of cAMP-phosphodiesterase) and to cholera toxin at 10 to 20 ng per ml of culture medium.

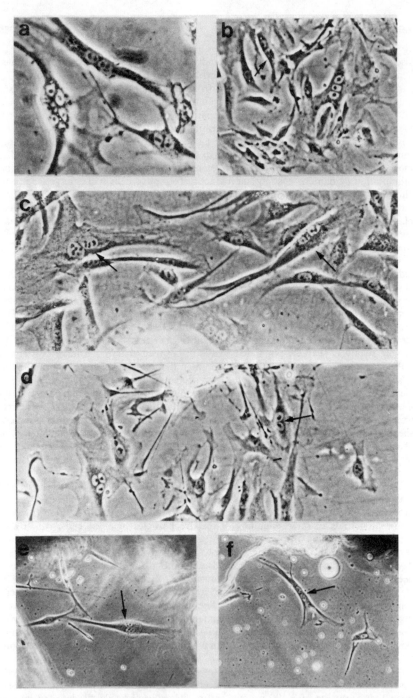

FIGURE 1. Examples of bi- and multinuclear cells in primary cultures from **a** and **b**, NF II; **c** and **e**, NF XV; **d**, NF XIV; **f**, NF V: **a, b, d,** and **f** are from conventional stem cultures, **c** and **e** from collagenase-dissociated material. Arrows point to the less obvious examples.

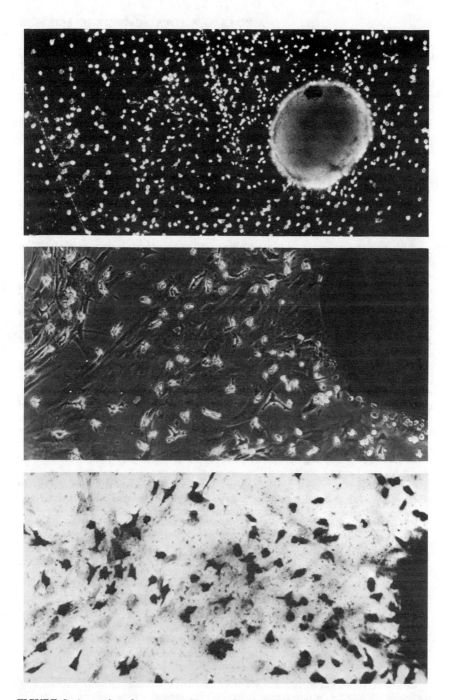

FIGURE 2. An explant from a neurofibroma of patient NF 21. Top: low-power dark field illumination showing only the shedding of numerous macrophages from this explant, which has completely rounded up. Center: 200 ×, phase contrast; macrophages on top of the adhering FLC. Bottom: same magnification, bright field, after cytochemical staining for unspecific esterase.

Despite persistent efforts we have not been able to stimulate continued proliferation of spindle cells. In several instances they have sustained transfer after local trypsinization; the cloning of cultures containing spindle cells has not, however, yielded any viable clone of this kind so far. This failure to obtain larger amounts of spindle cells from neurofibromas has greatly hampered the progress of cell culture studies on NF. The analysis of these cells and their comparison with normal Schwann cells in culture on all possible levels of scrutiny would certainly be one of the most promising approaches.

GROWTH PROPERTIES OF FLC FROM NEUROFIBROMAS

Although in our earlier study a high growth potential in the presence of 1% or 15% fetal calf serum, respectively, occurred more often among 11 NF strains than among 13 controls,[7] the most conservative interpretation of these results is that growth parameters of NF strains vary within the same wide range as those from normal strains. As far as serum requirement and final cell population densities are concerned, NF strains do not express properties of transformed cells in culture. We repeated this kind of experiment with 18 pairs of NF and control strains, determining growth for 150 hours and 300 hours, respectively, in the presence of 1% fetal calf serum. Rather than in sister cultures, initial cell densities were counted *in situ* with phase contrast optics, so that each culture flask provided a pair of determinations of initial and final cell densities, the latter being counted *in situ* after staining. The presentation of the results in TABLE 1 emphasizes the effectiveness of contact inhibition of growth: complete contact inhibition would yield no correlation whatsoever between initial and final cell densities ($r_{xy} = 0$); ineffectiveness of contact inhibition, on the other hand, would cause a high positive correlation. Hence, a significantly positive coefficient of correlation between final and initial cell densities would indicate relaxation of density-dependent growth regulation. The original results of this series of experiments were biased by two pairs of outlying values obtained with one particular pair of NF and control strain. After omitting these values to avoid spurious correlation within an inhomogenous sample, no significant correlation can be detected between final and initial cell densities in NF and control strains, respectively (TABLE 1). Although, like

TABLE 1. Coefficients of Correlation between Initial and Final Cell Densities[a]

		r	df	Probability of Error
NF strains	150 hour	+ 0.391	32[b]	$\alpha < 0.05$
NF strains	300 hour	+ 0.135	32[b]	$\alpha > 0.05$
Controls	150 hour	− 0.106	34	$\alpha > 0.05$
Controls	300 hour	− 0.291	34	$\alpha > 0.05$

[a]Cells were grown in Dulbecco's modification of Eagle's minimum essential medium (ED) containing 1% FCS for the time periods indicated. The 300 hour cultures received fresh medium at 150 hours. The figures are derived from comparisons of 18 NF strains with 18 control strains; each strain was used twice.
[b]Two outlyer values omitted to avoid inhomogeneity correlation.

TABLE 2. Determinations of the Average Weekly Cell Population Doublings and Highest Cell Densities Achieved during the Linear Phase of the *In Vitro* Proliferative Life Span

	NF Strains ($n = 15$)	Control Strains ($n = 13$)	Probability of Error
Average weekly CPD during linear phase	2.58 ± 0.48	2.18 ± 0.33	$0.05 > \alpha > 0.01$
Highest cell density achieved ($10^{-3}/cm^2$)	32.6 ± 13.7	26.2 ± 9.9	$\alpha > 0.05$

in our earlier experiments, the highest increments in cell numbers were achieved by NF strains, it must be concluded that the efficiency of density-dependent growth control varies within the same wide range in both kinds of strains.

Another growth parameter is the number of weekly cell population doublings (CPD) achieved during the linear phase of the *in vitro* proliferative life span (TABLE 2). There is no significant difference between the average weekly CPDs of the 15 NF and 13 control strains examined. Once again, the fastest growing strains occurred among our sample of NF strains. None of the strains has established itself as a permanent line.

A more rigorous measure of the growth potential is the colony-forming ability (CFA) or cloning efficiency. In the context of our comparative studies on the effects of x-ray irradiation and of mutagenic (cancerogenic) substances on CFA (see below), 12 NF strains and 13 control strains were cloned, most of them several times, on the thin homologous feeder layer of Cox and Masson.[8] In a total of 38 experiments performed so far, the following average CFAs were obtained: NF strains ($n=12$) 14.4% ± 6.2%; control strains ($n=13$) 16.7% ± 6.5%. The difference is not statistically significant. The lowest CFA observed was that of two NF strains, with 6.6% and 6.8% respectively. These data do not corroborate earlier claims of poor growth potential of NF cells.[9]

SENSITIVITY TO X-RAYS AND MUTAGENIC SUBSTANCES

Increased sensitivity against mutagenic agents is not only observed in some of the so-called chromosomal breakage syndromes with autosomal recessive inheritance. Decreased x-ray survival was observed in fibroblasts from some patients with retinoblastoma,[10] and there is some evidence for an enhanced sensitivity to ionizing radiation of cells from patients with tuberous sclerosis.[11,12] Paterson *et al.* reported a normal sensitivity of two strains of NF fibroblasts against γ-rays.[13]

FIGURE 3 summarizes the results of our experiments on x-ray survival of seven strains of NF cells and nine control strains derived from age- and sex-matched healthy donors.[14] The colony-forming ability was measured by the method of the thin homologous feeder layer according to Cox and Masson.[8] Fibroblasts derived from a patient with ataxia telangiectasia served as a positive control. There is no significant difference between the NF and the control strains in the range of dosages of x-rays

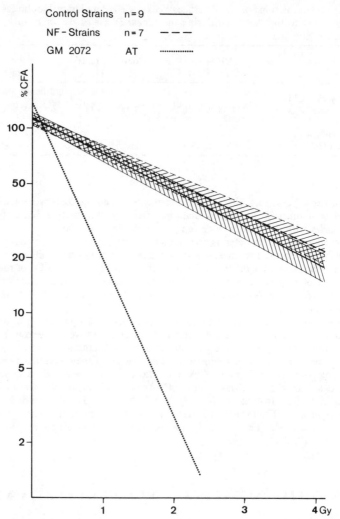

FIGURE 3. Summary diagram of a total of 22 clonal survival assays performed with the number of NF and control strains indicated. A strain from a patient with ataxia telangiectasia served as a positive control. The regression lines were computed from the averages of the survival data obtained in the various experiments performed with each strain.

applied. In a second series of experiments, performed with a sample of eight NF and control strains each, CFA was measured after exposure to the single higher dose of 4.75 Gy, and again, no difference was observed (data not shown). Similar results were recently reported by Schwenn et al.,[15] who also described normal sensitivity of NF cells to ultraviolet light and to the alkylating agent N-methyl-N'-nitro-N-nitroso-guanidine.

The sensitivity of six pairs of NF and control strains to the carcinogens 4-nitro-quinolin-*N*-oxide (4-NQO) and mitomycin C (MMC) was tested in a similar series of clonal survival assays. The substances were applied in serum-free medium before plating at 0.05, 0.1, and 0.2 μg/ml for 30 (4-NQO) and 60 (MMC) minutes, respectively. The average CFAs were lower in the NF strains than in the control strains at all concentrations of the carcinogens, the differences being larger after 4-NQO than after MMC treatment. Since the differences are not, however, significant statistically, the possibility of an enhanced sensitivity of NF strains to 4-NQO remains to be investigated with a larger series of strains.

COLLAGEN SYNTHESIS

It is well known that peripheral neurofibromas contain varying, sometimes large amounts of collagens.[16,17] Besides the collagens I and III forming an abundant extra-cellular network, the presence of collagens IV and V was detected by immunohisto-chemical methods in the basal laminas of the Schwann and endothelial cells, respectively, of neurofibromas.[18,19] The process of neoplastic transformation brings about alterations of qualitative as well as quantitative parameters of collagen syn-thesis.[20-23] It seems of interest to study these parameters in benign tumors and in cell cultures derived therefrom.

When suspensions of small fragments of unaffected skin, tumor-adhering skin, and tumor tissue were compared by the method of Peterkofsky and Diegelmann,[24] collagen synthesis amounted to about 1% of total protein synthesis during a 24 hour labeling period with radioactive proline (TABLE 3). A difference between these various samples could not be detected.

In cell culture the rate of collagen synthesis as a portion of the rate of total protein synthesis is influenced, among other things, by cell population density and by the concentration of fetal calf serum (FCS). A variety of NF and control strains were

TABLE 3. Collagen Synthesis in Tissue Fragments from Peripheral Neurofibromas (T), Adhering Skin (ST), and Unaffected Skin (S) from NF Patients

Patient	Tissue	Corrected Divisions per Minute in Total Proteins[a]	Divisions per Minute in Collagens	Percent Collagen Synthesis
NF V	T 1	7,610,400	79,200	1.0
NF V	T 2	5,521,300	50,900	0.9
NF V	S 1	1,118,700	10,600	0.9
NF V	S 2	1,543,600	12,200	0.8
NF XII	T	3,345,500	29,800	0.9
NF XII	ST	1,070,200	6,200	0.6
NF XIII	T	13,371,300	111,800	0.8
NF XIII	ST	7,143,000	75,000	1.1
NF III	T + ST	4,633,100	28,800	0.6

[a]Corrected according to the formula of Diegelmann and Peterkofsky.[50]

therefore compared at the concentrations of FCS indicated in TABLE 4. Although individual strains have shown a more pronounced optimum at 10% FCS, this effect levels off in the averages of both kinds of strains examined. There is no difference between NF and control strains with regard to the percentage of collagen synthesis.

The influence of cell population density on the rate of collagen synthesis was examined in comparative experiments set up with various initial cell densities, the actual cell densities at the time of labeling being determined by *in situ* counting of the stained cultures. The results of five experiments of this kind are presented in FIGURE 4. As described by other investigators, there is generally an increase of the rate of collagen synthesis with increasing cell density. The pattern of this dependence, however, varies between strains, some of them showing an apparently linear increase (e.g., NF II and NF VII), while others exhibit a plateau at high cell densities (e.g., NF VIII, Mm, and Go). A systematic difference between NF and control strains

TABLE 4. Collagen Synthesis as a Portion (%) of Total Protein Synthesis[a]

	Percent FCS	Culture Fluid	Cells
NF strains	0	9.4 ± 5.3 (n = 8)	1.7 ± 0.8 (n = 8)
	10	11.6 ± 2.9 (n = 8)	2.1 ± 0.7 (n = 5)
	20	7.5 ± 2.9 (n = 6)	1.3 ± 0.4 (n = 6)
Control strains	0	10.1 ± 5.4 (n = 7)	2.5 ± 0.6 (n = 7)
	10	12.4 ± 4.3 (n = 11)	1.6 ± 0.6 (n = 5)
	20	9.4 ± 2.9 (n = 6)	1.5 ± 0.5 (n = 6)

[a]Number of strains tested is shown in parentheses.

cannot be discerned. In view of the interindividual variability observed in other series of experiments where collagen synthesis was related to cell density (data not shown),[51] we do not attribute any significance to the fact that in four of the five experiments depicted in FIGURE 4 the control strain achieved higher rates of collagen synthesis than the NF strain at comparable cell densities. This rather seems to be a consequence of the choice of the particular pairs of strains compared.

An additional series of experiments was devoted to the question of whether or not NF influences in some way the ratio of synthesis of collagens type I and III. Five pairs of strains have been compared so far by the method of delayed reduction according to Sykes *et al.*[25] The proportion of collagen III varied in the control strains between 8% and 26%, and in the NF strains between 5% and 26%. Hence, the slightly elevated amount of collagen type III observed in peripheral neurofibromas in comparison with skin by Weber[26] does not seem to have an equivalent in cell cultures.

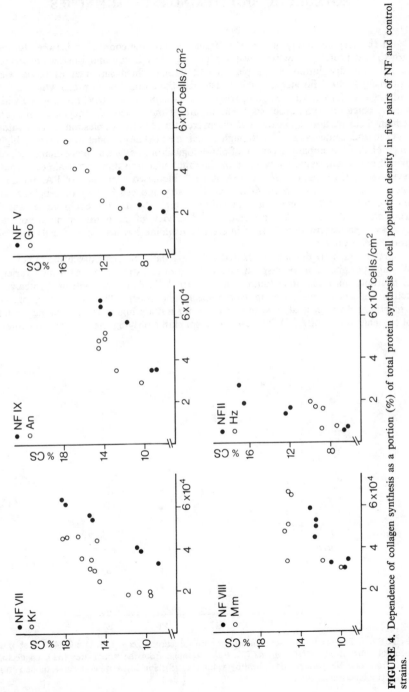

FIGURE 4. Dependence of collagen synthesis as a portion (%) of total protein synthesis on cell population density in five pairs of NF and control strains.

PROTEOLYTIC AND FIBRINOLYTIC ACTIVITIES

At the very beginning of the art of tissue culture, the connection between tumor growth and proteolytic activity was recognized when Carrel and Burrows observed in 1911 the dissolution of the plasma clot within which sarcomatous tissue was cultured.[27] In 1925 Fischer was able to establish the correlation of proteolytic activity with the transformed state by comparing Rous sarcoma virus (RSV) transformed with normal chick embryo fibroblasts.[28] The nature of the proteolytic enzymes, however, remained elusive until Unkeless *et al.* discovered the secretion of plasminogen activator (PA) in this same system.[29] Although it has meanwhile become evident that high levels of PAs accompany a variety of physiological processes which are characterized by cell migration, tissue remodeling, or the functional activation of certain cell types, reviewed by Christman *et al.*[30] and by Reich,[31] increased expression of PAs remains one of the interesting aspects of the biochemistry and cell biology of neoplasia. In some experimental systems the acquisition of high PA activity could be separated from other parameters of transformation.[32,33] In view of the multistep nature of the process of transformation, it is of interest to examine PA activities in cells derived from benign tumors.

Proteolytic activities were measured in homogenates of tumor tissue and of normal skin and peripheral nerve, respectively, and also in cell strains derived from a variety of neurofibromas and brain tumors, using normal fibroblasts as controls. Proteolytic activity in neurofibromas, as measured spectrophotometrically with a chromogenic tripeptide substrate, is at least one order of magnitude higher than in homogenates of normal skin (FIGURE 5). The samples from skin overlying the tumors show inter-

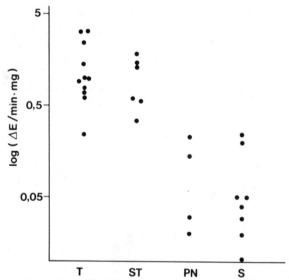

FIGURE 5. Proteolytic activities, measured with the chromogenic substrate S-2444 (Kabi), in neurofibromas from 11 NF patients (T), 6 skin samples from the tumor area (ST), unaffected skin from one NF patient and 7 healthy volunteers (S), and in peripheral nerve tissue (PN). Ordinate: logarithmic scale.

TABLE 5. Ratios of the Proteolytic Activities,[a] Measured with the Chromogenic Tripeptide Substrate S-2444 (Kabi), in the Culture Medium exposed for 24 Hours to NF and Control Cells in the Presence of 5% (v/v) Acid-Inactivated FCS

Patient	Control	Ratio
NF I	Me	1.7
NF III	Si	12.8
NF IV	Ke	2.8
NF VI	Gw	3.6
NF XVI	An	19.3
NF XVII	Ke	5.3

[a]The absolute activities were measured in ΔE_{405nm}/minute $\times$ mg protein.

mediate activities. The substrate (S-2444, Kabi, Stockholm) is specifically designed for the measurement of urokinase activity, but it is also hydrolyzed by trypsin. The proteolytic activities determined in the tumor homogenates cannot, however, be accounted for by urokinase alone which is presumably contributed by the macrophages. The potent inhibitor of PA, p-nitrophenylguanidinobenzoate (NPGB), reduces the proteolytic activity of the tumor homogenates more drastically than that of human urokinase. The same is true for the inhibition with sodium chloride. Furthermore, similar relationships between the activities of the various samples are obtained when leucine nitranilide is used as a substrate, with which urokinase does not react.

When serum-free medium was assayed by the spectrophotometric method after exposure to confluent cultures for 24 or 48 hours, no proteolytic activity could be detected. In the presence of 5% acid-inactivated FCS, both kinds of strains (NF and controls) showed highly variable activities, but most of the NF strains produced higher amounts of protease irrespective of absolute activity (TABLE 5). About half of this activity was dependent on the presence of plasminogen. In contrast to the neurofibroma-derived strains, cultures derived from a solitary peripheral schwannoma and those from an acousticus neurinoma secreted spectrophotometrically detectable amounts of proteolytic activity also into serum-free medium.

With the plasminogen-dependent fibrinolytic assay according to Unkeless et al.,[29] it was possible to detect activity also in serum-free culture medium. Individual strains of fibroblasts, however, secreted highly variable amounts of fibrinolytic activity into the medium. Therefore, the sum of the activities in the medium and in the cell lysate was used as a more reliable parameter for the comparison of NF and control strains. The data of TABLE 6 show that the relationship between NF and control strains concerning proteolysis (as measured spectrophotometrically) is also reflected in the level of fibrinolysis: most of the NF strains exhibit higher activities than the control strains. Also in this semiquantitative test, cell cultures derived from a variety of glial brain tumors (one astrocytoma, grade III; three glioblastoma multiforme; and one meningeoma) and those from a solitary peripheral schwannoma produce activities higher by at least an order of magnitude than the activities of the NF strains. Very high PA activity was also observed by Liepkalns et al. in a clonal cell line from a glioblastoma multiforme,[34] and Wilson et al. identified by electrophoretic and immunological methods the predominant type of PA produced by cell lines grown from a variety of glial brain tumors.[35]

The FLC growing from neurofibromas of NF patients thus exhibit proteolytic and fibrinolytic activities intermediate between those of cultures from other kinds of glial

TABLE 6. Ratios of the Fibrinolytic Activities[a] of NF and Control Strains

Patient	Control	Type of Culture Flask[b]	Ratio
NF II	Hz	N	5.90
NF II	Hz	P	1.11; 1.95
NF VII	Kr	P	2.47
NF VIII	Mm	P	1.89
NF IX	An	N	1.32
NF IX	An	P	1.05
NF XVII	Ke	N	3.63
NF XVII	Ke	P	2.24
NF VIII	To	P	1.64; 1.89
NF XIX	Gi	N	1.72
NF XIX	Gi	P	1.13
NF XX	Go	N	2.71
NF XX	Go	P	5.78

[a]The absolute activities were measured by the semiquantitative fibrinolytic assay and expressed as cpm per μg protein per hour; the values of the table are based on the sums of the activities of the serum-free culture medium and the cell lysate. Cultures were exposed for 24 hours to the serum-free medium.

[b]N, culture flasks from Nunc (Denmark); P, primaria flasks from Falcon, Becton Dickinson, Heidelberg.

tumors and those of normal fibroblasts. In view of the low rate of survival of Schwann cells during the early passages of our cultures and the inability of macrophages to divide under our conditions of cell culture, it seems unlikely that these cells contribute significantly to the increased PA activities of the NF cell cultures. This is only to be expected in primary cultures where, as described above, the rounding of the explants and areas of local detachment and contraction of the cell layer indicate proteolytic activity. We rather consider the elevated PA activity of the NF cells a biochemical corollary of their generally deviant properties, which are also expressed by their conspicuously altered morphology. Comparison with their normal counterparts which may be components of the endo- or the perineurium, respectively, would help to interpret our results. That the PA-plasmin system also functions in the normal nervous system has for instance been shown by Kalderon, who found a mitogenic response to plasminogen, elicited by its conversion to plasmin, in dissociated chick embryo spinal cord cells;[36] while Krystosek and Seeds, using the fibrin overlay assay, demonstrated the expression of PA in neurons and Schwann cells from mouse dorsal root ganglia.[37] With the same technique, Smokovitis and Astrup detected PA activity in the perineurium and the interfascicular epineurium of mammalian peripheral nerves.[38]

CYTOSKELETAL PROTEINS

The composition of the cytoskeleton manifests a certain degree of cell type specificity. This pertains particularly to the type of intermediary filament (IF) protein that is expressed.[39–41] Analysis of the components of the IF by immunocytochemical and/or electrophoretic methods has become a widely used means of identification of cell types and of the origin of tumors.[42-44] The discovery that a large part of the cytoskeletal proteins remains insoluble when cells are extracted with a nonionic detergent under carefully controlled conditions[45] has opened a relatively simple way to analyze the composition of the cytoskeleton by methods of protein separation. The most prominent bands on one-dimensional gradient gels of the so-called triton skeleton of FL cells are those of vimentin and actin (FIGURE 6). Among the less intense bands there are two heavier components migrating at 97 kD and 63 kD, respectively. Eleven of 14 cytoskeletal preparations of cultures grown from peripheral neurofibromas contain one or two additional bands at the molecular weights of 73 and/or 83 kD,

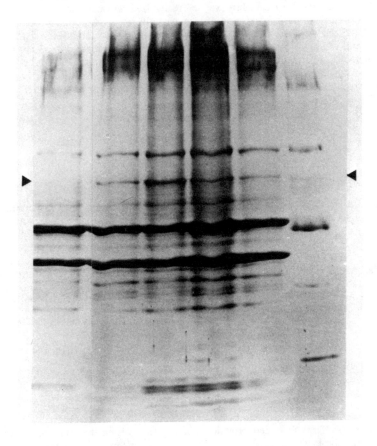

To   NF1   Gb1   NF10   NF10   MWS
(1/2)

FIGURE 6. Representative example of the separation of the components of the cytoskeleton on an exponential sodium dodecyl sulfate-polyacrylamide gradient gel. To, control (chosen from the few that shown the very faint band at 83 kD); NF1 and NF10, early passage cell cultures from neurofibromas of two NF patients; Gb1, culture from a glioblastoma multiforme; MWS, molecular weight standards.

respectively. To our surprise, one or both of these components could regularly be detected as comparatively conspicuous bands in the triton skeleton of cells growing from a variety of glial brain tumors. Cultures derived from a solitary peripheral schwannoma also exhibit one of these components. At comparable amounts of protein applied to the gels, a faint band corresponding to one or the other of these two components could also be detected in the cytoskeletal preparations from 5 of 16 control strains derived from healthy donors age and sex matched to the NF patients. Upon two-dimensional separation according to O'Farrell et al.,[46] the material can be located at the acidic side of vimentin; it does not seem to be a glycoprotein and thus is probably not homologous to the 85 kD glycoprotein shown recently to remain associated with the triton skeleton of baby hamster kidney (BHK) cells by Tarone et al.[47] Similar components can, however, be recognized on one- and two-dimensional gels prepared from the cytoskeleton of primary cultures of astrocytes of neonatal rat brain by Ciesielski-Treska et al.[48] The occurrence of these components of the cytoskeleton in most NF cell cultures and in cultures from astrocytomas, glioblastomas, neurinomas, and meningeomas suggests that these cultures have a type of cell in common which remains to be identified. We could not confirm the quantitative differences between the amounts of components of the cytoskeleton from skin fibroblasts and NF cells reported by Peltonen et al.[49]

TRANSFECTION ASSAYS

In order to test for the presence of an activated oncogene in neurofibromas, in other glial tumors, and in cell cultures derived therefrom, transfection assays were performed with the rat cell line 208F as a recipient. Among the DNA preparations from two glioblastomas, one oligodendroglioma, one acousticus neurinoma, one meningeoma, and one peripheral neurofibroma, only those from the two glioblastomas yielded transformed foci, part of which were propagated in soft-agar culture. None of the DNA preparations isolated from a total of 21 primary transfectants scored positive for the presence of a human Alu sequence when tested with the BLUR-8 probe by Southern blotting.

CONCLUSIONS

1. Most cell strains growing from neurofibromas differ morphologically from normal skin fibroblasts, but their growth properties vary within the same range as those of normal fibroblasts.

2. NF cells show normal sensitivity to x-ray irradiation and their colony-forming ability responds normally to treatment with mitomycin C. A slightly increased sensitivity to 4-nitroquinolin-N-oxide remains to be confirmed by more extensive experiments.

3. Collagen synthesis and its dependence on cell population density and on serum concentration are normal in NF cells, as is the ratio of synthesis of collagens type I to type III.

4. Many but not all NF strains (from neurofibromas) produce higher amounts of plasminogen activator than do fibroblasts from healthy donors.

5. Most strains of NF cells have additional components in their cytoskeleton (73 and/or 83 kD) which also occur in cultures derived from glial brain tumors.

6. Attempts at detecting by transfection assay a transforming gene in DNA from a neurofibroma, from a variety of other glial tumors, and from cell cultures of three neurofibromas are so far unsuccessful.

REFERENCES

1. BOVERI, T. 1914. Zur Frage der Entstehung maligner Tumoren. G. Fischer Verlag. Jena, Germany

2. JACKSON, J. L., K. K. SANFORD & P. B. DUNN. 1970. J. Nat. Cancer Inst. **45:** 11-21.

3. CRAVIOTO, H. & R. LOCKWOOD. 1969. Acta Neuropathol. Berlin **12:** 141-157.

4. ZELKOWITZ, M. 1980. Adv. Neurol. **29:** 67-75.

5. PELTONEN, J., H. AHO, U. K. RINNE & R. PENTTINEN. 1983. Acta Neuropathol. Berlin **61:** 275-282.

6. KRONE, W., G. JIRIKOWSKI, O. MÜHLECK, H. KLING & H. GALL. 1983. Hum. Genet. **63:** 247-251.

7. KRONE, W., S. ZÖRLEIN & R. MAO. 1981. Hum. Genet. **58:** 188-193.

8. COX, R. & W. K. MASSON. 1974. Int. J. Radiat. Biol. **26:** 193-196.

9. ZELKOWITZ, M. & J. STAMBOULY. 1981. Pediatr. Res. **15:** 290-293.

10. NOVE, J., J. B. LITTLE, R. R. WEICHSELBAUM, W. W. NICHOLS & E. HOFFMAN. 1979. Cytogenet. Cell Genet. **24:** 176-184.

11. SCUDIERO, D. A., A. N. MOSHELL, R. G. SCARPINATO, S. A. MEYER, B. E. CLATTERBUCK, R. E. TORONE & J. H. ROBBINS. 1982. J. Invest. Dermatol. **78:** 234-238.

12. PATERSON, M. C., B. M. SELL, B. P. SMITH & N. T. BECH-HANSEN. 1982. Radiat. Res. **90:** 260-270.

13. PATERSON, M. C., P. J. SMITH, N. T. BECH-HANSEN, B. P. SMITH & B. M. SELL. 1979. *In* Proceedings of the 6th International Congress of Radiation Research. S. Okada, M. Imamura, T. Terashima & H. Yamaguchi, Eds.: 484-495. Toppan Printing Co. Ltd. Tokyo, Japan.

14. MAO, R., W. KRONE, W. NOTHDURFT, A. REISACHER & H. GALL. 1985. Arch. Dermatol. Res. **277:** 439-443.

15. SCHWENN, M. R., R. R. WEICHSELBAUM & J. B. LITTLE. 1985. Mutat. Res. **142:** 55-58.

16. WEBER, K. & O. BRAUN-FALCO. 1972. Der Hautarzt **23:** 116-122.

17. JUNQUEIRA, L. C. U., G. S. MONTES, D. KAUPERT, K. M. SHIGIHARA, T. M. BOLONHANI & R. M. KRISZTAN. 1981. J. Neuropathol. Exp. Neurol. **40:** 123-133.

18. PELTONEN, J., H. AHO, T. HALME, K. NÄNTÖ-SALONEN, M. LEKTO, J.-M. FOIDART, V. DUANCE, A. VAHERI & R. PENTTINEN. 1984. Acta Pathol. Microbiol. Immunol. Scand. Sect. A **92:** 345-352.

19. WEBER, L. & T. KRIEG. 1984. Arch. Dermatol. Res. **276:** 335-337

20. HATA, R.-J. & B. PETERKOFSKY. 1977. Proc. Nat. Acad. Sci. USA **74:** 2933-2937.

21. SANDARRAJ, N. & R. L. CHURCH. 1978. FEBS Lett. **85:** 47-51.

22. KAMINE, J. & H. RUBIN. 1977. J. Cell. Physiol. **92:** 1-12.

23. PINNELL, S. R. 1982. J. Invest. Dermatol. **79:** 733-765.

24. PETERKOFSKY, B. & R. F. DIEGELMANN. 1971. Biochemistry **10:** 988-994.

25. SYKES, B., B. PUDDLE, M. FRANCIS & R. SMITH. 1976. Biochem. Biophys. Res. Commun. **72:** 1472-1480.

26. WEBER, L. Personal communication.

27. CARREL, A. & M. T. BURROWS. 1911. J. Exp. Med. **13:** 571-581.

28. FISCHER, A. 1925. Arch. Mikr. Anat. Entwicklungsmech. **104:** 210-261.

29. UNKELESS, J. C., A. TOBIA, L. OSSOWSKI, J. P. QUIGLEY, D. B. RIFKIN & E. REICH. 1973. J. Exp. Med. 137: 85-111.
30. CHRISTMAN, J. K., S. C. SILVERSTEIN & G. ACS. 1977. In Proteinases in Mammalian Cells and Tissues. J. C. Barrett, Ed.: 91-149. Elsevier. New York, N.Y.
31. REICH, E. 1978. In Biological Marker of Neoplasia: Basic and Applied Aspects. R. W. Ruddon, Ed.: 491-500. Elsevier. New York, N.Y.
32. BARRETT, J. C., B. D. CRAWFORD, D. L. GRADY, L. D. HESTER, P. A. JONES, W. F. BENEDICT & P. O. P. TS'O. 1977. Cancer Res. 37: 3815-3823.
33. PEARLSTEIN, E., R. O. HYNES, L. M. FRANKS, V. J. HEMMINGS, 1976. Cancer Res. 36: 1475-1480.
34. LIEPKALNS, V. A., C. ICARD-LIEPKALNS, A.-M. SOMMER & J. P. QUIGLEY. 1982. J. Neurol. Sci. 57: 257-264.
35. WILSON, E. L., M. L. B. BECKER, E. G. HOAL & E. B. DOWDLE. 1980. Cancer Res. 40: 933-938.
36. KALDERON, N. 1982. J. Neurosci. Res. 8: 509-519.
37. KRYSTOSEK, A. & N. W. SEEDS. 1984. J. Cell Biol. 98: 773-776.
38. SMOKOVITIS, A. & T. ASTRUP. 1983. Haemostasis 13: 136-144.
39. LAZARIDES, E. 1980. Nature 283: 249-256.
40. LAZARIDES, E. 1981. Cell 23: 649-650.
41. OSBORN, M & K. WEBER. 1982. Cell 31: 303-306.
42. MOLL, R., W. W. FRANKE & D. L. SCHILLER. 1982. Cell 31: 11-24.
43. OSBORN, M. & K. WEBER. 1983. Lab. Invest. 48: 372-394.
44. MOLL, R., J. MOLL & W. W. FRANKE. 1984. Arch. Dermatol. Res. 276: 349-363.
45. OSBORN, M. & K. WEBER. 1977. Exp. Cell Res. 106: 339-349.
46. O'FARRELL, P. Z., H. G. GOODMAN & P. H. O'FARRELL. 1977. Cell 12: 1133-1142.
47. TARONE, G., R. FERRACINI, G. GALETTO & P. COMOGLIO. 1984. J. Cell Biol. 99: 512-519.
48. CIESIELSKI-TRESKA, J., J.-F. GOETSCHY & D. AUNIS. 1984. Eur. J. Biochem. 138: 465-471.
49. PELTONEN, J., K. NÄNTÖ-SALONEN, H. J. AJO, T. KOURI, I. VIRTANEN & R. PENTTINEN. 1984. Acta Neuropathol. 63: 269-275.
50. DIEGELMANN, R. F. & B. PETERKOFSKY. 1972. Dev. Biol. 28: 443-453.
51. MÜHLECK, O. S., W. KRONE, R. MAO & L. WEBER. 1986. Arch. Dermatol. Res. 278: 232-237.

Hormonal Modulation of Schwann Cell Tumors[a]

I. The Effects of Estradiol and Tamoxifen on Methylnitrosourea-Induced Rat Schwann Cell Tumors

JEFFREY R. JAY,[b] DAVID T. MacLAUGHLIN,[c]
THOMAS M. BADGER,[c] DOUGLAS C. MILLER,[d]
AND ROBERT L. MARTUZA[b,e]

Neurofibromatosis Clinic
Massachusetts General Hospital Cancer Center
and
[b] *Department of Surgery (Neurosurgical Service)*
[c] *Department of Gynecology*
[d] *Department of Pathology (Neuropathology)*
Massachusetts General Hospital
Boston, Massachusetts 02114

Tumors of Schwann cell origin represent the most common clinically important manifestation of neurofibromatosis (NF).[1,2] Prior studies have noted that neurofibromas may develop or enlarge during puberty and pregnancy and that acoustic neuromas and neurofibromas contain cytoplasmic and nuclear binders for sex steroid hormones.[3,4] We postulated that the growth of Schwann cell tumors could be modulated by hormonal manipulation.[4] Since no naturally occurring animal model for NF is presently available, we studied the effects of castration, 17-β-estradiol (E_2), and the antiestrogen Tamoxifen on the onset and growth of Schwann cell tumors induced in rats by parental administration of N-methyl-N-nitrosourea (MNU).

[a] Supported in part by grants from the National Institutes of Health (NS20025, R.L.M.), the National Neurofibromatosis Foundation (R.L.M.), and the Vincent Research Fund (D.T.M. and T.M.B.). Dr. Martuza is the recipient of the Teacher-Investigator Development Award (NS00654) from the National Institute of Neurologic and Communicative Disorders and Stroke.

[e] Author to whom correspondence should be addressed, at ACC 312, Massachusetts General Hospital, Boston, Mass. 02114.

METHODS

Pharmacology of Hormone Administration

In order to determine the optimum method of hormone administration, 48 castrated male CDF rats (Charles River Breeding Laboratories, Kingston, Mass.), 12 weeks of age weighing approximately 225 grams, were injected daily in the nape of the neck with 4 μg E$_2$ (Sigma Chemical Co., St. Louis, Mo.) per 100 g body weight. Corn oil (Fleischmann's, Nabisco Brands Inc., East Hanover, N.J.) was the solvent for half of the group; a 1:1 mixture of 5% ethanol and 0.9% NaCl solution was the solvent for the others. Animals were decapitated at various times after injection, and blood was collected. The serum was extracted twice with 5 volumes of methylene chloride. The organic phase was dried under nitrogen and resuspended in phosphate-buffered saline, containing 0.1% gelatin. Recovery of tritiated E$_2$ during extraction was greater than 80%. Serum E$_2$ levels were determined by radioimmunoassay as previously described.[5]

Tumor Induction

Seventy-one male CDF rats 12 weeks of age were divided into five groups. Sixty animals were castrated; 11 were not. Starting at age 16 weeks, all 72 rats received twice weekly tail vein injections of 10 mg/kg MNU for 9 weeks. All MNU solutions were freshly prepared (5 mg/ml) in 14 volumes saline/1 volume phosphate citrate buffer (pH 4.2).

Hormonal Manipulation

The rats that were not castrated represented the uncastrated control (UC) group. The castrated animals were divided into four groups: castrated controls (CC), E$_2$-treated rats (CE), Tamoxifen (Stuart Pharmaceuticals, Wilmington, Del.) treated rats (CT), and those receiving E$_2$ and Tamoxifen (CET). From the time of the first MNU treatment, both control groups (UC, CC) had daily subcutaneous saline injections. The other groups received the following daily subcutaneous injections according to body weight: CE, 4 μg E$_2$/100 g body weight; CT, 400 μg Tamoxifen/100 g body weight; CET, 4 μg E$_2$ plus 400 μg Tamoxifen/100 g body weight. The rats were housed in individual cages, fed lab chow (Ralston Purina, St. Louis, Mo.) and water *ad libitum*, examined daily, and weighed weekly for the duration of the experiment.

The onset of neurologic deficit was noted, and animals were sacrificed when death was imminent from tumor growth. A complete autopsy was performed. For hormone-binding studies, portions of tumors were immediately frozen at $-80°C$. Other portions of tumor were fixed in 10% formalin, embedded in paraffin, sectioned at 6 μ, and stained with hematoxylin and eosin for histologic study. Some animals died unobserved. These were autopsied, but no hormone-binding studies were done.

Preparation of Cytosol Fractions

Estrogen- and progestin-binding studies (EBc, PBc) were performed on tumor samples. Rat tumors were collected and frozen at $-80°C$. The tissue was homogenized at 40°C in a hand-held tissue grinder containing 2.5 ml of 10 mM Tris HCl, 1.5 mM EDTA, 10% glycerol (w:v), and 10 mM sodium molybdate at pH 8.0. The homogenate was then placed on a 2.5 ml pad of 1.2 M sucrose in an ultracentrifuge tube and centrifuged for 120 minutes at 8900 $\times$ g at 4°C essentially as described by Kelner *et al.*[6] The supernatant was aspirated from the sucrose and recentrifuged at 105,000 $\times$ g in a model L8-50 Beckman Ultracentrifuge for 60 minutes at 4°C. The resulting supernatant was used as cytosol in subsequent receptor assays. The protein content of the cytosol fraction was measured according to the method of Lowry *et al.*[7]

Hormone-Binding Assays

Cytosol from each tumor (0.5 mg/ml protein final incubation concentrations) was incubated for 18 hours at 4°C 20 nM with ^3H-E_2 (91 Ci/mM) or the synthetic progestin R5020 (Promegestone) (87 Ci/mM) in duplicate in the absence or presence of a 200-fold molar excess of unlabeled diethylstilbestrol (DES), or R5020. (All isotopes were purchased from New England Nuclear Corp.) At the end of the incubation period, the cytosols were kept at 4°C in an ice bath and unbound steroid was removed by the addition of dextran-coated charcoal (500 μl of 0.0025% and 0.25% respectively) for 10 minutes with shaking at 4°C. Aliquots (0.5 ml) of the resulting supernates were counted for radioactivity. Specific binding is defined as total binding minus nonspecific binding where nonspecific binding is that seen in the presence of an excess of unlabeled competitor.

Statistical Analysis

The time to death, number of tumors per animal, and the hormone-binding levels were statistically compared between the test groups using a Wilcoxon rank test.[8]

RESULTS

Hormonal Administration

In order to determine an appropriate route of administration of E_2, 24 rats received E_2 dissolved in corn oil and 24 received E_2 dissolved in ethanol-saline. TABLE 1 demonstrates that E_2 in corn oil achieved higher and more sustained blood levels than E_2 administered in EtOH-saline. Therefore, corn oil was used as the solvent for the rest of the study.

Tumor Pathology

Overall, 100 Schwann cell tumors developed in the MNU-treated rats. No animal died of or with such a tumor prior to day 177 of the study. The 100 tumors developed in 50/54 rats surviving longer than 150 days; the four rats not developing tumors were distributed between all of the groups except the noncastrates. Thus, tumors occurred in 93% of the rats surviving 150 days or more.

Schwann cell tumors occurred in characteristic locations. The largest number (53) were found attached to cranial nerves or dorsal roots within the spinal canal or within the nerve foramina; some of the latter had a typical "dumbbell" configuration (FIGURE 1). We termed all of these tumors "central." The 12 benign tumors in central locations were well encapsulated and did not invade the spinal cord, although some cord compression was noted in a few cases. The 41 malignant tumors in central locations all invaded and partially replaced the brain stem or spinal cord parenchyma. While

TABLE 1. Pharmacology of Estradiol Administration[a]

Day	Hour	Corn Oil	EtOH/Saline
1	0	Not done	6.5 ± 2
1	4	903.1 ± 162	36.0 ± 10
1	8	632.4 ± 40	16.5 ± 10
6	0	32.2 ± 14	20.8 ± 14
6	4	776.4 ± 164	38.8 ± 10
6	8	372.9 ± 35	12.9 ± 10
7	0	24.2 ± 10	12.7 ± 3

[a]Castrated male CDF rats were injected daily with E_2 (4 µg/100 g body weight) in corn oil or in ethanol-saline, starting on day 0, hour 0. The first samples were collected 24 hours later, immediately prior to the second injection (day 1, hour 0). Other samples were collected 4 and 8 hours after the second injection. Specimens were also tested before the seventh daily injection (day 6, hour 0) and sequentially afterward. Serum E_2 levels were determined by radioimmunoassay and are expressed in pg/ml as the mean $\pm$ standard error of the mean (SEM).

many of these tumors were recognizable schwannomas, with Antoni A tissue with nuclear palisades, they all had an increased mitotic rate and were more cellular than the benign schwannomas and neurofibromas.

The next largest group of Schwann cell neoplasms (33) was that occurring in peripheral nerves. These presented either as a paresis of one limb, as a subcutaneous mass, or were found during the thorough autopsies as focal mass expansions on major nerves. Those presenting with limb symptoms had nodular masses attached to and enlarging major nerves, especially the sciatic nerve; the skin masses were often large and tended to have cystic, necrotic centers. Tumors were termed malignant if they exhibited markedly increased cellularity, a high mitotic rate, and areas of necrosis; there were 22 of these, 1 of which was associated with an axillary lymph node metastasis. Benign peripheral Schwann cell tumors (11) had the characteristic histological pattern of schwannomas or neurofibromas without these malignant features.

The third group of Schwann cell tumors occurred in viscera. Except for one mediastinal mass, all 14 of these were in kidneys or the urinary tract. All were highly

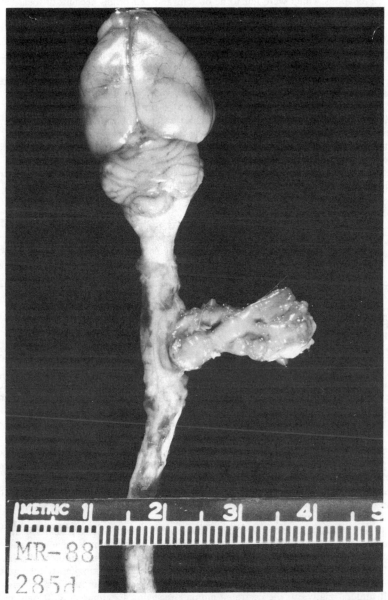

FIGURE 1. This specimen of a normal rat brain and spinal cord demonstrates an MNU-induced Schwann cell tumor of the brachial plexus.

malignant and anaplastic, and were diagnosed as being of Schwann cell origin because of their close resemblance to some of the malignant tumors in central or peripheral nerve locations which were felt to be of Schwann cell origin because of focal better-differentiated areas and their origin from peripheral nerve tissue.

The malignant Schwann cell tumors were found in rats dying or sacrificed from day 177 until day 413. Two of the malignant schwannomas (one peripheral nerve, one central) had focal rhabdomyosarcomatous differentiation ("Triton tumor"). Benign tumors occurred (or were found) with a delayed onset, between days 275 and 413. In all there were 23 benign tumors and 77 malignant tumors, including 14 visceral malignancies.

Other tumors were also noted. One animal in the E_2 group developed a malignant salivary gland tumor at day 10 but had no other tumors at autopsy. Five animals developed brain tumors: two were in the Tamoxifen group at day 111 (grade III astrocytoma) and day 314 (grade III astrocytoma); three were in the E_2-Tamoxifen group at day 268 (grade III astrocytoma), day 332 (grade III astrocytoma), and day 413 (glioblastoma multiforme). One animal had a meningioma; one had a thyroid follicular adenoma; one had a breast fibroadenoma.

TABLE 2. Schwann Cell Tumors Induced by Methylnitrosourea[a]

Test Group	Number Surviving Past Day 150	Average Number of Schwann Cell Tumors per Animal
UC (uncastrated control)	10	2.7
CC (castrated control)	10	2.2
CE (castration + E_2)	11	1.8
CT (castration + Tamoxifen)	11	1.7
CET (castration + E_2 + Tamoxifen)	12	1.0

[a]The average number of Schwann cell tumors developing in each group is shown for animals surviving at least 150 days. There are significantly fewer tumors in the castrated animals receiving E_2 plus Tamoxifen (CET) than in comparable castrated animals receiving only E_2 ($p < 0.004$) or the comparable castrated control group (CC) ($p < 0.04$).

Several nontumor deaths also occurred. One rat in the uncastrated group died of a postinjection hemorrhage on day 28. A similar event occurred to one castrated animal on day 52. A castrated animal died of pneumonia on day 146, and an E_2-Tamoxifen animal died of pneumonia on day 161. Two animals died of unknown causes and had normal autopsies. One was in the castrated group (day 353), and one was in the E_2 group (day 275).

Some animals had more than one Schwann cell tumor. TABLE 2 demonstrates the number of Schwann cell tumors that developed in those animals surviving past 150 days. There was no statistically significant difference between the numbers of Schwann cell tumors developing in the uncastrated, castrated, E_2, or Tamoxifen-treated groups. In contrast, the castrated E_2-Tamoxifen-treated group had significantly fewer Schwann cell tumors relative to the castrated animals receiving E_2 alone ($p < 0.004$) and to the castrated control groups ($p < 0.04$). There were less than in the castrated-Tamoxifen group as well, but this difference was not significant ($p < 0.12$).

The time of development of Schwann cell tumors did not significantly differ between the groups. The median time was 10.1 months for the uncastrated group, 10.6 months for the castrated group, 9.6 months for the E_2 group, 8.7 months for the Tamoxifen group, and 10.6 months for the E_2-Tamoxifen group. There was no difference in distribution of tumors (spinal vs. peripheral nerve), or in the time of death between the groups.

Steroid Hormone Binding

Estrogen and progestin binding were measured only in tumors of sufficient size removed immediately after sacrifice of the animal. Tumors found at autopsy in animals that died unobserved were not analyzed for steroid binding. Sufficient material was present for analyses in 24 malignant Schwann cell tumors and in 5 benign Schwann cell tumors (TABLE 3). Four malignant Schwann cell tumors were sufficiently large to allow testing of several sections of the same tumor. Among the malignant Schwann cell tumors, the castrated control group contained 7 tumors with an average EBc = 30 fmol/mg and with 4/7 (57%) having EBc > 10 fmol/mg. The uncastrated control group had only 3 malignant specimens adequate for testing (EBc = 0, 0, 52.28 fmol/mg), and the E_2 group had only 2 (EBc = 5.482, 26.52 fmol/mg). The Tamoxifen-treated group had an average EBc = 6 fmol/mg with 2/7 (29%) having EBc > 10 fmol/mg. In contrast, those treated with E_2 plus Tamoxifen had a higher average EBc = 32 fmol/mg with all 5/5 (100%) malignant specimens having EBc > 10 fmol/mg.

No cytosolic progestin binding was noted in any of the 3 malignant tumors in the uncastrated control group. In the castrated controls, 4/7 (57%) of the malignant Schwann cell tumors had PBc > 10 fmol/mg; the average PBc for the group was 15.86 fmol/mg. The E_2-treated group had only 2 testable specimens, but both had high levels of PBc (61.33, 176.7 fmol/mg). Both groups receiving Tamoxifen had the least percentage of tumors with PBc > 10 fmol/mg. In those receiving only Tamoxifen, 2/7 (29%) malignancies had PBc > 10 fmol/mg; the average PBc = 8 fmol/mg. In those receiving E_2 plus Tamoxifen, 2/5 (40%) malignancies had PBc > 10 fmol/mg. While the average PBc = 40 fmol/mg, this is heavily weighted by the one specimen with PBc = 175.0 fmol/mg.

DISCUSSION

Neurofibromatosis is a common autosomal dominant human genetic disorder which causes multiple Schwann cell tumors.[9] While most of these are benign, malignant degeneration occurs in 2-29% of patients and is usually fatal.[10,11] Spontaneous neurofibromas have been identified in various animal species,[12,13] but no comparable transmissible genetic disorder has been identified. In contrast, various chemical agents have been used to produce Schwann cell tumors in animals. The most effective of these have been alkylnitrosoureas.[14] Ethylnitrosourea (ENU), when administered to pregnant female rats, crosses the placenta and is carcinogenic to the offspring. While various tumor types may be produced, careful selection of the animal strain, ENU dose, and time of administration in embryogenesis allows the production of predom-

TABLE 3. Cytosolic Estrogen and Progestin Binding by Schwann Cell Tumors[a]

Test Group	Day of Death	Benign (B) or Malignant (M)	Tumor Location	EBc (fmol/mg)	PBc (fmol/mg)
Uncastrated	316	M	Abdominal wall	0	0
Control		M	Abdominal wall	0	0
	323	M	Abdominal wall	55.28	0
		B	Intercostal nerve	5.56	17.84
	337	B	Intercostal nerve	33.28	5.132
Castrated	217	M	Sciatic nerve	0	0
Control	224	M	Abdominal wall	0	0
	241	M	Abdominal wall	0.1130	10.20
	245	M	Lumbar cord	5.462	19.36
	332	M	Chest wall:		
			Edge*	12.19	5.69
			Center*	11.51	20.49
	332	M	Kidney	181.13	0
		M	Chest wall	13.25	68.37
	345	B	Sciatic nerve	3.27	0
Castration +	261	M	Mediastinum	5.482	61.33
Estradiol	337	M	Cauda equina	26.52	176.7
Castration +	177	M	Dorsal root	0	0
Tamoxifen	210	M	Chest wall	0	0
	247	M	Chest wall:		
		M	Edge*	11.806	0
			Center*	0	1.826
	346	M	Back	28.73	21.30
		B	Brachial plexus	7.27	54.65
	317	M	Kidney	0	0
		M	Lumbar cord	0	32.00
		M	Abdominal wall	0	0
Castration +	303	M	Back	12.12	18.53
Estradiol +	318	M	Thoracic cord	101.74+	0
Tamoxifen	323	B	Chest wall:		
			Edge*	3.10	38.93
			Center*	1.96	28.17
		M	Kidney	20.22	175.0
	323	M	Kidney	18.83	1.50
	332	M	Thoracic:		
			Necrotic center*	9.72	6.42
			Edge*	11.24	4.18

[a]Steroid hormone binding was measured in 24 malignant and in 5 benign schwannomas. Four large tumors had more than one sample tested and are marked with asterisks. Neither EBc nor PBc levels differed significantly between the groups.

inantly Schwann cell tumors. Most develop in the trigeminal ganglion and are invasive with malignant characteristics.[15,16] Methylnitrosourea is not effective transplacentally. However, chronic administration in certain rat strains will allow the production of predominantly Schwann cell tumors. These tumors are generally more benign than those induced with ENU, although both benign and malignant schwannomas can develop.[17,18] A comparison of our results with previous studies using MNU indicates a higher percentage of malignant tumors in our rats.[17,18] However, this is largely due to our use of different pathological criteria for malignancy. We termed "malignant" many tumors that were recognizably either schwannomas or neurofibromas but that exhibited mitotic counts and invasive behavior that fit the criteria for malignancy in human examples of Schwann cell tumors.[19] Thus, many of the benign tumors reported in the literature would fall into our "malignant" category.

For our studies, we chose to use MNU-induced rat tumors for three reasons: (1) the development of benign tumors plus malignant tumors more closely resembles human NF than do the very invasive tumors produced by ENU; (2) most MNU-induced tumors occur on dorsal spinal roots and peripheral nerves, similar to human NF; and (3) adult animals of one sex (male) could be used, making hormone administration and determinations more consistent.

In human NF, we had previously hypothesized that female sex steroid hormones might be involved in the modulation of tumors developing in this disorder because (1) neurofibromas usually first appear or become numerous at the time of puberty;[1,2] neurofibromas and vestibular schwannomas (acoustic neuromas) have been noted to enlarge with pregnancy;[2,3] and (3) Schwann cell tumors preferentially develop in the dorsal spinal roots rather than in the ventral roots, and the dorsal spinal cord has been shown to be able to bind estrogen.[20] Therefore we sought to test the effects of estradiol and the antiestrogen Tamoxifen on the development of MNU-induced rat Schwann cell tumors. Female rats were not used because the early production of breast malignancies by MNU can obscure the later development of Schwann cell tumors. Although prior studies of MNU-induced Schwann cell tumors had used intact male rats, we used castrated males to eliminate endogenous gonadal hormones. We therefore had two control groups and found no difference in tumor number or distribution between the uncastrated and the castrated groups.

We found no increase in tumor number after daily administration of E_2, nor did we find that Tamoxifen alone had any effect on tumor number in castrated male rats. However, in those rats receiving E_2 plus Tamoxifen, we found a significant reduction ($p < 0.004$) in number of Schwann cell tumors compared with the group treated with E_2 alone. In comparison with the castrated control group, the reduction of tumor number was greater. We conclude from this study that Tamoxifen reduces the number of Schwann cell tumors when it is administered to E_2-treated castrated male rats, but has no effect in castrated male rats not receiving simultaneous estradiol treatment.

These results are comparable to those of Beniashvili *et al.*[21] Their study differs from ours in several ways. They used albino female rats, administered 10 mg/kg MNU per week throughout the study, and administered estrogen by monthly subcutaneous implant. Yet they found that estrogen did not significantly increase tumor number, but oophorectomy significantly reduced tumor number and prolonged the latency of tumor development.[21] The mechanism of action of estradiol and Tamoxifen in our study is uncertain. We demonstrated significant levels of estradiol and progestin binding in the cytosolic fractions of tumors in all test groups. There were too few benign tumors to analyze. In the castrated control group, seven malignant Schwann cell tumors had an average cytosolic estrogen binding of 30 fmol/mg. In contrast, the Tamoxifen-treated group had an average cytosolic estrogen binding of 6 fmol/

mg. While this suggests a reduction in EBc values in the Tamoxifen group, comparison of the two groups was not statistically significant (p = 0.10).

The group treated with estradiol plus Tamoxifen had an average cytosolic estrogen binding of 32 fmol/mg with 5/5 (100%) of the malignant tumors having EBc > 10 fmol/mg. This was not statistically different from either the castrated control group (p = 0.99) or the Tamoxifen group (p = 0.09). Constraints on tumor size and freshness minimized the number of tumors that could be studied. This was particularly evident in the uncastrated control group (n = 3) and the estradiol-treated group (n = 2). Thus, the statistical comparisons of EBc levels in the malignant schwannomas suggest that lower levels are found in the Tamoxifen-treated group; however, the numbers of tumors assayed were too small in this study to reach levels of statistical significance. Also, too few benign schwannomas could be assayed to comment on hormone-binding levels.

The results of the progestin-binding assays were similarly hampered by the numbers of tumors that could be analyzed. No treatment group significantly differed from another in the level of PBc. However, it is notable that both groups receiving Tamoxifen had the fewest numbers of tumors with PBc > 10 fmol/mg. The Tamoxifen-treated group had the lowest average EBc, the lowest percentage of tumors with EBc > 10 fmol/mg, the lowest average PBc, and the lowest percentage of tumors with PBc > 10 fmol/mg. Yet the number of tumors in the Tamoxifen-treated group did not differ from the number in the castrated control group, suggesting that Tamoxifen, in the absence of E_2, has little effect on tumor growth. In contrast, the E_2 plus Tamoxifen group showed EBc > 10 fmol/mg in all 5 malignant specimens tested, had the highest average EBc level, but only 2/5 malignant schwannomas had PBc > 10 fmol/mg. It is this group that had significantly fewer Schwann cell tumors than the other groups. Thus, in this system it would appear that E_2 must be present for Tamoxifen to reduce tumor number effectively. Moreover, the lower PBc levels in the groups receiving Tamoxifen suggest the possibility that some of the Tamoxifen effect may be through its interaction with the estrogen-estrogen receptor system. However, other possibilities and other interactions of E_2 and Tamoxifen could be considered. For example, E_2 might induce the production of an antiestrogen receptor and Tamoxifen could act via this route. Suggestions for a similar mechanism have been put forth in other systems,[22] and in our results this could explain the necessity for cotreatment with E_2 in order to show the Tamoxifen effect.

A further consideration should be that Tamoxifen may interact with other growth-regulating factors. For example, Vinores et al. have recently shown that infusion of 2.5 S nerve growth factor (NGF) can reduce the number of ENU-induced rat Schwann cell tumors.[23] The possibility that E_2 may interact with NGF is suggested by studies showing an alteration in cells that produce NGF after E_2 treatment.[24]

An additional growth factor that may be important in the development of Schwann cell tumors is glial growth factor (GGF), which is a known mitogen for rat sciatic nerve Schwann cells.[25,26] Recent studies demonstrate high levels of GGF activity in human Schwann cell tumors (Brockes et al., unpublished data). To date, levels of GGF activity have not been reported for MNU-induced rat Schwann cell tumors; however, the possibility that E_2 and Tamoxifen may interact with GGF on rat Schwann cells is worthy of further study.

We conclude that methylnitrosourea produced both benign and malignant Schwann cell tumors in 70% of the male CDF rats in the study and in 93% of CDF male rats surviving 150 days or more, making this an excellent animal model for the study of these neoplasms. Daily administration of Tamoxifen plus estrogen significantly decreased the number of tumors that developed.

REFERENCES

1. CROWE, F. W., W. J. SCHULL & J. V. NEEL. 1956. A Clinical, Pathological and Genetic Study of Multiple Neurofibromatosis. Charles C. Thomas. Springfield, Ill.
2. MARTUZA, R. L. & R. G. OJEMANN. 1982. Bilateral acoustic neuromas: clinical aspects, pathogenesis, and treatment. Neurosurgery 10: 1-12.
3. SWAPP, G. H. & R. A. MAIN. 1973. Neurofibromatosis and pregnancy. Br. J. Dermatol. 80: 431-435.
4. MARTUZA, R. L., D. T. MacLAUGHLIN & R. G. OJEMANN. 1981. Specific estradiol binding in schwannomas, meningiomas, and neurofibromas. Neurosurgery 9: 665-671.
5. CROWLEY, W. F., I. Z. BEITINS, W. VALE, B. KLIMAN, J. RIVIER, C. RIVIER & J. W. McARTHUR. 1980. The biologic activity of a potent analogue of gonadotropin-releasing hormone in normal and hypogonadotropic men. N. Engl. J. Med. 302: 1052-1057.
6. KELNER, K. L., A. L. MILLER & E. J. PECK, JR. 1980. Estrogens and the hypothalamus: nuclear receptor and RNA polymerase activation. J. Recept. Res. 1: 215-237.
7. LOWRY, O. H., N. J. ROSEBROUGH, A. L. FARR, *et al.* 1951. Protein measurement with the Folin phenol reagent. J. Biol. Chem. 193: 265-275.
8. HOLLANDER, M. & D. A. WOLFE. 1973. Nonparametric Statistical Methods: 68-74. Wiley & Sons. New York, N.Y.
9. MARTUZA, R. L. 1984. Genetics in neuro-oncology. Clin. Neurosurg. 31: 417-440.
10. HOPE, D. G. & J. J. MULVIHILL. 1981. Malignancy in neurofibromatosis. Adv. Neurol. 29: 33-56.
11. SORDILLO, P. P., L. HELSON, S. I. HAJDU, G. B. MAGILL, C. KOSLOFF, R. B. GOLBEY & E. J. BEATTIE. 1981. Malignant schwannomas: clinical characteristics, survival, and response to therapy. Cancer 47: 2503-2509.
12. GOEDEGEBUURE, S. A. 1975. A case of neurofibromatosis in the dog. J. Small Anim. Pract. 16: 329-335.
13. MONLUX, A. W., W. A. ANDERSON & C. L. DAVIES. 1956. A survey of tumors occurring in cattle, sheep, and swine. Am. J. Vet. Res. 14: 646-677.
14. ZELLER, W. J., S. IVANOVIC, M. HABS & D. SCHMAHL. 1982. Experimental chemical production of brain tumors. Ann. N.Y. Acad. Sci. 381: 250-263.
15. KOESTNOR, A., J. A. SWENBERG & W. WECHSLER. 1971. Transplacental production with ethylnitrosurea of neoplasms of the nervous system in Sprague-Dawley rats. Am. J. Pathol. 63: 37-50.
16. GROSSI-PAOLETTI, E., P. PAOLETTI, D. SCHIFFER & A. FABIANI. 1970. Experimental brain tumors induced in rats by nitrosourea derivatives. II. Morphological aspects of nitrosoethylurea tumors obtained by transplacental injection. J. Neurol. Sci. 11: 573-581.
17. DENLINGER, R. H., A. KOESTNER & J. A. SWENBERG. 1973. An experimental model for selective production of neoplasms of the peripheral nervous system. Acta Neuropathol. 23: 219-228.
18. SWENBERG, J. A., A. KOESTNER & W. WECHSLER. 1972. The induction of tumors of the nervous system with intravenous methylnitrosourea. Lab Invest. 26: 74-85.
19. TROJANOWSKI, J. Q., G. M. KLEINMAN & K. H. PROPPE. 1980. Malignant tumors of nerve sheath origin. Cancer 46: 1202-1212.
20. STUMPF, W. E. & M. SAR. 1979. Steroid hormone target cells in the extra hypothalamic brain stem and cervical spinal cord: neuroendocrine significance. J. Steroid Biochem. 11: 801-807.
21. BENIASHVILI, D. S., N. G. TURKIIA & V. I. LIAMTSER. 1979. Development of experimental peripheral nerve tumors with hormonal imbalance. Zh. Neuropatol. Psikhiatr. 79(5): 571-575.
22. SUTHERLAND, R. L., L. C. MURPHY, M. S. FOO, *et al.* 1980. High affinity anti-oestrogen binding site distinct from the oestrogen receptor. Nature 228: 273-275.
23. VINORES, S. A. & A. KOESTNER. 1982. Reduction of ethylnitrosourea-induced neoplastic proliferation in rat trigeminal nerves by nerve growth factor. Cancer Res. 42: 1038-1040.

24. PEREZ-POLO, J. R., K. HALL, K. LIVINGSTON & K. WESTLUND. 1977. Steroid induction of nerve growth factor synthesis in cell culture. Life Sci. **21:** 1535-1544.
25. BROCKES, J. P. 1984. Mitogenic growth factors and nerve dependence of limb regeneration. Science **225:** 1280-1287.
26. LEMKE, G. E. & J. P. BROCKES. 1984. Identification and purification of glial growth factor. J. Neurosci. **4:** 75-83.

Clinical Diagnosis of von Recklinghausen's Neurofibromatosis

THOMAS B. FITZPATRICK[a] AND ROBERT L. MARTUZA[b]

[a] Department of Dermatology
[b] Department of Surgery (Neurosurgical Services)
Harvard Medical School
Massachusetts General Hospital
Boston, Massachusetts 02114

The Neurofibromatosis Clinic at the Massachusetts General Hospital has been active now for more than four years. It is quite clear that the problem in diagnosis of von Recklinghausen's neurofibromatosis (VRNF) is the young child with three or more café-au-lait macules. In children, the most reliable diagnostic finding—the Lisch nodules in the iris—is not yet present; these appear after the age of six years and are present in more than 96% of adult patients, as reported by Carey and co-workers.[1,2] Clearly the need for establishing the diagnosis of VRNF is in children when early genetic counseling is most helpful in family planning.

In a study of the genetics of neurofibromatosis, Carey and associates of the University of Utah reviewed the recent data on the criteria for diagnosis of NF in a clinical evaluation of 55 familial cases in 12 Utah kindreds.[1,2] In more than 90% of NF patients five or more café-au-lait macules were present. Of the 45 patients older than age six years, 43 (96%) had multiple Lisch nodules of the iris, which confirmed the value of this physical finding in establishing the diagnosis of NF.

Recent studies on a cell marker for VRNF have disclosed that the so-called macromelanosome is not in fact a large melanosome but an autophagosome merged with a secondary lysosome.[3] This organelle has been renamed a *melanin macroglobule* (MMG). These MMG are present in a large number of diverse disorders (TABLE 1). Nevertheless it has been possible to quantitate the number of MMG in whole amounts of skin incubated with dopa. It has been determined that whole mounts from café-au-lait macules that contain more than 10 MMG per five high-power fields are present only in VRNF patients.[4] Unfortunately this study comprised only VRNF patients older than 15 years of age; thus the question is still unsettled—only in adolescents and adults is the quantitation of MMG proved. A study of VRNF in patients younger than 15 is now under way and this should answer the question, Is the presence of more than 10 MMG per five high-power fields a reliable criterion for establishing the diagnosis of VRNF in children? (See TABLE 2.)

TABLE 1. Melanin Macroglobule in Various Disorders

HUMAN
   Neoplastic
     Dysplastic melanocytic nevus
     Melanocytic nevi (junctional & compound)
     Lentigo simplex
     Lentigo maligna
     Nevus spilus
     Dermal melanosis associated with metastatic malignant melanoma
     Vitiligo-like leukoderma associated with malignant melanoma
     Melanocytoma of the optic disc and the uvea
   Genetic
     von Recklinghausen's neurofibromatosis (in café-au-lait macules and "normal" skin)
     X-Linked ocular albinism (including carriers)
     Hermansky-Pudlak syndrome (oculocutaneous albinism + hemorrhagic diathesis)
     Multiple lentiginous syndrome (Moynahan's syndrome)
     Xeroderma pigmentosum
   Chemical/Drug
     Lentigines following oral PUVA photochemotherapy
   Developmental
     Becker's hairy nevus
   Microbiologic
     Tinea versicolor
   Normal Skin
ANIMAL
   Normal
     Mouse—pallid (hair)
     Rat—scrotum
     Bovine—tapetum lucidum
   Experimental
     Gerbil—DMBA-induced dermal hyperpigmentation and blue nevus-like tumors

TABLE 2. Tentative Criteria for the Diagnosis of von Recklinghausen's Neurofibromatosis[a]

1. Café-au-lait macules
   > 6 lesions with diameter of 1.5 cm or more (adults) *or*
   > 5 lesions with diameter of 0.5 cm or more (younger than five years of age) and melanin macroglobules, > 10 per 5 high-power fields in "split" dopa specimens (white adults)
2. Pigmented nodules of the iris (Lisch nodules)
3. Cutaneous neurofibromata (> 3)

   [a] Any one of the three.

REFERENCES

1. SØRENSEN, S. A., *et al.* On the natural history of von Recklinghausen neurofibromatosis. Ann. N.Y. Acad. Sci. (This volume.)
2. CAREY, J. C., *et al.* The genetic aspects of neurofibromatosis. Ann. N.Y. Acad. Sci. (This volume.)
3. NAKAGAWA, H., *et al.* 1984. The nature and origin of the melanin macroglobule. J. Invest. Dermatol. **83:** 134.
4. MARTUZA, R., *et al.* 1985. Melanin macroglobules as a cellular marker of neurofibromatosis: a quantitative study. J. Invest. Dermatol. **85:** 347-350.

Neurofibromatosis in the Bicolor Damselfish (*Pomacentrus partitus*) as a Model of von Recklinghausen Neurofibromatosis[a]

MICHAEL C. SCHMALE,[b] GEORGE T. HENSLEY,[c]
AND LANNY R. UDEY[d]

[b] Division of Biology and Living Resources
Rosenstiel School of Marine and Atmospheric Science
University of Miami
4600 Rickenbacker Causeway
Miami, Florida 33149-1098

[c] Department of Pathology
[d] Department of Microbiology and Immunology
School of Medicine
University of Miami
Miami, Florida 33136

Von Recklinghausen neurofibromatosis (NF) has been reported to have an incidence of 1 in 3000 individuals.[1] Although NF is established to be an autosomal dominant disorder, fully half of the known cases are attributed to new mutations.[2] In spite of the high incidence and the extensive clinical experience with NF, little is known about the etiology, early patterns of development, or the reasons for malignant transformation of associated tumors in this disease. An understanding of the variability in expression and rates of progression of the disease has been particularly elusive. A major limitation on experimental research on NF is the absence of a suitable animal model of this disease.[2]

Although Schwann cell-derived tumors have been observed sporadically in various mammalian species, none appears regularly or at high incidence.[3] The induction of Schwann cell tumors in mice via transplacental exposure to ethylnitrosourea[4] and the examination of several types of heritable Schwann cell disorders, such as dystrophia muscularis,[5] have contributed to the understanding of irregularities in Schwann cell development and function, yet none of these lesions is comparable to those of neurofibromatosis.

A wide variety of neoplastic diseases have been reported in fishes.[6] Perhaps the most common of these are peripheral nerve sheath tumors.[7] The majority of tumors represent isolated occurrences. However, several examples of high incidences of such

[a] This research was supported by an institutional grant from the American Cancer Society, a contract from the Sanctuary Programs Division of the National Oceanic and Atmospheric Administration (NA82-AAA02794), and a grant from the National Institute of Neurological and Communicative Disorders and Stroke of the National Institutes of Health (NS21997).

lesions have been reported in fish populations. Schlumberger described both neurofibromas and schwannomas from a population of goldfish in a pond in Cleveland, Ohio.[8] Lucké reported a high incidence of neurofibromas in several species of snapper (lutjanidae) from Florida reefs.[9] In addition, several types of pigment cell tumors have been reported in fishes,[10,11] some of which may also involve proliferating Schwann cells.

In the past five years we have investigated the histopathology, development, and geographic distribution of Schwann cell tumors in the bicolor damselfish, *Pomacentrus partitus*, from Florida reefs. A major objective of this research has been to determine the applicability of these tumors to basic research on neoplastic diseases, particularly NF. An initial step in evaluating the potential usefulness of this disorder as a model of NF was to document the patterns and rates of development of the lesions in affected fish.

SPECIES AND DISEASE CHARACTERISTICS

The bicolor damselfish is a common species on reefs throughout Florida, the Bahamas, and the Caribbean. Individuals reach sexual maturity at a total length of 60-70 mm and obtain a maximum size of about 85 mm. These fish are omnivores, feeding primarily on zooplankton, phytoplankton, and benthic algae. Both adults and juveniles are highly territorial and rarely move more than about 10 m from the centers of their territories. The social behavior of this species has been extensively studied.[12,13]

Numerous bicolor damselfish on Florida reefs were observed to exhibit multiple pigmented and nonpigmented lesions of the skin and fins. Histological examinations demonstrated that these fish were affected with multiple, widely disseminated Schwann cell tumors.[14] The pattern of proliferation of most of these tumors was identical to that observed in neurofibromas. They were characterized by an enlargement of the diameter of the nerve as a result of Schwann cell proliferation throughout the nerve.[15] This proliferation was accompanied by excessive collagen production and a decrease in detectable myelin concentrations.

A survey of all major reef populations of *P. partitus* in South Florida demonstrated a high prevalence of the disease in adult fish. Only about 1% of the diseased fish observed were considered to be sexually immature (subadult). Prevalence rates of the disease ranged from 0.3 to 24% of the adults in these populations, with the exception of one disease-free population.[15]

METHODS

Field and laboratory studies were conducted to document the patterns and approximate rates of development of this disease. The gross anatomy of the development of these lesions was monitored in affected fish both in the laboratory and in the field. Histological changes were investigated in tumors at various points in disease development

A disease-staging system was developed in order to characterize the severity of the disease in individual fish. Grouping cases into discrete categories, or stages, facilitated quantification of the progression of the disease, both within individuals and through populations.

Laboratory observations of disease development were conducted using 92 diseased *P. partitus* collected on Florida reefs. Fish were collected using an anesthetic mixture of 10% quinaldine and 90% ethanol. The anesthetic had no detectable side effects and significantly reduced the trauma of capture. Fish were maintained in 37 liter aquaria that were either open systems with flowing seawater or closed systems with undergravel filtration. Salinity was maintained at 30-38 ppt and temperature at 21-27°C. Fish were fed frozen brine shrimp daily.

These individuals were closely observed and photographed so that changes in the external appearance of tumors could be documented until death. These observations were essential to developing a disease-staging system that could be used in the field.

Several fish were also sacrificed for histological studies at various points in disease development. Fish were cut into blocks by making several cross-sectional cuts. This allowed preparation of complete cross-sections at various levels of the fish so that the orientation of tissues and internal organs was undisturbed. Preservation, decalcification, paraffin embedding, and hematoxalin and eosin staining of sections were conducted using standard techniques.[16]

Additional information on the orientation of tumors to specific branches of the peripheral and cranial nervous systems was provided by clearing and staining whole or hemisectioned fish. This technique utilized digestion in a buffered trypsin solution with subsequent glycerol impregnation to render the fish transparent. Before final clearing, Sudan Black B was used to stain the entire central and peripheral nervous systems.[17]

The disease-staging system developed for the present study utilized a scoring system based on the size and location of externally visible tumors on specific areas of the body. The body surface was subdivided into six areas: the head region (forward of the pectoral fins), the caudal peduncle, the remaining body surface, the caudal fin, the dorsal and anal fins, and the pectoral and pelvic fins. The choice of subdivisions was based on ease of rapid categorization of the tumors. Each of the body areas was scored as having either no visible tumors, few tumors (less than 10% of the area involved), or numerous tumors (TABLE 1). An increase in the numbers of body areas or tumor score subdivisions would have provided more information but would have required an unacceptable increase in observation time to score accurately each diseased fish, when used in the field. Body-area scores were then summed to provide a composite score for each fish that reflected the portion of the body affected with externally visible tumors. These composite scores were then used to group affected fish into discrete categories, or disease stages.

A long-term monitoring program, termed the cohort survival study, was conducted to determine the natural pattern and rate of progression of the disease in fish in the field. For this study two groups of *P. partitus* containing diseased individuals were selected on different reefs in the Florida Keys (Molasses Reef and Grecian Rocks). These two study groups were observed at approximately monthly or bimonthly intervals over a two-year period from September 1981 to October 1983. During each observation period diseased fish were identified and photographed underwater by the senior author. The relocation of such fish was feasible due to their extreme territoriality. The identity of individual diseased fish was confirmed from month to month by detailed comparison of the distinct patterns of tumors visible in the photographs. The photographs were used to evaluate and score the patterns of externally visible tumors.

Two measures of the rate of disease progression were used in the present study, the survival time of fish in a given disease stage and the time spent in each disease stage (termed the stage duration). Calculation of survival functions utilized the Survival/Life Table Analysis program from the Statistical Package for the Social Sciences,[18] which is based on the actuarial method of Berkson and Gage.[19]

Fish observed in the cohort survival study were included in the analysis of disease development and survival times only if they could be considered to be residents on the study sites. Residency was defined as presence on a given site for a minimum of three observation periods (thus, at least three months residence). Most fish that met this residence requirement remained on the sites for a relatively long period of time (usually in excess of six months) indicating that the emigration rates of diseased fish on these sites were quite low. Studies of healthy *P. partitus* populations have also suggested low rates of emigration.[12,13]

Deaths of diseased fish could not be directly documented due to the efficiency of predators and scavengers on the reef. A reasonable alternative was to equate disappearance of a resident individual from the study site with death. These disappearances were carefully documented by exhaustively searching areas outside of as well as within

TABLE 1. Disease-Staging System for Schwann Cell Tumors in *P. partitus*

A. Six body areas scored for presence of tumors (see text for description of body areas).

Score	Condition
0	No tumors visible
1	Tumors present on less than 10% of body area
2	Tumors present on greater than 10% of body area

B. Body-area scores summed to obtain composite tumor score used to classify disease stage.

Stage	Description	Composite Tumor Score
0	Healthy fish: no signs of tumor development	0
1	Potentially tumored: a single sign of *possible* tumor development	1
2	Early stage: several small but definite tumors	2-3
3	Mild stage: small numbers of tumors on several body areas	4-6
4	Moderate stage: large numbers of tumors on several body areas or small numbers of tumors over the entire body	7-8
5	Severe stage: large numbers of tumors over the entire body	9-12

the study site for the fish in question. Because of the high degree of territoriality in this species, the area searched was large enough that the possibility of emigration beyond it was small.

The time of death was estimated as being midway between the time a fish was last observed and when it was determined to be missing. Time of death could not be determined for those fish still alive at the end of the study. These individuals were included in the analysis as censored observations. For the purposes of calculating survival functions, censored observations were considered to have been withdrawn from the study at the time when the study ended.

The majority of fish were not observed in all five possible disease stages. Many fish were either beyond the earliest stages when first observed or not yet in advanced stages by the end of the study or at their time of death. Survival times were calculated for all fish observed in a given disease stage. A population estimate of this value was calculated as the median time until death for these fish. This parameter was defined as the time at which the cumulative proportion of fish in the group surviving reached 0.50.

A comparison of survival times for each disease stage was made using the Lee-Desu statistic.[20] This statistic is based on calculation of sums of rankings of the survival time of an individual versus that of all the other individuals in a population.

Time spent in each disease stage was calculated for all fish observed in that stage and was termed the stage duration. For an individual fish, time spent in a disease stage was measured from the time a fish entered a stage or was first observed in a stage until the fish died or entered into a higher disease stage. Fish still alive at the end of the study were considered censored observations for calculation of time spent in the stage in which they were last observed.

The disease-staging system was also used in the field to classify the relative severity of tumors in affected fish in different reef populations. A previous study on the prevalence of this disorder on 19 Florida reefs[15] provided an opportunity to classify the disease severity and tumor patterns of 516 diseased fish encountered in the field during that study. Comparisons of disease-stage distributions were made between low and high disease prevalence populations, as these were previously defined by Schmale.[15]

RESULTS

Developmental Stages

Laboratory and field observations of diseased fish demonstrated that the disease is progressive, irreversible, and essentially always fatal. Although some affected individuals showed periods of little change in tumor development, no cases of remission or recovery were observed. In addition, all fish held in the laboratory eventually died from the direct effects of the neoplastic process or from its complications.

The disease was first detectable as one or more hyperpigmented nodules on the skin or fins. As the disease progressed the lesions both enlarged and increased in number, appearing at discrete sites on the body. These spots typically coalesced, forming large areas of rugose, hyperpigmented epithelium.

Affected fish were classified into five disease stages as outlined in TABLE 1, based on the composite body-area scores. Although this grouping system was somewhat arbitrary, it appeared to reflect important changes in the severity of this disease as it progressed from first diagnosis until death.

Fish classified as disease stage 1 were those that showed any abnormal marking that might indicate a site of initial tumor development. These fish showed insufficient symptoms to be diagnosed confidently as being diseased, as these tiny marks could have resulted from other causes such as injuries or parasite infestations. Thus, for the purpose of field assessments of disease prevalence, stage 1 fish were considered to be healthy rather than diseased and were listed as potentially tumored. Only in the cohort survival study, where all such fish were observed over time, could those stage 1 fish that eventually developed diagnosable symptoms be identified. For these fish, stage 1 could be considered the earliest detectable stage of the disease.

Excepting these cohort survival study fish, disease stage 2 was considered the first diagnosable stage of disease development. This stage was defined by the appearance of one or two small, but identifiable, lesions. Disease stages 3, 4, and 5 represented an increasing coverage of the body and fins by the lesions. Stage 5 fish were those in which virtually the entire body was covered with pigmented lesions.

The sequence of development of tumors in one fish from the cohort survival study is shown in FIGURE 1. This individual illustrates a relatively complete progression of disease stages, from the point at which tumors have become visible (stage 2) to the time when the disease has become severe and the tumors widely disseminated (stage 5).

The hyperpigmented lesions produce erosion and distortion in the adjacent bony scales. This process also occurs in affected areas of the fins resulting in conspicuous fin erosion and distortion of the bony fin rays (FIGURES 1 and 2). These lesions were somewhat destructive of cranial bones and connective tissue immediately below the dermis. However, pigmented tumors did not invade more internal areas of the body.

During the early stages of the disease, small neurofibromas also form in peripheral nerves in areas below the dermis (FIGURE 3). In contrast to the tumors that develop in the dermal and epidermal layers, these are typically unpigmented. These unpigmented Schwann cell tumors sometimes reached relatively large size (exceeding 1 cm^3 in volume) and often showed malignant growth patterns. Tumor cells could be seen invading muscle, internal organs, and skeletal structures.[14,15]

The pattern of distribution of both nonpigmented tumors and the larger pigmented lesions could be observed in the hemisectioned, cleared fish stained with Sudan Black B (FIGURE 4a). Detailed examination of small tumors in the dermal areas (FIGURE 4b) as well as larger, subcutaneous neurofibromas demonstrated the nerves of origin of these lesions. Both pigmented and nonpigmented tumors were stained to varying degrees by the Sudan Black B, indicating the presence of some myelin or related compounds in the lesions. The early stages of formation of neurofibromas could be seen as irregular thickening and elongation of affected nerves using this technique.

Unpigmented tumors often erupted through the dermal layers resulting in discrete, externally visible nodules during the later stages of the disease (FIGURE 5). These lesions were observed on all areas of the body except the fins. Such tumors were typically more damaging to individuals than the hyperpigmented ones due to their location and invasive behavior. For this reason, each disease stage was also classified as to the presence or absence of externally visible, unpigmented tumors. Fish without such lesions were termed type A while those showing such erupting nodules were labeled type B.

Because this disorder in the bicolor damselfish involves multiple Schwann cell tumors, including neurofibromas, as well as abnormal pigmentation, we have proposed that the disease be designated as damselfish neurofibromatosis (DNF).

Development Rates and Survival Functions

During the two-year period of the cohort survival study, 67 tumored fish were observed on the study sites. Forty-six of these fish satisfied the minimum residency criterion; 26 at Molasses reef and 20 at Grecian Rocks. Throughout the study period on both reefs, fish that met the residency criterion maintained stable territory locations. There was no indication that fish altered their territory locations as the disease progressed.

A comparison of the survival-time distributions calculated separated for Molasses Reef and Grecian Rocks fish indicated that there was no significant difference (using

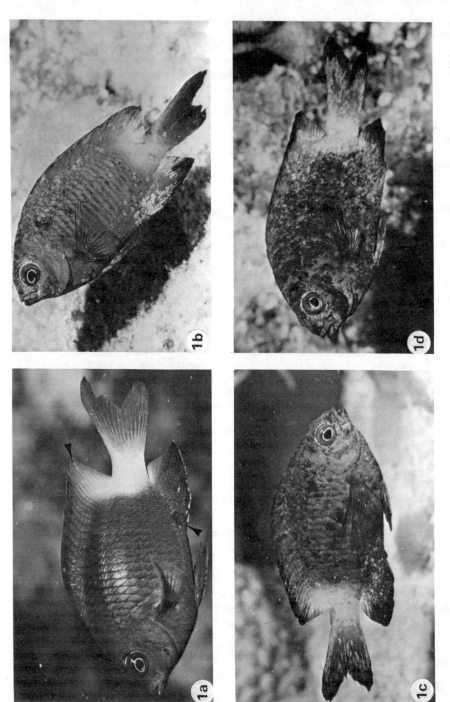

FIGURE 1. Photodocumentation of tumor development in fish no. LMI-32. Photographs taken on Molasses Reef, Florida: (**a**) October 3, 1984—stage 2, note small pigmented lesions (arrows); (**b**) May 25, 1983—stage 3; (**c**) July 21, 1983—stage 4; (**d**) October 16, 1983—stage 5 (all stages were type A—no unpigmented, nodular tumors present).

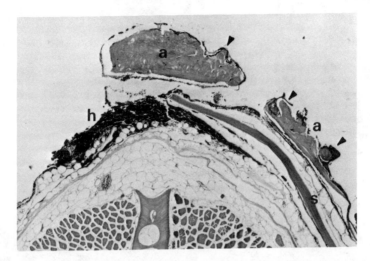

FIGURE 2. Cross-section of body surface and underlying musculature in the area of a hyperpigmented lesion. An area of hyperpigmentation (h) can be seen adjacent to several grossly abnormal scales (a). These scales have been distorted both by erosion and excess deposition (arrows) of bony material. A normal scale (s) can also be seen. H&E, × 100.

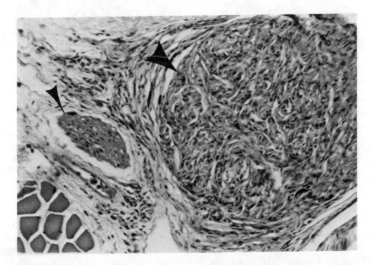

FIGURE 3. Formation of a neurofibroma in a branch of the trigeminal nerve. This illustrates an abnormal proliferation of Schwann cells throughout the abnormal nerve (large arrow), producing an overall enlargement of the nerve's diameter. A relatively normal branch of this nerve (small arrow) can also be seen here. H&E, × 1300.

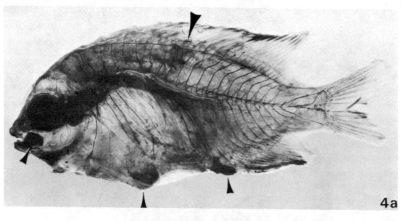

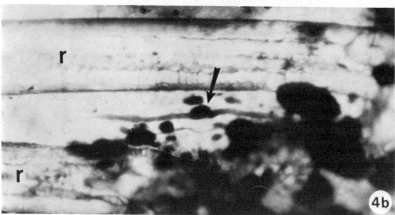

FIGURE 4. Specimen of *P. partitus*, cleared with trypsin digestion, myelinated nerves stained with Sudan Black B. (a) Sagittal section of fish with DNF (1.3×). Note three large, well-stained neurofibromas (small arrows), including one in the buccal cavity originating from the trigeminal nerve. Large arrow indicates region of numerous small neurofibromas. (b) Higher magnification (35×) of area near large arrow in a showing a small neurofibroma (arrow) arising from an abnormally thickened nerve between two bony rays (r) of the dorsal fin. Numerous other small neurofibromas are visible in this area as darkly stained masses.

the Lee-Desu statistic) in these two groups of data. Thus, pooling of the survival and stage-duration times of these two populations was justified for further analysis.

Patterns of mortality were analyzed as the decrease in the cumulative proportion surviving for fish observed in a given disease stage as shown in FIGURE 6. The median survival time can be calculated from these data as the point at which, for each disease stage, the cumulative proportion surviving was 0.50. The sharp drop in survival for stage 1 fish after about 450 days was largely an artifact of the high occurrence of censored observations in this group. Half of the fish that were initially observed in stage 1 were still alive at the end of study and were thus lost to follow-up.

Pairwise comparisons of median survival times were conducted to determine the significance of the disease stages defined in this study in predicting survival times. Significant differences in calculated survival times for different disease stages would indicate that these stages represented meaningful distinctions in the progression of the disorder. This analysis showed that survival times estimated from each disease stage were significantly different from those of the other stages, with the exception of stage 2 (Lee-Desu statistic; $p < 0.05$, TABLE 2). Disease stage 2 showed some overlap

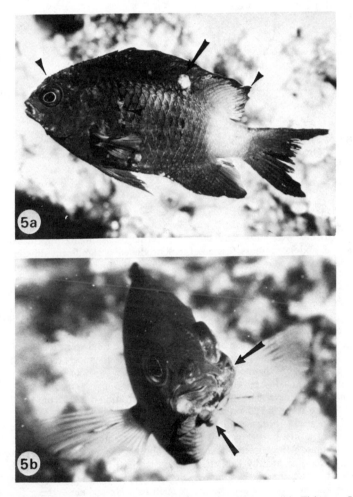

FIGURE 5. Photodocumentation of nodular tumor development: **(a)** Fish no. LM1-02 (Molasses reef, Fla.) showing a single unpigmented, nodular tumor (large arrow) and several small pigmented tumors (small arrows). **(b)** Frontal view of fish no. LG1-22 (Grecian Rocks, Fla.) showing a large number of erupting nodular tumors (arrows), some with overlying hyperpigmented lesions. Note distortion of bones surrounding the left eye as well as the displacement of the eye.

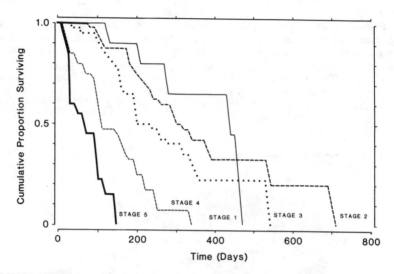

FIGURE 6. Survival times for fish from the cohort survival study observed in the five disease stages. This demonstrates the decrease in the proportion of fish surviving over time in each disease stage.

with both stage 1 and stage 3. This may have been due to a high degree of variability in the survival times recorded for stage 2.

Comparisons were also conducted to determine if utilizing information on the presence of nodular tumors (disease type) produced a significant difference in the survival estimations for each disease stage. Survival times were significantly shorter for type B than for type A fish in stages 3 and 4 (Lee-Desu statistic; $p < 0.05$). Consideration of nodular tumors did not significantly alter calculated survival times for fish in stage 1, 2, or 5. The findings suggest that nodular tumors are predictive of a shorter survival time when they occur at intermediate stages of the disease.

Median stage durations were also calculated as a measure of the relative amount of time spent in each disease stage (TABLE 2). The total duration of disease was defined as the median survival time from first possible diagnosis to death. This value could be estimated as the median survival time of stage 1 fish, or it could be calculated as the sum of the median survival time for a given stage and the median stage durations of all preceding stages. These estimates of total duration varied from median values of 364 to 446 days, based on the data in TABLE 2. The total range in individual survival times was from a minimum value of about 200 days for a fish to progress from stage 2 to death in stage 5 to a maximum of about 700 days.

Unfortunately, because no data are available on the average life span or normal mortality rates for healthy fish, there is no standard for comparison with diseased individuals. Thus, the higher apparent mortality rates of fish in stages 4 and 5 may be an artifact of a greater average age of such fish. Nevertheless, these data indicate that the majority of affected fish did reach the more advanced stages, at a rate indicated by the stage durations, before dying. Of the 46 fish in the study, 63% died when they were in either stage 4 or 5, 11% died while in stage 3, 6% in stage 2, and 20% of the fish were lost to follow-up (alive at the end of the study) while in stages 2 or 3 (TABLE 2).

Relative Prevalence of Disease Stages

Evaluation of relative disease severity conducted on the 516 diseased (or potentially tumored) fish observed in the field during a disease-prevalence survey[15] established that the majority of these fish were present in the more advanced stages of the disease (FIGURE 7). These results also confirm that nonpigmented, nodular tumors (type B fish) were more abundant in fish in stages 4 and 5. However, in rare individuals large nodular tumors developed in early stages.

The study of disease prevalence determined that reef populations of *P. partitus* could be divided into two distinct groups based on disease prevalence: low-disease reefs, having less than 3% of adult fish affected, and high-disease reefs.[15] A comparison of disease severity in these two population groups demonstrated a highly significant difference in the relative abundance of the five disease stages (chi-square; $p < 0.001$; FIGURE 8). The relative proportions of fish with nonpigmented, nodular tumors (type B) within stages 2, 3, 4, and 5 were also higher, although not significantly, in the high-disease populations.

DISCUSSION

Neurofibromatosis has been termed a complex neurocristopathy because of the origins of its cardinal lesions, café-au-lait spots and neurofibromas, in dysgenetic neural crest cells.[21] The disorder described here in the bicolor damselfish also involves abnormalities in neural crest derivatives, the Schwann cells of the peripheral nervous system and the pigment cells of the skin. DNF may also originate from a defect in embryonic development. However, it is also likely that the fish lesions are caused by a mutagenic process occurring in much of the peripheral nervous system subsequent to embryonic development.

No etiologic agents have as yet been discovered for DNF. The primary agents that might produce DNF are a defective gene or genes, chromosomal rearrangements,

TABLE 2. Median Survival Times and Disease Stage Durations for Cohort Survival Study

Disease Stage	Number of Fish[a]	Median Survival Time (days)	Median Stage Duration (days)	Number of Fish Dying in a Stage	Number of Fish Lost to Follow-up[b]
1	10	446	75	NA[c]	NA
2	33	308	79	3	2
3	40	210	115	5	7
4	29	117	70	8	3
5	18	74	74	15	3

[a]Number of fish observed while in a given stage; total number of individuals included in study was 46. Includes fish classified as type A and type B.
[b]Censored observations, alive at the end of the study.
[c]Not applicable—by definition, only fish that were observed to progress beyond stage 1 were considered as diseased and included in the study.

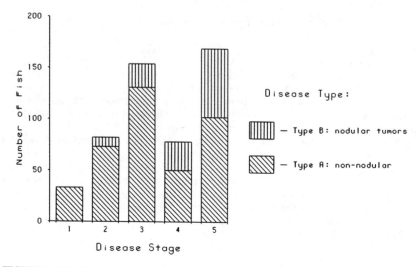

FIGURE 7. Distribution of disease stages for 516 diseased (and potentially tumored) fish observed in a survey of 19 Florida reefs.[15] Disease stages and types as described in TABLE 1.

a chemical carcinogen, or an oncogenic virus. Preliminary field and laboratory studies have suggested that carcinogens are unlikely to be an important factor.[15]

We believe that this disease in the bicolor damselfish may be a useful model of neurofibromatosis regardless of its etiology. In DNF we have the opportunity to investigate all stages in the development of multicentric, disseminated Schwann cell neoplasms. The involvement of neoplastic pigment-producing cells, whether they originate as melanocytes (sometimes termed chromatophores in fishes) or Schwann cells, makes this model additionally applicable to NF.

Teleost fishes have the ability to regenerate damaged or amputated fins rapidly. Diseased *P. partitus* typically exhibit tumors on the fins. Preliminary studies have indicated that diseased fins regenerate with tumors following surgical amputation.[15] This provides a unique opportunity to examine the development of Schwann cell tumors in a regenerating appendage. This will also permit a variety of experimental approaches to the questions of how local nerve supplies and growth factors, such as nerve growth factor and glial growth and differentiating factors, affect the pattern and rate of growth of neurofibromas. Such experiments can be repeated on the same fish because fins will be repeatedly regenerated after each amputation (unless the local nerve supply is destroyed). The potential also exists to examine the effects of experimental denervation on the growth of existing neurofibromas in the fish.

Previous studies have suggested similar structures and cross-reactivity of certain of these growth factors (such as fibroblast growth factor) between mammals and amphibians.[22,23] Thus, the prospect of obtaining useful data on growth factors in these fish using assays developed for mammals seems promising.

Teleost fishes have been repeatedly shown to have strong allograft rejection abilities.[24,25] Further, first-set and accelerated second-set allograft rejection has been demonstrated in this family of fish, the pomacentridae.[26] Thus, this is a potentially useful system for attempting to stimulate cell-mediated rejection of isografted as well as allografted (or xenografted into a related species) tumor tissue. Initial rejection of foreign tissues might be overcome using chemically immunosuppressed fish. Naturally occurring tumors in DNF do not elicit any detectable cellular response.[15] Thus, such studies may indicate if type I and type II major histocompatibility complexes (MHC) determinants are expressed on these cells.

Many of the tumors in DNF are highly invasive of surrounding tissues. Most of these lesions retain the elongate, spindle-shaped cells, oriented in parallel or in whorling fasicles, typical of human neurofibromas.[14] However, some tumors also become very anaplastic and are dominated by relatively plump, pleomorphic cells typical of a malignant schwannona or a neurofibrosarcoma.[15] Any data that could be obtained on the circumstances associated with such transformations might be useful in predicting the course of human lesions because malignant transformation is an important feature of NF.

The involvement of excessive pigment production in DNF is not completely homologous to that in the human disease because the pigment in the fish is found in neoplastic cells in the skin. Nevertheless, the factors responsible for this overproduction of pigment may be very similar in man and in this fish. The rapid spread of hyper-pigmented lesions in DNF may provide an excellent opportunity to investigate mechanisms that control pigment production.

Most cases of NF in man can be diagnosed at birth or shortly thereafter.[27] In contrast, the disorder in *P. partitus* is not detectable until after sexual maturity in these fish, at an age of about 1 to 1½ years. This time of onset may be due to several factors. Lesions could be present from the time of "birth" (hatching), but not be of detectable size. Subsequent development could be a simple result of tumor growth over time or growth stimulated by hormones released during sexual maturation, analogous to the accelerated NF progression during puberty that has been reported

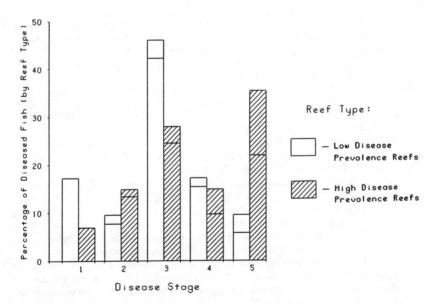

FIGURE 8. Comparison of the relative abundance of disease stages observed on high and low disease prevalence reefs. Horizontal lines on bars (except for stage 1) subdivide each stage into type A individuals without (below line) and type B fish with (above line) unpigmented, nodular tumors.

in man.[2] Alternatively, the lesions may be induced later in life by some oncogenic events.

The genetic features of DNF have not been investigated. Regardless of the initial source of the mutation(s) involved, these may prove to be vertically transmitted. There are several important advantages in studying genetic or vertical transmission in the bicolor damselfish. These animals breed readily in laboratory aquaria, and a single spawning can produce 2000 to 20,000 eggs. The large number of potential offspring from each cross would greatly simplify genetic studies. In addition, it is probable that this fish, as with many other fish species, can be induced to develop from unfertilized eggs providing a source of genetically similar offspring.[28]

The eggs of this fish develop outside of the female and have transparent membranes. These properties allow the easy observation of developing embryos. Such a system also permits the manipulation of embryos by chemical or biological agents at various stages of development. Such procedures have been useful in investigating the relationship of embryonic neural crest development to the occurrence of inherited melanomas in platy-swordtail hybrids.[29]

One potential difficulty in the use of this species for genetic studies is that the larvae are not easy to raise. There is a critical period during the first four to five weeks posthatching when meeting the water quality and food specificity requirements of the larvae is a labor-intensive task. In preliminary experiments, we have been successful in rearing larvae to an age of three weeks. Additional research will be required to maximize the efficiency of raising the fish through this critical stage.

There are several additional aspects of the natural history of this species and the occurrence of the disorder, in addition to the histology of the tumors, that make this a potentially useful model system:

1. *Pomacentrus partitus* are easily maintained in the laboratory because of their small size, simple dietary requirements, and high resistance to disease and trauma.
2. This species is very common on tropical reefs, and virtually all reefs observed in the Florida Keys have shown some incidence of tumored fish. Thus, specimens of affected fish are easily obtainable.
3. The tumor incidence varies greatly from reef to reef with some populations having prevalence rates in the range of 20%. These variations should facilitate the elucidation of factors, such as genetic markers, that may be associated with occurrence of tumors.
4. The variation in relative abundance of severely diseased fish in high and low disease prevalence populations may provide a useful point of comparison to determine factors that affect the rate of development of these tumors.
5. The hyperpigmented epidermal areas appear very early in the disease process so that diseased fish are quite conspicuous at an early stage of tumor development.
6. The restriction of diagnosable DNF to sexually mature fish in nature suggests that hormonal mediation of tumor development may be important in this disorder. This question, as well as questions involving the mechanisms of such a response, could be addressed experimentally using this model.
7. The strongly territorial behavior of this species provides a unique opportunity to document the development of tumors in individual fish in natural populations.
8. The relatively rapid course of development of this disease (approximately one year duration) makes this system particularly suitable for laboratory studies.

Preliminary studies in the laboratory and in the field have indicated that an infectious agent may be involved in this disease.[15] Experiments are currently in progress to test the hypothesis that an oncogenic virus may be involved in the initiation of these lesions. If such a virus could be isolated in DNF, this might allow identification of a new, neural-crest-specific oncogene. *C-onc* genes tend to have highly conserved sequences through evolution.[30,31] Therefore, a damselfish NF gene may be useful as a probe for its human counterpart. This approach with avian *v-onc* and *c-onc* genes has been very successful.[32]

ACKNOWLEDGMENTS

We wish to thank Wade Sheldon for his assistance in preparing the specimens that were cleared and stained with Sudan Black.

REFERENCES

1. CROWE, F. W., W. J. SCHULL & J. R. NEEL. 1956. A Clinical, Pathological, and Genetic Study of Multiple Neurofibromatosis. C. C. Thomas. Springfield, Ill.
2. RICCARDI, V. N. 1981. Neurofibromatosis: an overview and new directions in clinical investigations. Adv. Neurol. **29:** 1-10.
3. MOULTON, J. E., Ed. 1978. Tumors in Domestic Animals. 2nd edit. University of California Press. Berkeley, Calif.
4. SPENCE, A. M., L. J. RUBINSTEIN, F. L. CONLEY & M. M. HERMAN. 1976. Studies on experimental malignant nerve sheath tumors maintained in tissue and organ culture systems. III. Melanin pigment and melanogensis in experimental neurogenic tumors: a reappraisal of the histogenesis of pigmented nerve sheath tumors. Acta Neuropathol. **35:** 27-41.
5. SIDMAN, R. L. & S. V. O'GORMAN. 1981. Cellular interactions in Schwann cell development. Adv. Neurol. **29:** 213-236.
6. DAWE, C. J. & J. C. HARSHBARGER. 1975. Neoplasms in feral fishes: their significance to cancer research. *In* The Pathology of Fishes. W. E. Ribelin & G. Migaki, Eds.: 871-894. University of Wisconsin Press. Madison, Wis.
7. MAWDESLY-THOMAS, L. E. 1975. Neoplasia in Fish. *In* The Pathology of Fishes. W. E. Ribelin & G. Migaki, Eds.: 805-870. University of Wisconsin Press. Madison, Wis.
8. SCHLUMBERGER, H. G. 1952. Nerve sheath tumors in an isolated goldfish population. Cancer Res. **12:** 890-899.
9. LUCKÉ, B. 1942. Tumors of the nerve sheaths in fish of the snapper family (Lutjanidae). Arch. Pathol. **34:** 133-150.
10. TAKAYAMA, S., T. ISHIKAWA, P. MASAHITO & J. MATSUMOTO. 1981. Overview of biological characterization of tumors in fish. *In* Phyletic Approaches to Cancer. C. J. Dawe, *et al.*, Eds.: 3-17. Japan Science Society Press. Tokyo, Japan.
11. KIMURA, I., N. TANIGUCHI, H. KUMAI, I. TOMITA, N. KINAE, K. YOSHIZAKI, M. ITO & T. ISHIKAWA. 1984. Correlation of epizootiological observation with experimental data: chemical induction of chromatophoromas in the croaker, *Nibea misukurii.* Nat. Cancer Inst. Monogr. **65:** 139-154.
12. MYRBERG, A. A. 1972. Ethology of the bicolor damselfish, *Eupomacentrus partitus:* a comparative analysis of laboratory and field behavior. Anim. Behav. Monogr. **5**(3): 197-283.
13. SCHMALE, M. C. 1981. Sexual selection and relative reproductive success in males of the bicolor damselfish *Eupomacentrus partitus.* Anim. Behav. **29:** 1172-1184.
14. SCHMALE, M. C., G. HENSLEY & L. R. UDEY. 1983. Multiple schwannomas in the bicolor damselfish, *Pomacentrus partitus.* Am. J. Pathol. **112**(2): 238-241.

15. SCHMALE, M. C. 1985. Histopathology, distribution, and development of a neoplastic disease in the bicolor damselfish (*Pomacentrus partitus*) from Florida reefs. Ph.D. Dissertation. University of Miami. Miami, Fla.

16. LUNA, L. G. 1968. Manual of Histologic Staining Methods of the Armed Forces Institute of Pathology. 3rd edit. McGraw-Hill. New York, N.Y.

17. FILIPSKI, G. T. & M. V. WILSON. 1984. Sudan Black B as a nerve stain for whole cleared fish. Copeia: 204-208.

18. HULL, C. H. & N. H. NIE. 1981. SPSS Update; New Procedures and Facilities for Releases: 7-9. McGraw Hill Co. New York, N.Y.

19. BERKSON, J. & R. GAGE. 1950. Calculations of survival rates for cancer. Mayo Clin. Proc. 25: 270-286.

20. LEE, E. & M. DESU. 1972. A computer program for comparing K samples with right-censored data. Comp. Prog. Biomed. 2: 315-321.

21. BOLANDE, R. P. 1981. Neurofibromatosis—the quintessential neurocristopathy: pathogenic concepts and relationships. Adv. Neurol. 29: 67-76.

22. GOSPODAROWICZ, D & A. L. MESCHER. 1980. Fibroblast growth factor and the control of vertebrate regeneration and repair. Ann. N.Y. Acad. Sci. 339: 151-174.

23. SCHWARTZ, M., M. BELKIN, A. HAREL, A. SOLOMON, V. LAVIE, M. HADANI, I. RACHAILOVICH & C. STEIN-IZSAK. 1985. Regenerating fish optic nerves and a regeneration-like response in injured optic nerves of adult rabbits. Science 228: 600-603.

24. HILDEMANN, W. H. 1957. Scale homeotransplantation in goldfish (*Carassius auratus*). Ann. N.Y. Acad. Sci. 64: 775-791.

25. ANDERSON, D. P. 1974. Fish Immunology. T.F.H. Publications Inc. Neptune, N.J.

26. HILDEMANN, W. H. 1972. Transplantation reactions of two species of Osteichthyes (Teleostei) from South Pacific coral reefs. Transplantation 14: 261-267.

27. RICCARDI, V. N. 1981. Von Recklinghausen neurofibromatosis. N. Engl. J. Med. 305: 1617-1627.

28. PURDOM, C. E. & R. F. LINCOLN. 1973. Chromosome manipulation in fish. *In* Genetics and Mutagenesis of Fish. J. H. Schroder, Ed.: 83-89. Springer-Verlag. New York, N.Y.

29. VIELKIND, J., H. HAAS-ARDELA, U. VIELKIND & F. ANDERS. 1982. The induction of a specific pigment cell type by total genomic DNA injected into the neural crest region of fish embryos of the genus *Xiphophorus*. Mol. Gen. Genet. 185: 879-389.

30. DEFEO-JONES, D., E. M. SCOLNICK, R. KOLLER & R. DHAR. 1983. *ras*—Related gene sequences identified and isolated from *Saccharomyces cerevisiae*. Nature 306: 707-709.

31. GALLWITZ, D. C., C. DONATH & C. SANDER. 1983. A yeast gene encoding a protein homologous to the human c-*has*/*bas* proto-oncogene product. Nature 306: 704-707.

32. WEISS, R., N. TEICH, H. VARMUS & J. COFFIN. 1982. RNA Tumor Viruses. Cold Spring Harbor Publ. Cold Spring Harbor, N.Y.

Enhanced Sensitivity of Skin Fibroblasts from Neurofibromatosis Patients to Transformation by the Kirsten Murine Sarcoma Virus[a]

A Potential Laboratory Assay for Individuals at Risk of Cancer

JACK W. FRANKEL,[b,c] PASCUAL BIDOT,[c] AND
LEVY KOPELOVICH[c,d]

[b] Tampa Branch Laboratory
State Department of Health and Rehabilitative Services
Post Office Box 2380
Tampa, Florida 33601

[c] Cancer Genetics and Cancer Prevention Laboratory
Medical Research (151)
Veterans Administration Medical Center
Bay Pines, Florida 33504

INTRODUCTION

Recent evidence suggests that cellular genes, or protooncogenes, are involved in the malignant transformation of human cells. This evidence is based largely on the identification and isolation of DNA sequences and RNA transcripts from human cells that show homology with oncogenes of tumor viruses, the transforming activity of these genes in the NIH/3T3 transfection assay, and their effect on neodifferentiation.[1-6] For instance, a significant proportion of human tumor cells contain activated *ras* genes.[1,3,5] However, little is known about how either the transforming or the normal *ras* gene regulates the expression of tissue-specific differentiation genes.[6-9]

Perturbation of human cells by tumor viruses has been used to examine genetic determinants associated with cancer predisposition. Enhanced viral transformation of cultured skin fibroblasts (SF) has been demonstrated in individuals with certain autosomal dominant disorders that predispose to cancer. For example, individuals

[a] This work was supported in part by Grants CA 31597 (L.K.) and CA 29277 (J.W.F.) from the National Cancer Institute, and by funds from the Veterans Administration, VAMC, Bay Pines, Florida.

[d] To whom correspondence should be addressed.

with hereditary adenomatosis of the colon and rectum (ACR), its variant the Gardner's syndrome (GS), bilateral retinoblastoma (RB), and neurofibromatosis (NF) all show increased sensitivity to transformation by the Kirsten murine sarcoma virus (KiMSV).[9–16] Cultured SF from individuals with lung cancer are also more susceptible to transformation by KiMSV.[17] In addition, SF from ACR, GS, and NF were shown to have increased sensitivity to transformation by Simian virus 40 (SV40) (NF; Kopelovich, L., unpublished).[11,18,19] In contrast, SF from individuals with Huntington's disease, which is an autosomal dominant trait without predisposition to cancer, are not abnormally sensitive to transformation by KiMSV.[20] Thus, considerable specificity has been demonstrated through the use of viral probes, the k-*ras* oncogene in particular, for the cancer trait in heritable forms of cancer and in the general population.

It would appear, therefore, that cancer traits can be diagnosed at present through the use of cells derived from cancer-prone individuals.[21–27] The ability to detect persons predisposed to cancer actually implies that in such instances individuals whose clinical symptoms are unclear or gene carriers who are otherwise clinically asymptomatic can, nevertheless, be identified through laboratory probes. The characterization of cells derived from cancer-prone individuals provides a measure of the extent to which such cells differ from the normal phenotype (cancer initiation).[21–27] Properly selected biological and biochemical traits, while presumably not specific for a given form of cancer, represent the highest possible amplification level of the cancer trait. This approach facilitates the monitoring of interacting cancer-causing genes in all premutations as well as their modulation by other genes as it might occur *in situ*.[24–27] Implicit in these observations is the fact that predisposition to cancer, *at present*, can best be detected as a global syndrome at the phenotypic level.[24–28] Therefore, studies on specific forms of cancer should be conducted in the context of pedigrees known to express the cancer trait strongly for a given type(s) of cancer. They include autosomal dominant syndromes that predispose to cancer, familial aggregates for cancer, and a fraction of the sporadic forms of cancer as well.[24–27]

Neurofibromatosis is an autosomal dominant trait with both developmental and neoplastic features.[29] Although it occurs with high incidence, gene expression is variable and the clinical symptoms are phenotypically complex.[29] There is also a high fraction of new NF mutations. Therefore, problems exist in diagnosing NF. Preliminary results from this laboratory showed increased sensitivity of cultured cells from NF patients to transformation by KiMSV.[15,16] Here, we have summarized results on the differential sensitivity of about 150 SF cultures to transformation by KiMSV. We have demonstrated that SF from symptomatic gene carriers and a fraction of the clinically asymptomatic members within NF pedigrees were abnormally sensitive to transformation (about 10- to 1000-fold) by KiMSV. We suggest that this laboratory assay, together with the clinical data, could be used in NF kindreds to further ascertain the NF genotype, including NF cases presumed to represent a spontaneous mutation.

THE EXPERIMENTAL SYSTEM

In the present study we have used cultured cells obtained from cutaneous biopsies of clinically uninvolved skin. By using only cultured skin fibroblasts, we were able to examine a single cell type under reproducible laboratory conditions for presumptive differences between NF patients, their clinically asymptomatic progeny, and normal individuals. Since NF cell strains appear to senesce relatively early (Kopelovich and

Wallace, in preparation), they were regularly passaged at a 1:3 split ratio and used, in general, between the 4th and no later than the 10th passage. This observation may be responsible, in part, for results suggesting a slower growth rate for NF cells,[29] while in fact faster than normal rates have been seen in early passage NF cells (Kopelovich and Wallace, in preparation). The preparations of KiMSV stock virus and viral transformation protocols have been described in detail elsewhere.[10] It is imperative that the virus used in these studies be a KiMSV (KiMuLV). This virus provides well-defined, easily identifiable foci consisting of refractile spindle-shaped and round cells which grow on top of the monolayers, exhibiting cytoplasmic vacuoles.[10] Laboratories using the KiMSV (BaEV) often find it difficult to identify and quantitate the number of transformed cell cultures.[30,31] The KiMSV (BaEV)-induced foci in human cell cultures are small, consisting primarily of fusiform cells barely visible even on day 14 postinfection.[31] Here, the results on virus transformation were obtained at 14 days postinfection and are given as either end-point titration[16] or as log titers (number of foci × dilution factor per ml of original stock virus).[10]

TABLE 1. KiMSV Transformation by End-Point Titration[a] of Cultured SF from Unrelated NF Patients and from Patients in NF Families

Phenotypic Classification	Total Number Tested	< 1	1	2	3	4	Total Positive Transformants 1 and > 1
Symptomatic NF Clinically	37	6 (16)[b]	11 (30)	13 (35)	5 (14)	2 (5)	31 (84)
Asymptomatic NF	46	33 (72)	6 (13)	4 (9)	2 (4)	1 (2)	13 (28)
Normal controls[c]	29	28 (96)	0	0	1 (4)	0	1 (4)

[a]Highest KiMSV dilution (reciprocal $\log_{10}$) inducing transformation.
[b]Figures in parenthesis denote percent positive transformed cultures.
[c]Families without hereditary disorders, or cancer.

RESULTS

TABLE 1 summaries previous experiments carried out on both unrelated and related NF patients, their clinically asymptomatic progeny, and normal controls.[15,16] We were unable to distinguish between the various genotypes at less than 10-fold dilution of the stock virus. In contrast, viral dilutions of 10-fold and greater appeared to give increasingly better resolution, consistent with the increased sensitivity of NF cells to transformation by KiMSV. In fact, through end-point titration by serial dilutions, a relatively narrow cut-off point is reached that identifies cells from NF patients (84% positive transformants) and a fraction of their asymptomatic progeny (28% positive transformants), compared with those presumably free of disease (72% nontransformants) and normal control (4% positive transformants). Given the number of individuals tested and gene expression in NF,[29] the occurrence of 28% positive transformants in the clinically asymptomatic group at the time of assay is, in general, consistent with the expected distribution of an autosomal dominant trait. The incidence of 4% positive transformants is probably related to background transformation frequency found in the general population, notwithstanding the possibility that some of these cells might have been obtained from persons with extensive history for cancer. In fact, the incidence of a positive assay result in the general population could, at times, be as high as about 8% (Kopelovich, L., unpublished).

Current studies on the utility of the KiMSV probe in NF patients using log-titer determinations are shown in TABLE 2. In these experiments the total number of foci per dish was counted and corrected for dilution per ml of original stock virus. As shown in TABLE 2, a value of 4.4 has been found in cells from 10 unrelated NF patients. This value is similar to that obtained in cells from 4 unrelated ACR patients (e.g., 4.6) who were previously shown to be sensitive to transformation by KiMSV[10] and were, therefore, used as positive controls. A value of 3.0 has been observed in SF from a group of 7, age-matched, control persons. Thus using log titers, a difference of about 50-fold appears to segregate between affected NF or ACR patients and normal persons. This margin is, in general, lower than that previously reported to exist in a study of ACR patients (100- to 1000-fold).[10] We have recently found, however, that the extent to which normal SF are segregated from cells taken from ACR or NF patients can be modulated through the potency of the virus (in preparation). We are currently analyzing the genetic determinants associated with potency of the KiMSV (KiMuLV) probe in order to arrive at the best possible resolution for the present assay.

To demonstrate the utility of the KiMSV probe in the context of a known family history, several NF pedigrees were studied (TABLE 3). In pedigree 0 (FIGURE 1), the virus sensitivity test was carried out on clinically diagnosed NF patients only, showing values (log titers) up to 1000-fold above control (TABLE 2). A similar pattern is indicated in a simple example of pedigree F (TABLE 1, FIGURE 2) in which the F1 progeny segregated as would be anticipated from a dominant trait, with the exception of one "false negative" (II F8). Individuals II F3 and II F4 who are positive by the virus assay will be followed closely for any clinical manifestations. Pedigree 11 shows the differential sensitivity of a child (IINF 11) who is supposed to represent a spontaneous case, since both parents are apparently free of clinical symptoms for NF. Thus, cells from the affected child did show high sensitivity to transformation by KIMSV (e.g., 4.3), while SF from the mother who was clinically asymptomatic at the age of 34 (INF 13) also showed considerable sensitivity to the virus probe (TABLE

TABLE 2. KiMSV Transformation of SF from Unrelated NF Patients and Age-Matched Normal Controls

Phenotypic Classification	Number of Individuals	Log Titers[b]
NF	10	4.4 (3.8-4.8)[c]
ACR	4	4.6 (4.0-4.7)
Normal	7	3.0 (2.7-3.2)

[a]Results are given as average of 2-3 experiments in duplicates.
[b]The titer on human SF was expressed as focus forming units per milliliter of original virus stock.
[c]Figures in parenthesis show range.

TABLE 3. KiMSV Transformation of SF from Persons in NF Kindreds

Generation	Individual	NF Phenotype	Age	Sex	Other Cancer	Comments	Log Titer
Pedigree 0							
III	NF 1	+	45	F	—	—	3.5
	NF 7	+	63	F	—	—	5.5
IV	NF 10	+	42	F	—	—	4.5
V	NF 1	+	23	F	—	—	6.1
	NF 5	+	9	M	—	—	3.6
Pedigree F[a]							
I	NF 01	+	—	F	—	—	(1 & > 1)
II	NF 01	−	—	F	—	—	(< 1)
	NF 02	−	—	F	—	—	(< 1)
	NF 03	−	—	F	—	—	(1 & > 1)
	NF 04	−	—	F	—	—	(1 & > 1)
	NF 05	+	—	F	—	—	(1 & > 1)
	NF 06	+	—	M	—	—	(1 & > 1)
	NF 07	+	—	M	—	—	(1 & > 1)
	NF 08	+	—	M	—	—	(< 1)
	NF 09	−	—	M	—	—	(< 1)
Pedigree 11							
I	NF 11	−	38	M	—	—	2.7
	NF 13	−	34	F	—	—	4.7
II	NF 12	+	12	F	—	spontaneous?	4.3
Pedigree 30							
I	NF 31	+	43	F	—	3 stillborn children	4.5
II	NF 32	−	21	F	—	—	4.0
	NF 33	−	26	F	—	—	4.7

[a]Results in this instance are given as positive or negative according to end-point titration; positive (1 & > 1); negative (< 1).[16]

3). These results may suggest that at the time of this study the mother conceivably may have represented a latent case of NF. Another example is pedigree 30 in which the mother (INF 31) at age 43 has been diagnosed as a positive NF both clinically and through the virus assay, while her daughters, ages 21 and 26, who at the time of this study were free of clinical symptoms, were highly positive by the virus probe. They are currently under observation.

These few examples point out the advantage of studying the sensitivity to transformation by KiMSV in the context of a known family history for NF and, indeed, other families at risk of cancer.[23–28] A study within a pedigree provides a better baseline for the differential response of cells from normal family members as compared with those from known patients. In addition, certain cases diagnosed as spontaneous mutation may, at times, represent the lack of expression of the cancer trait by clinical criteria. Certainly, high sensitivity to the virus assay of a progeny to a parent diagnosed as positive NF, both clinically and through the virus assay, warrants follow-up observations of these clinically asymptomatic children. Many such NF pedigrees are currently under extensive investigation in this laboratory.

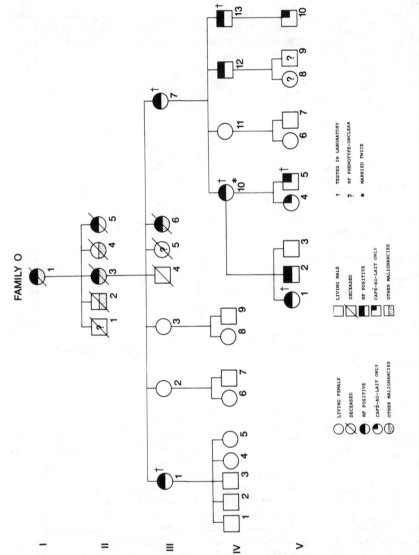

FIGURE 1

DISCUSSION

The mechanisms responsible for the differential susceptibility of NF cells to KiMSV and, indeed, to SV40 are not well understood. The fact that other dominant traits such as ACR, GS, and RB share this property suggests that predisposition to cancer through a dominant mutation is not restricted to a specific clinical form of this disease.[21–27] This observation applies to other laboratory correlates for cancer predisposition as well.[25–28] The role of c-*ras*[ki] or v-*ras*[ki] appears to be related, at least in the case of human fibroblasts, to the effect on "silent" differentiation genes, i.e., other than the gene(s) responsible for the phenotypic expression of a normal, fully differentiated cell type.[6] The number and quality of "silent" genes that are presumably turned on by an activated *ras* gene, and the type of cancer that might ultimately be expressed in a fraction of such cells, will depend on the target tissue and the hormonal milieu (both agonists and antagonists) that regulates this tissue.[6]

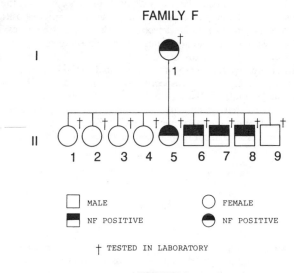

FAMILY F

MALE □
NF POSITIVE ■

FEMALE ○
NF POSITIVE ◐

† TESTED IN LABORATORY

FIGURE 2

The effect of the *ras* oncogenes is apparently not an early one,[6,26,27] since initiated cells taken from cancer-prone individuals do not contain the activated form of this gene.[26,27,32] The increased sensitivity of these cells to v-*ras*[ki] suggests that genetic information, probably in the form of a relatively limited and specific number of DNA sequences associated with the dominant mutation (cancer trait), contributes to the effects by v-*ras*[ki] on initiated cells at higher than normal probability. This type of information, if identified, might represent the earliest event in cancer development.[24–27]

The apparent correlation between SV40 and KiMSV suggests a common site of control and/or interaction at the level of host DNA in initiated cells. In this regard, human DNA fragments with nucleotide sequences homologous to SV40 have been detected in human cells. The existence of such enhancer elements in human cell DNA raises the possibility that families of these sequences may regulate the expression of a variety of human genes, including the NF mutation, much the same way as has been described for SV40 mutants.[33] Whether initiated cells are enriched for, or are more susceptible to, such sequences remains to be established. This presumably can also be illustrated through the overproduction of the transformation-associated host cell coded p53 in unperturbed NF and ACR cells (Kopelovich and Deleo, in preparation).[34] Overproduction of this protein has been previously shown to occur in cells infected with KiMSV or SV40 and in spontaneously occurring human tumor cells.[35–37] The overproduction of p53 in initiated cells prior to any alteration in c-*ras* genes suggests that it might represent an early stage in oncogenesis. Another example is the ability to form tumorigenic human cells *in vitro* through the sequential application of SV40 and KiMSV. Although this was demonstrated for both human fibroblasts[19,27] and epithelial cells,[38] tumorigenicity in the former case was not associated with the acquisition of immortality. In addition, while fibroblasts transformed by these two viruses did form large tumors (1 cm in diameter) subcutaneously, their malignant potential (progressive growth that will result in the death of the host animal) is still under investigation.

Thus, molecular biological considerations support the concept about the utility of oncogenic viruses to understand genetic determinants of cancer predisposition and to establish a role for such probes for the detection of the cancer trait in cancer-prone families. The basic assumptions and strategies for the screening of individuals genetically at risk of cancer have been discussed in detail.[24–27] In our view the ability to distinguish a cancer-predisposed person from a normal individual in a well-defined pedigree (both prospectively and retrospectively) should qualify a test as "cancer specific." This group of individuals should also include follow-up of children and adults who have been treated systemically for cancer and might, therefore, be at an increased risk of developing secondary neoplasms.[26,27] Further refinements in deployment of the virus probes as a laboratory assay for cancer traits are currently under consideration.[6]

SUMMARY

The present work describes a laboratory assay for individuals predisposed to cancer within NF pedigrees. The assay is based on the association between the increased sensitivity of human skin fibroblasts to transformation by the Kirsten murine sarcoma virus and predisposition to cancer in clinically affected patients and in otherwise apparently healthy individuals within NF pedigrees. The more sensitive the cells are to transformation by KiMSV, the greater the probability that a person from whom such cells have been derived will develop cancer. The results show a strong correlation with the NF trait. Together with the clinical data this laboratory assay could, therefore, be used to ascertain the NF genotype.

ACKNOWLEDGMENT

We thank Ms. A. Wallace and Mr. R. F. Rich for technical assistance and Ms. Sue McMahan for typing the manuscript.

REFERENCES

1. SHIH, C., B.-Z. SHILO, M. P. GOLDFARB, A. DANNENBERG & R. A. WEINBERG. 1979. Passage of phenotype of chemically transformed cells via transfection of DNA and chromatin. Proc. Nat. Acad. Sci. USA **76:** 5714-5718.
2. COOPER, G. M. 1982. Cellular transforming genes. Science **217:** 801-808.
3. SHIH, C., L. C. PADHY, M. MURRAY & R. A. WEINBERG. 1981. Transforming genes of carcinomas and neuroblastomas introduced into mouse fibroblasts. Nature **290:** 261-264.
4. KRONTIRIS, T. G. & G. M. COOPER. 1981. Transforming activity of human tumor DNA. Proc. Nat. Sci. Acad. USA **78:** 1181-1184.
5. PERUCHO, M., M. GOLDFARB, K. SHIMIZU, C. LAMA, J. FOGH & M. WIGLER. 1981. Human-tumor-derived cell lines contain common and different transforming genes. Cell **27:** 467-476.
6. KOPELOVICH, L., R. F. RICH & A. L. WALLACE. 1986. Hydrocortisone promotes the neodifferentiation of Kirsten murine sarcoma virus transformed human skin fibroblasts to adipose cells; relevance to oncogene mechanism. Exp. Cell Biol. **54:** 25-33.
7. MARX, J. C. 1984. Oncogenes linked to cell regulatory system. Science **226:** 527-528.
8. McGARTH, J. P., D. J. CAPON, D. V. GOEDDEL & A. D. LEVINSON. 1984. Comparative biochemical properties of normal and activated human ras p21 protein. Nature **310:** 644-649.
9. SWEET, R. W., S. YOKOYAMA, T. KAMATA, J. R. FERAMISCO, M. ROSENBERG & M. GROSS. 1984. The product of ras is a GTPase and the T24 oncogenic mutant is deficient in this activity. Nature **311:** 273-276.
10. PFEFFER, L. & L. KOPELOVICH. 1977. Differential genetic susceptibility of cultured human skin fibroblasts to transformation by kirsten murine sarcoma virus. Cell **10:** 313-329.
11. RASHEED, S. & M. GARDNER. 1981. Growth properties and susceptibility to viral transformation of skin fibroblasts from individuals at high genetic risk for colorectal cancer. J. Nat. Cancer Inst. **66:** 43-49.
12. MIYAKI, M., N. AKAMATSU, M. ROKUTANDA, T. ONO, H. YODHIKURA, M. SASAKI, A. TONOMURA & J. UTSUNOMIYA. 1980. Increased sensitivity of fibroblasts of skin from patients with adenomatosis coli ad Peutz-Jeghers' syndrome to transformation by murine sarcoma virus. Gann **71:** 797-803.
13. RHIM, J. S., R. TRIMMER & R. J. HUEBNER. 1982. Differential susceptibility of human cells to transformation by murine and avian sarcoma viruses. Proc. Soc. Exp. Biol. Med. **170:** 350-358.
14. MIYAKI, M., M. AKAMATSU & T. ONO. 1983. Susceptibility of skin fibroblasts from patients with retinoblastoma to transformation by murine sarcoma virus. Cancer Lett. **18:** 137-142.
15. FRANKEL, J. W., V. V. BERGS, H. V. SAMIS, P. BIDOT & L. KOPELOVICH. 1984. Skin fibroblasts from humans with neurofibromatosis are abnormally sensitive to transformation by kirsten murine sarcoma virus. Proc. Int. Am. Soc. Ther. **1:** 15.
16. BIDOT-LOPEZ, P. & J. W. FRANKEL. 1983. Enhanced viral transformation of skin fibroblasts from neurofibromatosis patients. Ann. Clin. Lab. Sci. **13:** 27-31.
17. FRANKEL, J. W., P. BIDOT, H. SAMIS, F. MacFARLAND, J. COTELINGAM & J. ZIMBLE. 1982. Feasibility study of a diagnostic test to identify individuals at risk for cancer. *In* Advances in Comparative Leukemia Research (1981). D. S. Yohn & J. R. Blakesless, Eds.: 555-556. North Holland, Elsevier. Amsterdam, Holland.
18. KOPELOVICH, L. & S. SIRLIN. 1980. Human skin fibroblasts from individuals genetically predisposed to cancer are sensitive to an SV40-induced T antigen display and transformation. Cancer **45:** 1108-1111.
19. KOPELOVICH, L. 1984. Skin fibroblasts from humans genetically predisposed to colon cancer are abnormally sensitive to SV40. Cancer Invest. **2(5):** 333-338.
20. MILLER, C. A. & S. RASHEED. 1981. Viral susceptibility of skin fibroblasts from patients with Huntington disease. Am. J. Hum. Genet. **33:** 197-202.
21. KOPELOVICH, L. 1977. Familial polyposis: a model of tumor progression. *In* Workshop on Cancer Invasion and Metastasis Biologic Mechanisms and Therapy. S. Day, Ed.: 375-387. Raven Press. New York, N.Y.
22. KOPELOVICH, L. 1980. Hereditary adenomatosis of the colon and rectum: recent studies

on the nature of cancer promotion and cancer prognosis. *In* Progress in Cancer Research. S. J. Winawer, P. Sherlock & D. Shottenfeld, Eds.: 91-108. Raven Press. New York, N.Y.

23. KOPELOVICH, L. 1982. Hereditary adenomatosis of the colon and rectum: relevance to cancer promotion and cancer control. Cancer Genet. Cytogenet. **5:** 333-351.

24. KOPELOVICH, L. 1982. Adenomatosis of the colon and rectum: relevance to inheritance and susceptibility mechanisms in human cancer. Cancer Surv. **1:** 72-91.

25. KOPELOVICH, L. 1982. Genetic predisposition to cancer in man: in vitro studies. Int. Rev. Cytol. **77:** 63-88.

26. KOPELOVICH, L. 1982. Prevention of hereditary large bowel cancer: tissue culture assays and logistics. *In* Prevention of Hereditary Large Bowel Cancer: 131-145. Alan R. Liss. New York, N.Y.

27. KOPELOVICH, L. 1985. Recent studies, observations and considerations in hereditary adenomatosis of the colon and rectum. *In* Biomarkers, Genetics and Cancer. A. H. Guirgis & H. T. Lynch, Eds.: 50-80. Van Nostrand Reinhold Co., Inc. New York, N.Y.

28. RIDER, S. H., H. A. MAZZULLO, M. B. DAVIS & J. D. A. DELHANTY. 1986. Familial polyposis coli: growth characteristics of karyotypically variable cultured fibroblasts, response to epidermal growth factor and the tumour promoter 12-*O*-tetradecanoyl phorbol-13-acetate. J. Med. Genet. **23:** 131-144.

29. RICCARDI, V. M. & J. J. MULVIHILL. 1980. Neurofibromatosis. Adv. Neurol. **29.**

30. RASHEED, S. 1980. Paper presented at the National Cancer Institute Conference on Cancer Biomarkers, Bethesda, Md., January.

31. RHIM, J. S., R. TRIMMER, R. F. HUEBNER, T. S. PAPAS & G. JAY. 1980. Differential susceptibility of human cells to transformation by murine and avian sarcoma viruses. Proc. Soc. Exp. Biol. Med. **170:** 350-358.

32. NEEDLEMAN, S. W., Y. YUASA, S. SRIVASTAVA & S. A. AARONSON. 1983. Normal cells of patients with high cancer risk syndromes lack transforming activity in the NIH/3T3 transfection assay. Science **222:** 173-174.

33. WEINER, H., M. KONIG & P. GRUSS. 1982. Multiple point mutations affecting the simian virus 40 enhancer. Science **219:** 626-631.

34. KOPELOVICH, L. & A. DELEO. 1984. Fibroblasts from humans genetically predisposed to colon cancer show abnormal levels of the transformation associated cellular p53 protein. Proc. Am. Assoc. Cancer Res. **25:** 254.

35. DELEO, A. B., G. JAY, E. APPELLA, *et al.* 1979. Detection of a transformation related antigen in chemically induced sarcomas and other transformed cells of the mouse. Proc. Nat. Acad. Sci. USA **76:** 2420-2424.

36. CRAWFORD, L. V., D. C. PIM, E. G. GURNEY, *et al.* 1981. Detection of a common feature in several human tumor cell lines: a 53,000 dalton protein. Proc. Nat. Acad. Sci. USA **78:** 41-45.

37. KLEIN, G. 1982. The transformation-associated cellular p53. *In* Viral Oncology **2:** 1-180. Raven Press. New York, N.Y.

38. RHIM, J. S., G. JAY, P. ARNSTEIN, F. M. PRICE, K. K. SANFORD & S. A. AARONSON. 1985. Neoplastic transformation of human epidermal keratinocytes by AD12-SV40 and kirsten sarcoma virus. Science **227:** 1250-1252.

Index of Contributors

413